# ALTERNATIVE MEDICAL APOCRYPHA

## BODY-MIND CORRELATIONS

### Dr. Stewart A. Swerdlow

with Janet Diane Mourglia-Swerdlow

Research Compiled by

Clifton E. Davis

Expansions Publishing Company, Inc.
Saint Joseph, Michigan
USA

Copyright © 2020 Expansions Publishing Company, Inc.

Published by: Expansions Publishing Company, Inc.
P.O. Box 12
Saint Joseph, Michigan 49085 USA
269-519-8036
Skype: eventsatexpansions
customersupport@expansions.com
www.expansions.com

ISBN: 978-1-7343408-0-8

Cover Photo by Jonathan J. Swerdlow
www.jonathanswerdlow.com

All rights reserved. Printed in the United States of America. No parts of this book may be used or reproduced in any manner whatsoever without written permission except in the case of brief quotations embodied in critical articles and reviews.

## Medical Disclaimer

The information provided in this publication is not an attempt to practice medicine or provide specific medical advice, nor is it a substitute for medical care.

We always recommend consulting with a healthcare professional before starting any diet, exercise, supplementation, or medication program.

You assume full responsibility for using any information provided and agree that we are not responsible or liable for any claim resulting from its use by you or any user.

# Books by Stewart A. Swerdlow & Janet Diane Mourglia-Swerdlow

*13-Cubed: Case Studies in Mind-Control & Programming*

*13-Cubed Squared: More Case Studies in Mind-Control & Programming*

*1099 Daily Affirmations for Self-Change*

*Alternative Medical Apocrypha: Body-Mind Correlations*

*Blue Blood, True Blood: Conflict & Creation*

*Decoding Your Life: An Experiential Course in Self-Reintegration*

*Healer's Handbook: A Journey Into Hyperspace*

*Healing Archetypes and Symbols*

*Heights of Healing*

*Hyperspace Helper*

*Hyperspace Plus*

*King Bee, Queen Bee*

*Little Fluffs Series for Children*

*Montauk: Alien Connection*

*Revelations of Space & Time, History and God*

*Stewart Says…*

*Template of God-Mind*

*True Reality of Sexuality*

*True World History: Humanity's Saga*

*White Owl Legends: An Archetypal Story of Creation*

# Dedication & Gratitude

I started this work in 2003. In a matter of a few weeks, I thought I was done. Ha! So many years later, and *finally* this book is as complete as it can be... for now. Since that time, I have traveled through all 50 States of the USA and to all 7 continents, learning new alternative methods and holistic technologies.

I studied at Panamerican University School of Medicine where I received a Doctorate in ***Alternative Healing & Deprogramming***, my medical license in ***Indigenous Medicine***, and became an Associate Professor. I now teach on their campuses in Tampa, Nevis, Quito, and San Juan. In addition I am honored to have been adopted into the Taino Tribe of Puerto Rico.

Through it all, I was encouraged to pursue my goals because of the unconditional love of my incredible wife, Janet. In Arabic, her name means, "paradise." She is that and more to me. I dedicate this work, and ***all*** my work, to her. I would not be here without her unending, unwavering, unconditional support and love.

I want to state my gratitude to all my children and their spouses who keep me on my toes with questions, comments, criticisms, and humor that keep me humble and focused.

I thank all of my incredible grandchildren for making me laugh and bringing me unceasing joy in my intense life. Thinking of them always makes me smile and laugh.

A special thank you to my friend, Clifton E. Davis of Utah, who spent copious hours transcribing videos and webinars as well as researching to enhance my words and work.

Much gratitude to our Customer Service Specialist, Patricia L. O'Bryant, for her dedication, patience, and customer support that keeps Expansions going onward at all times.

I cannot express in human words the gratitude and blessing of my father-in-law, Robert Austin Mourglia, who has supported us on every level imaginable for decades. Without him, I do not know where we would be now. He is our blessing from heaven.

Above all, I dedicate all of my work in The Name of the Absolute-God-Mind, Metatron, and all the Archangels who have guided me and saved me from myself. I am truly blessed.

Finally, I am grateful for my Yakutian Laika dogs, Jade and Jasmine; and for my Maine Coon cats, Solomon and Q. They always turn Grumpy Stew into Happy Pappy!

# Contents

Introduction ... 9

**Part I**

Mind-Pattern & DNA ... 15

Levels ... 19

Systemic Anatomy ... 21

Regional Anatomy ... 37

Anatomy Chakra System Correlations ... 49

General Chakra Mind-Pattern Correlations ... 51

Specific Chakra Mind-Pattern Correlations ... 57

Body Energy & Exercise ... 107

Body Movement ... 111

Muscular Movement ... 113

Blood Pressure ... 115

Healing Archetypes for Mind/Body Correlations ... 119

Flowchart of the Human Body and Digestive System ... 121

Spine and Nervous System ... 125

Skeletal System ... 129

Muscular System ... 147

Cancer ... 161

Regeneration vs. Removal and Cryopreservation ... 169

**Part II**

Health Conditions & Treatments ... 177

General Supplements with General Information ... 323

The Top 8 Herbs for Andropause ... 335

**Part III**
    Addicted to Addictions ................................................................ 341
**Part IV: Articles by Janet**
    Body Follows Mind ..................................................................... 393
    Mind Builds Body ....................................................................... 395
    Increasing Your Frequency .......................................................... 409
    Free Permanent Weight Loss—No Gimmicks! ........................... 421
    Parasites ....................................................................................... 423
    Victim Mentality ......................................................................... 429
    Can Money Buy Happiness? ...................................................... 433
**Appendices**
    Complete Body Scan .................................................................. 440
    A Compilation of Interesting Notes
        Accumulated Through the Years ........................................ 441
    Glossary ...................................................................................... 511
    Index .......................................................................................... 519

# Introduction

Health and Healing. These are the biggest challenges that you face. No one wants to hurt, become ill, or have a chronic health condition. Many people even say that once you are born, your body begins dying. With this in mind, "aging" as currently defined is avoided at all cost—at least superficially.

This book gives you the Missing Link to Permanent Health & Healing:

Mind-Pattern Analysis.

Your body always follows your Mind. Change your mind to change your health…permanently!

This book is an in-depth analysis of the various body systems and the mind-patterns that create the body. Use it as a guide to understand your life, which in turn affects the greatest, deepest, and most importantly, permanent, healing that you have never-before imagined or known existed.

Because no matter what you do, where you go, or what you take, permanent healing can only happen when you go directly to the point of origin of dis-ease—your MIND.

In addition, body systems correlate to the chakra system, which has a biological basis. Within the physical body, there are bunches of nerves called "ganglions" that coordinate within each chakra band. Mind creates your chakra bands, which in turn animate your physical body.

Many members of the medical community who have attended Expansions' seminars say that they learned more in two days than in their four years of medical school and beyond. As you read, prepare to have your boundaries stretched, which is important to changing your foundational mind-patterns upon which your entire life is built.

All things come from One Source. You can combine whatever you need to boost your mind-pattern to get you to your goal. Learning to align with what is most correct and beneficial for your personal situation is a key element to permanent Health & Healing.

Stewart and Janet have both healed their mind-patterns of a variety of mental and emotional conditions, which in turn allowed their bodies to heal.

Stewart has healed his mind-pattern and therefore his body of:
- Anorexia
- Crohn's Disease
- Allergies
- Migraine Headaches
- Chronic Body Pain
- Eye Issues
- Irritable Bowel Syndrome

Janet has healed her mind-pattern and therefore her body of:
- Anorexia
- Cervical vertigo
- Dry Eye
- Chronic bronchitis
- Walking pneumonia
- Edema
- Eczema
- Allergies
- Mononucleosis
- Near-sightedness
- Sinus Infections

- Post Nasal Drip
- TMJ
- Lower back injury

Together, Janet and Stewart have taught their unique techniques to thousands of people who have healed their mind-patterns and healed their bodies, thus healing their lives. Their combined work is the Missing Link that you need for permanent and effective Health & Healing.

Janet and Stewart give you a new standard of Health as well as the tools to attain and maintain the Mind and Body that you deserve!

# Part I

# Mind-Pattern & DNA

Your physical body literally "goes with the flow" of your thoughts. Your thoughts create mind-pattern that in turn pulls the molecular arrangement of your specific physical body. This is why there are no two physical bodies exactly alike. Even twins have physical differentiations because their thoughts are unique to each individual. Even twins each have unique cellular structures and DNA, including fingerprints and retina scans. This is very important to understand because it is the individual mind-pattern within the species that causes this.

No one person thinks in the same way that another person thinks. This is why you must learn to analyze your own mind-pattern—in this way, you understand who you are and why your physical body is uniquely formed around you.

The mind is electromagnetic. Your thought waves can be measured with an electro-encephalogram. In the space around you, there is no such thing as a vacuum. What appears to be empty space is actually full of billions and trillions of free-floating molecules and atomic structures. They are not attached to anything and can be used to materially manifest anything at all.

As your electromagnetic mind-pattern enters into dense physical energy, your mind-pattern acts like a magnet that attracts the atomic particles. These then form into the four protein bases: cytosine, thiamine, adenine, and guanine. There is a fifth protein base but it is not part of your DNA.

The protein bases form the DNA structure, which is literally the blueprint for your body and creates your physical body, which is only an outpicturing of your mind-pattern. Mind-pattern attracts atomic structure in the environment, which forms around the mind-pattern, which in turn physically manifests.

The atomic structure forms the four protein bases that form the basis of your DNA. This is the blueprint that creates the body.

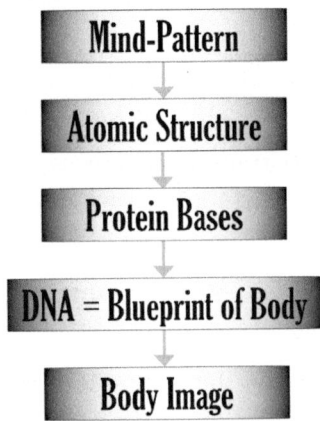

Always remember that what you think is what you are and what you will become.

Whatever you hold in your mind physically manifests in your body.

97% of all DNA is identical, whether a human, alien, amoeba, or elephant. This means that only 3% of DNA differentiates species as well as individuals within that species. When you hear that the "human genome has been mapped," this is a reference to this 3%.

You may hear that 97% of DNA is "junk DNA," but this is not true.

Humans as a group have a species mind-pattern that creates similar DNA for similar DNA patterning. This species group mind-pattern is the foundational mind-pattern for all individuals within the human species. In other words, there is a species group mind-pattern that is the foundational mind-pattern for all the individuals in the particular species.

It is your unique individual experiences within the species group mind that differentiates your specific body.

You might wonder, "If one person has exactly the same issue with his/her knee as another person, do they have the same mind-pattern?"

When two people have the same physical issue, they do have the same mind-pattern about that specific issue, which then causes the physical outpicturing. However, there are many differences in their individual personalities or they would be the same person.

So, if there are two identical mind-patterns, would they create more than one body?

No, they cannot. For example, think about Simultaneous Existence. Every point in time and space has a unique vibration and frequency. When two points match, there is an instantaneous connection and immediate cohesion; the two points become one.

There cannot be two individuals with identical mind-patterns or they would be "one" individual, not "two." It is the commonalities of individuals that create a species group mind-pattern. These commonalities explain why each species generates common physical bodies, yet no two bodies within the species are identical.

# Levels

| HYPERSPACE | — | ASTRAL | — | PHYSICAL |
|---|---|---|---|---|
| Vapor | | Water | | Ice |
| Superconscious | | Subconscious | | Conscious |
| Right Brain | | Pineal Gland | | Left Brain |
| Meditation | | Visualization | | Prayer |
| Thought | | Emotions | | Body |
| Linear Past | | Linear Present | | Linear Future |

The levels of manifestation are represented in Hyperspace by the archetype/symbol of an equilateral triangle.

The levels of manifestation have three components. They are not in any specific order because they are all equal in importance. The various "levels" are only referenced in correlation to linear time for better understanding.

## PAST — PRESENT - FUTURE

From a linear perspective, the physical body, consciousness, and physical reality relate to the future. How could this be when the superconscious, right brain, and Hyperspace relate to the past? At first glance, you might think that conceptually, this conflicts. But why? Because most people have the opinion that the future is better and higher while the past is old and no longer necessary.

When you view the physical body from a linear time perspective, the body is the future because thought came first. Thought is the past as shown in the flowchart. In True Reality, past, present, and future occur simultaneously. In True Reality, time is an illusion because everything exists within the Eternal Now. For purposes of understanding this reality and ultimately, your mind-pattern, your physical body must be viewed as the end result.

## Physical Body Issues

| Left Side | Right Side |
|---|---|
| Issues with Females including Self if Female | Issues with Males including Self if Male |
| Logical Issues | Emotional Issues |
| Issues with Physical Reality | Issues with Spirituality, Spiritual Figures & Ideas |

Any time you have an issue on the Left Side of your body, keep these background ideas in mind.

Any time you have an issue with the Right Side of the body, keep these background ideas in mind.

Knowing these mind-patterns deepens your understanding of contributing factors to any body issue that you or your loved ones have.

In addition, it is important to live in a geographic location that matches the frequency of your genetics and personal configuration.

The Earth emanates its own frequency and you need to live in a location that best matches the frequency of your own body.

For example, the genetics of a cactus match in a desert environment while the genetics of a fern best match in a forest environment. You may be able to transplant them to different locations, but each will optimally thrive in its location of genetic origin. The same is true for your physical body.

# Systemic Anatomy

In medical terms "systemic anatomy" stands for the various systems of the body. There are seven basic systems or parts of Systemic Anatomy.

These are the seven Systemic Anatomy levels you will learn about, as well as correlating them to the chakra system and mind-patterns:

**1- Integumentary**

**2- Skeletal**

**3- Muscular**

**4- Nervous**

**5- Circulatory/Vascular**

**6- Visceral**

**7- Endocrine**

These are globally accepted medical systems. Chinese, Indian, and Eastern medicine modalities have different terminologies and groupings since those systems are geared to energetic levels.

Eastern medicine connects the various parts of the body in ways that Western medical science refutes. Acupuncture and acupressure work with sympathetic and energetic systems not accepted by Western medicine. A Western medical professional must accept and practice conventional Western medicine for legal recognition.

## INTEGUMENTARY SYSTEM

The integumentary system consists of the skin, sweat/oil glands, hair, and nails. The skin is the largest organ of the body and protects from external contaminants such as microbes, bacteria, and viruses. The skin also defends the body from harmful cosmic and ultraviolet radiations.

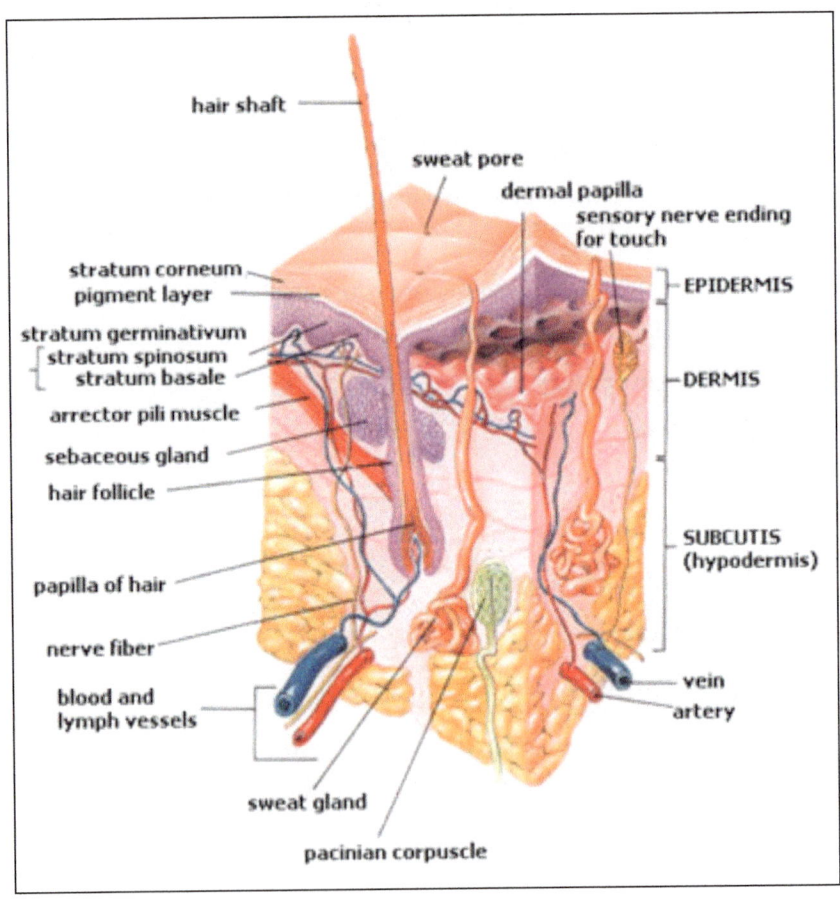

## SKELETAL SYSTEM

The skeletal system is the support and mobility structure of the body. Bones provide the support structure and protect vital organs. Joints allow for movement within the body. The upper axial skeleton maintains the upright posture and is comprised of the skull, spinal column, and the rib cage. The axial skeleton distributes weight from the upper extremities to the lower extremities. The appendicular skeleton makes movement possible and protects the major organs of digestion, reproduction, excretion, and locomotion. It consists of the upper and lower limbs, pelvic, and pectoral girdles.

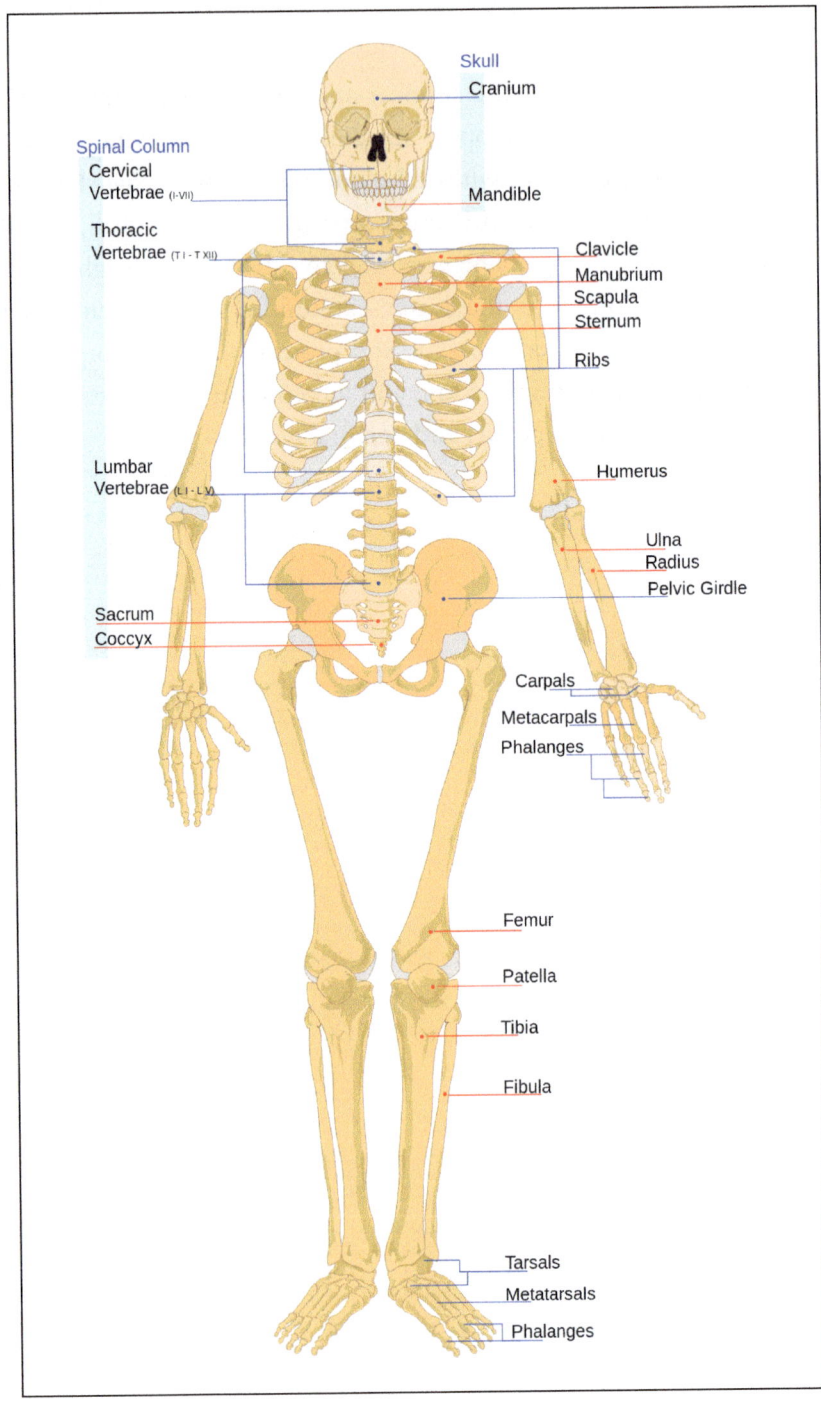

## Muscular System

The muscular system is composed of muscles, cartilage, and specifically connective tissues like ligaments and tendons that move the joints. Sometimes the muscular and skeletal systems are considered together as the "musculoskeletal system." It is also called the "locomotor system," involving the parts that move the body. The muscular system's main function includes protecting vital organs, providing motion, and supporting the body. There are over 600 muscles in the human body.

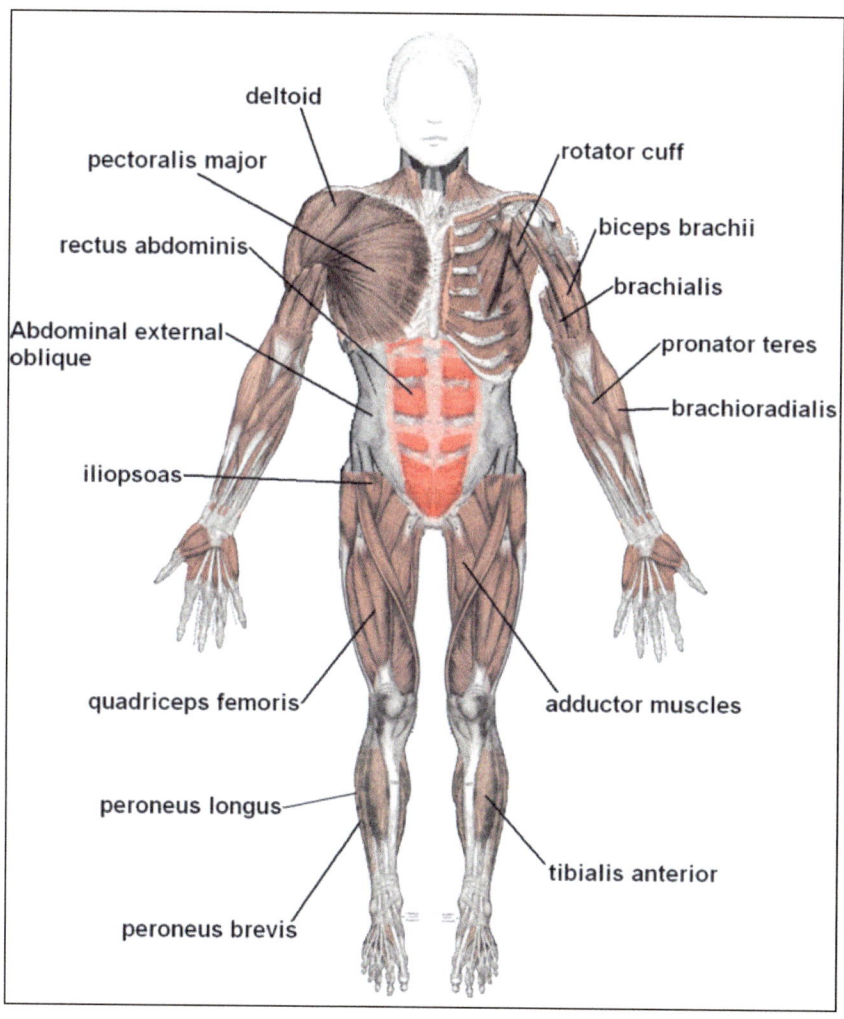

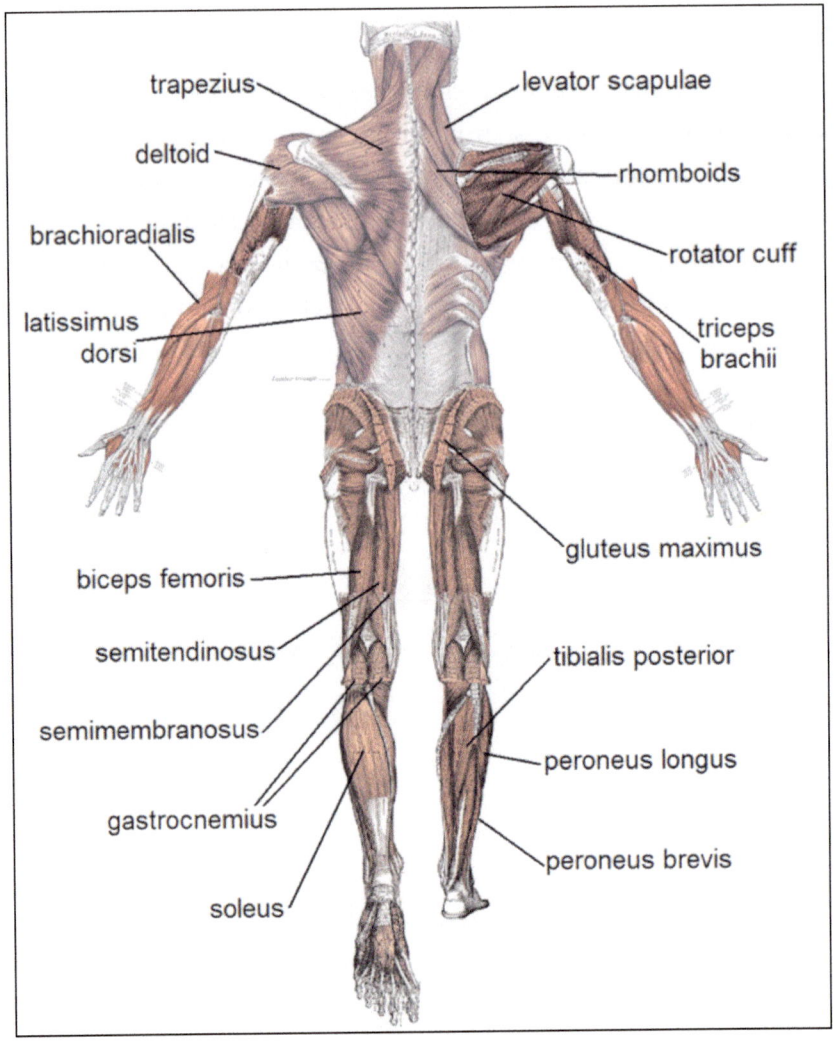

## Nervous System

The nervous system includes the nerves, brain, spinal cord, and all the coverings/sheathings that protect the nerves, brain, and the spinal cord. Most of the brain's function is misunderstood. This is why you are told that humans only use 10% or less of their brains' capacity.

Does this mean that only 10% or less of the brain is used or active?

In fact, close to 100%, if not all of it is used all of the time. However, the 90% corresponds to the functions conventional medical science does not fully understand or want you to know about. In actuality, this portion of the brain relates to nonphysical reality and correlates to interdimensional and Oversoul information/communication. You are learning to develop this with your Hyperspace/Oversoul methodologies. Even opening up a small percentage of the unused capacity of the brain/mind can give you amazing abilities.

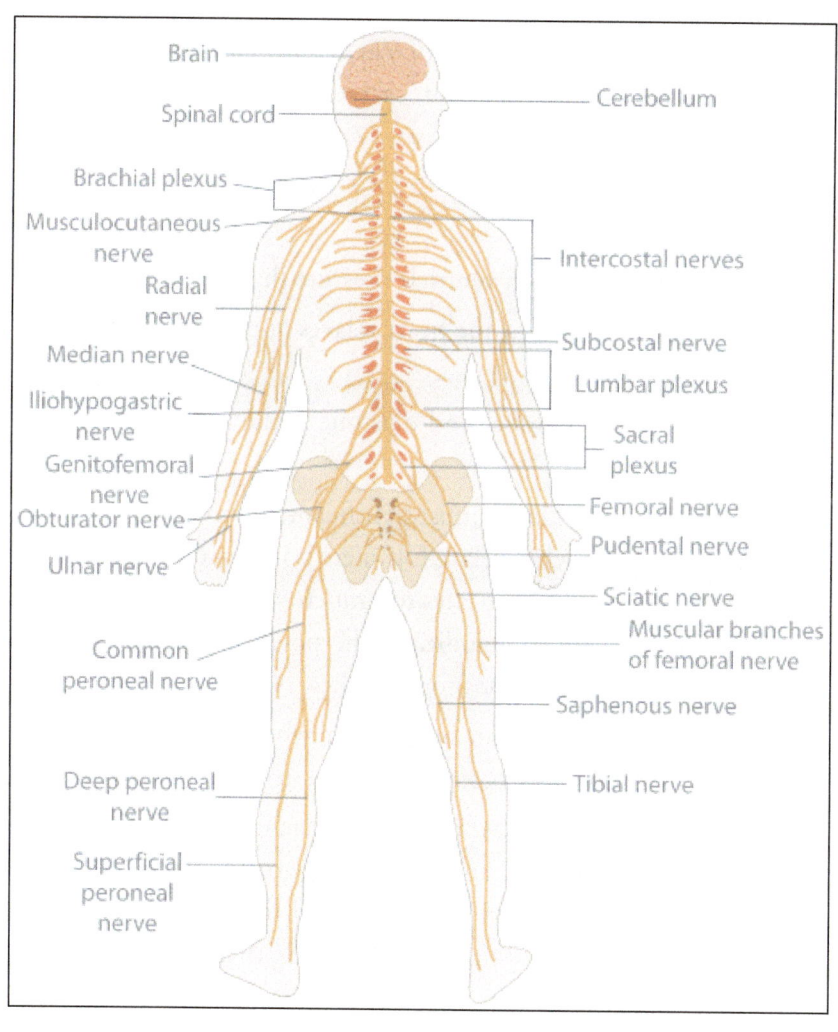

## Circulatory/Vascular System

The circulatory/vascular system includes the heart, blood vessels, and the lymphatic system. The lymphatic system includes lymph nodes and lymph vessels. This is sometimes referred to as the "cardiovascular system." The reason the lymph nodes and lymph vessels are included in this system is because the lymph system has capillaries, which are ducts and arteries that feed into the circulatory system. Everything is connected. This is why cancer cells that are draining off of an organ get caught up in the bloodstream to be carried elsewhere so the individual may be cured of cancer in a particular organ. The cure allows the lymph system to drain the cells out, carrying it elsewhere in the body; this is why/how cancer metastasizes.

### Blood Pressure

Systolic represents the left ventricle pressure that propels your blood.

Diastolic pressure is after the heart relaxes and is the "in-between" beats of the heart.

Systolic is the top number and diastolic is the bottom number of blood pressure results.

The bottom number is the most significant. This number indicates the state of your heart while relaxed. If there is increased pressure when your heart is relaxed, this indicates too much pressure in your arteries and capillaries. In turn, this indicates the potential for an aneurysm (blood vessel bubbles and pops) or a stroke.

Strokes and aneurisms can happen anywhere in the body. Even purple spots in the legs are basically a mini-stroke in a blood vessel.

Blood pressure is tricky because of the machines used. You do not know who calibrated them and how long ago. In addition, what is normal for some people may not be normal for someone else. Your blood pressure can increase simply by knowing that someone is going to take it.

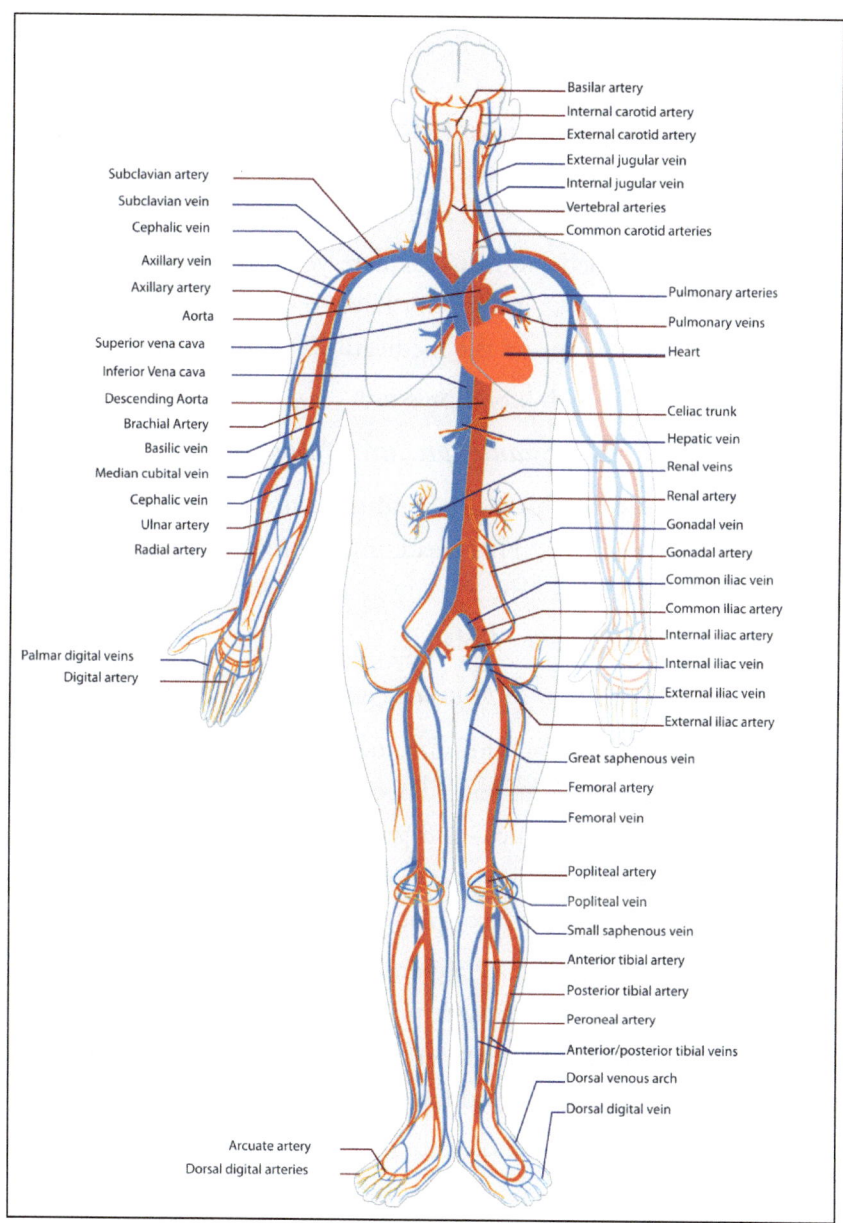

You can purchase your own blood pressure monitor that you wear around your wrist. This monitor takes readings over many days and nights to help you determine what is normal for you.

Hypertension, or high blood pressure, until recently was considered 140/90 or higher.

In 2019, blood pressure is considered high at 120/80. This means more people have "high blood pressure" simply because the numbers have changed. More people can, and will, be put on medication.

When you take medication to regulate your blood pressure, your body's intelligence thinks it does not have to do the job. Then, your body becomes dependent on the medication.

Mind-pattern for high blood pressure:

*I feel constantly pressured in my life.*

Your body translates this into a condition where cholesterol/plaque builds up in your arteries. This creates more pressure, which can lead to a heart attack or stroke.

Insulating with cholesterol/plaque:

*I need to protect myself in life.*

To herbally treat blood pressure, take red yeast rice, garlic, red wine—Pinot Noir is recommended because it has the highest capacity to reduce cholesterol/plaque—and wild rice, which is really a grass seed with a nutty taste. Using the Color Code of Purple to flush the arteries also dissolves cholesterol/plaque.

Vitamin B-3/Niacin, Calcium, and Vitamin D pull cholesterol/plaque out of the system and build your skeletal structure at the same time. This combination is also helpful to dissolve fibroids, cysts, kidney stones, and gallstones.

In general, to remove cholesterol/plaque, begin with 100 mg of Niacin for two weeks. If you do not have a flush, increase to 200 mg. As soon as you experience the flush, stop taking the Niacin.

Niacin loosens the cholesterol/plaque from your arterial walls, literally allowing it to slide out of the veins and the arteries. A Niacin flush is the sensation you feel when the cholesterol/plaque slides out of your circulatory system. This is why you must stop taking the Niacin, or the vascular walls may collapse.

Once this happens, replace the Niacin with odorless garlic, which scrubs the arteries, helping to keep them clean and clear.

Cayenne pepper is also helpful to lower blood pressure and remove cholesterol/plaque.

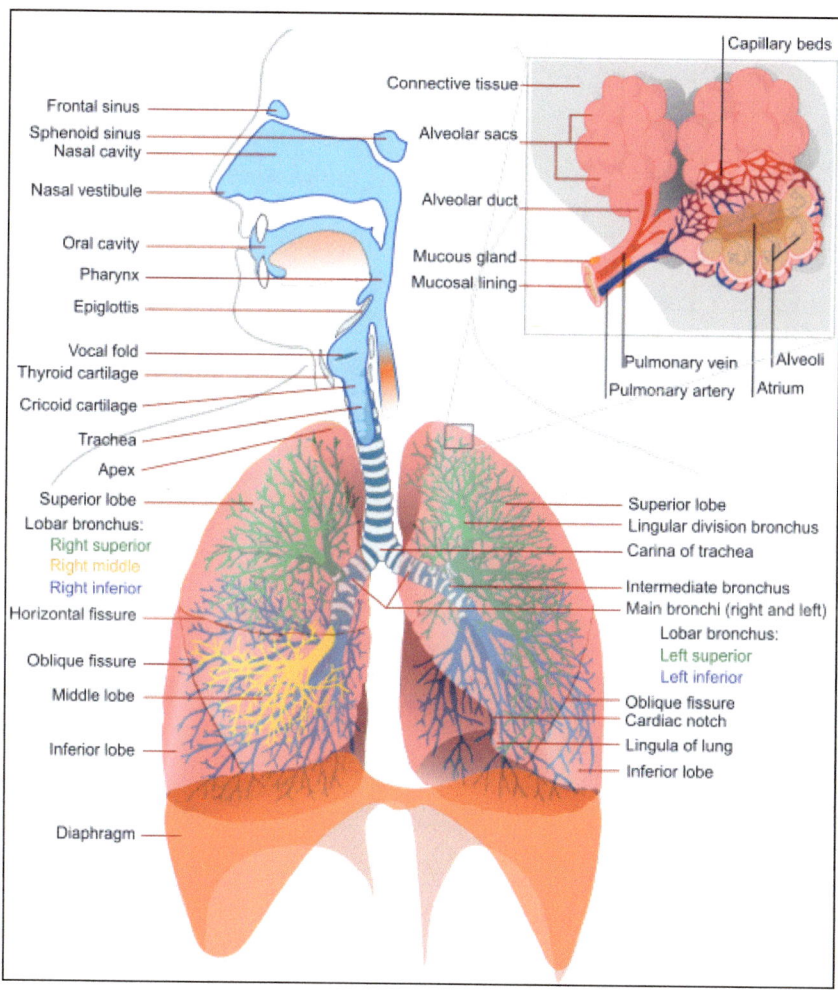

## Visceral System

The medical term for the visceral system is the "alimentary/digestive system." The visceral system includes the respiratory system, urinary system, and the genital system. The last two are medically referred to as the "urogenital systems."

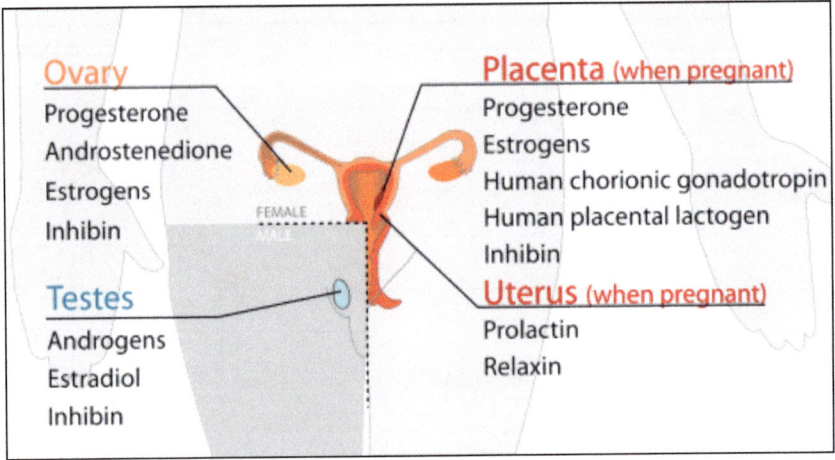

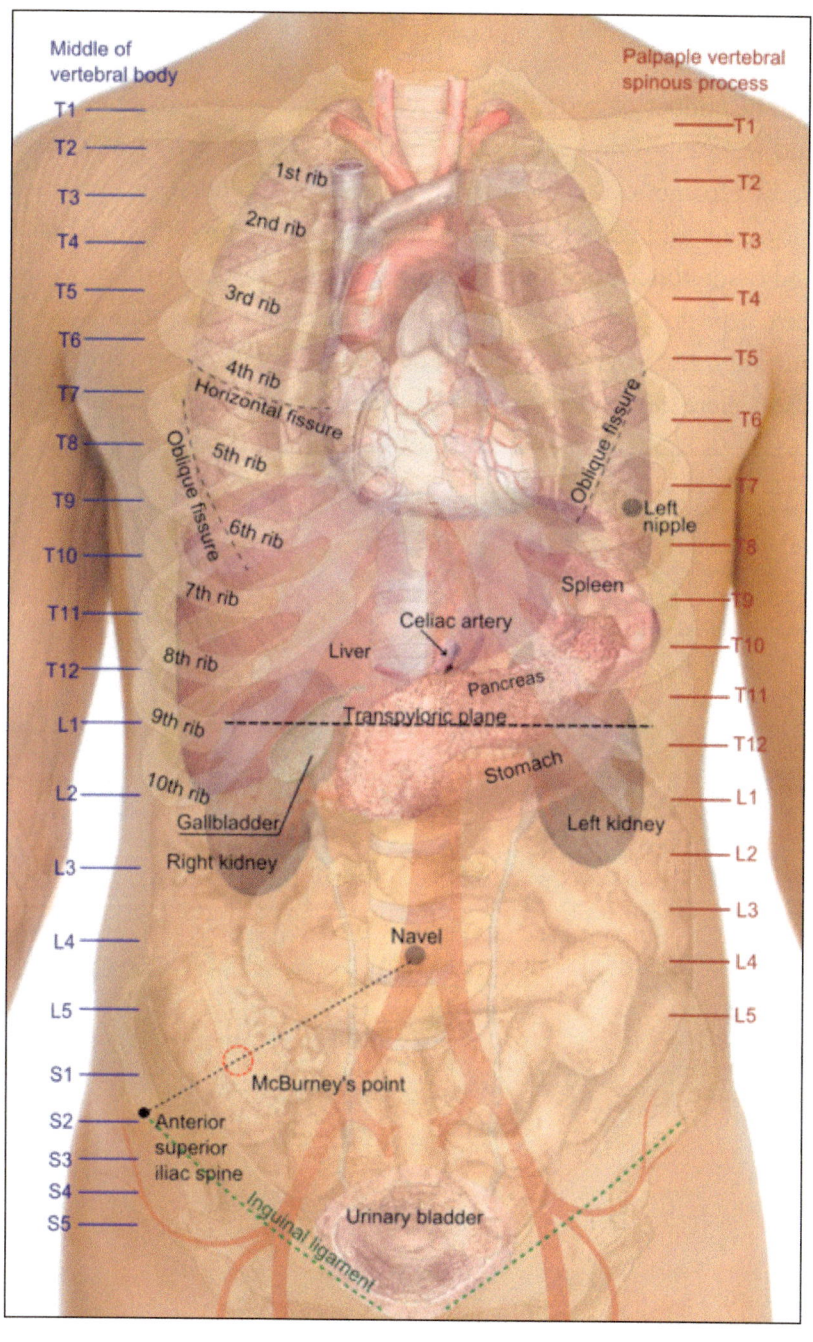

## Endocrine System

The endocrine system is a network of ductless glands that produce and secrete hormones into the circulatory system for all parts of the body. Hormones are chemical mediators that generate a response in the organs and tissues. Hormones regulate mood, growth, metabolism, and tissue function. The endocrine system's effects initiate slowly and have a prolonged response. The two main endocrine glands are the pituitary and thyroid glands. The heart, liver, kidneys, and gonads also secrete hormones and have secondary endocrine functions.

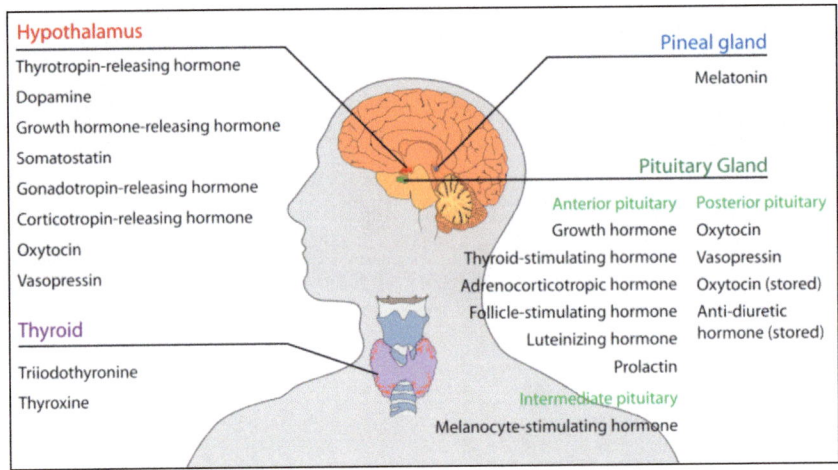

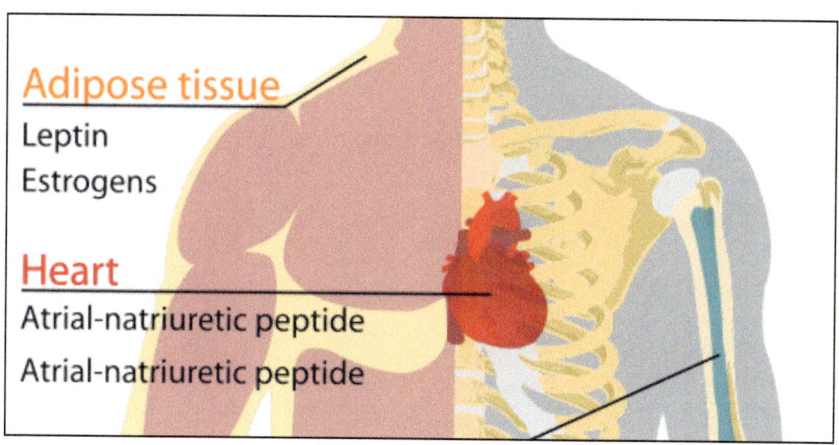
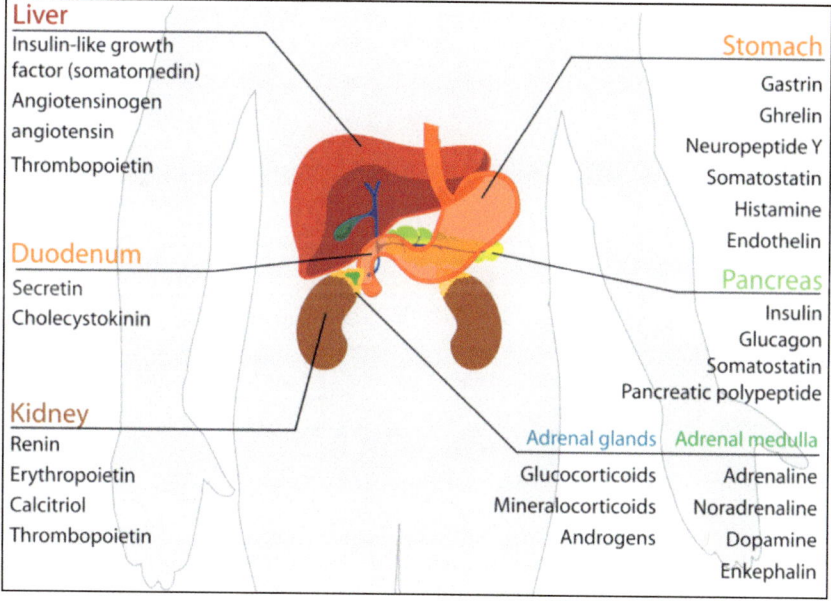

# Regional Anatomy

While Systemic Anatomy provides the basics to recognize the systems of the human body, Regional Anatomy breaks it down even further. Regional Anatomy is the study of the regions of the human body and their various locations, also known as "Topographic Anatomy." Medical professionals use these generally accepted terminologies.

These are the nine generally accepted medically segments of Regional Anatomy:

    **1- Thorax**

    **2- Abdomen**

    **3- Perineum with Pelvis**

    **4- Back**

    **5- Upper Limb**

    **6- Lower Limb**

    **7- Head**

    **8- Cranial Nerves**

    **9- Neck**

## THORAX

1
2
3
4
5
6
7
8
9
10
Cardiac notch
Lower margin of lung
Lower margin of pleura

Transversus thoracis
Internal mammary vessels
Sternum
Left phrenic nerve
Pulmonary pleura
Costal pleura
Heart
Sympathetic trunk
Thoracic duct
Azygos vein
Vagus nerves

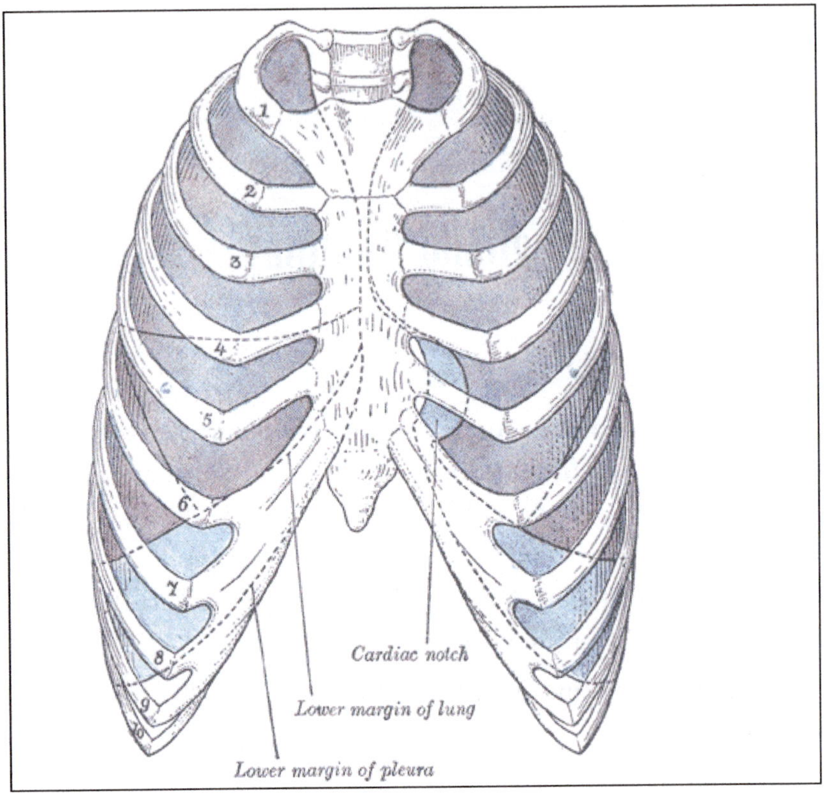

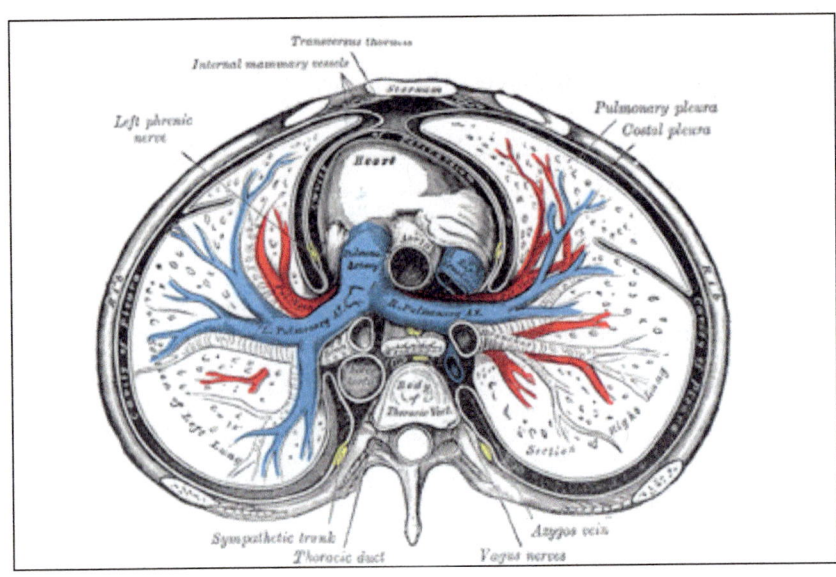

## ABDOMEN

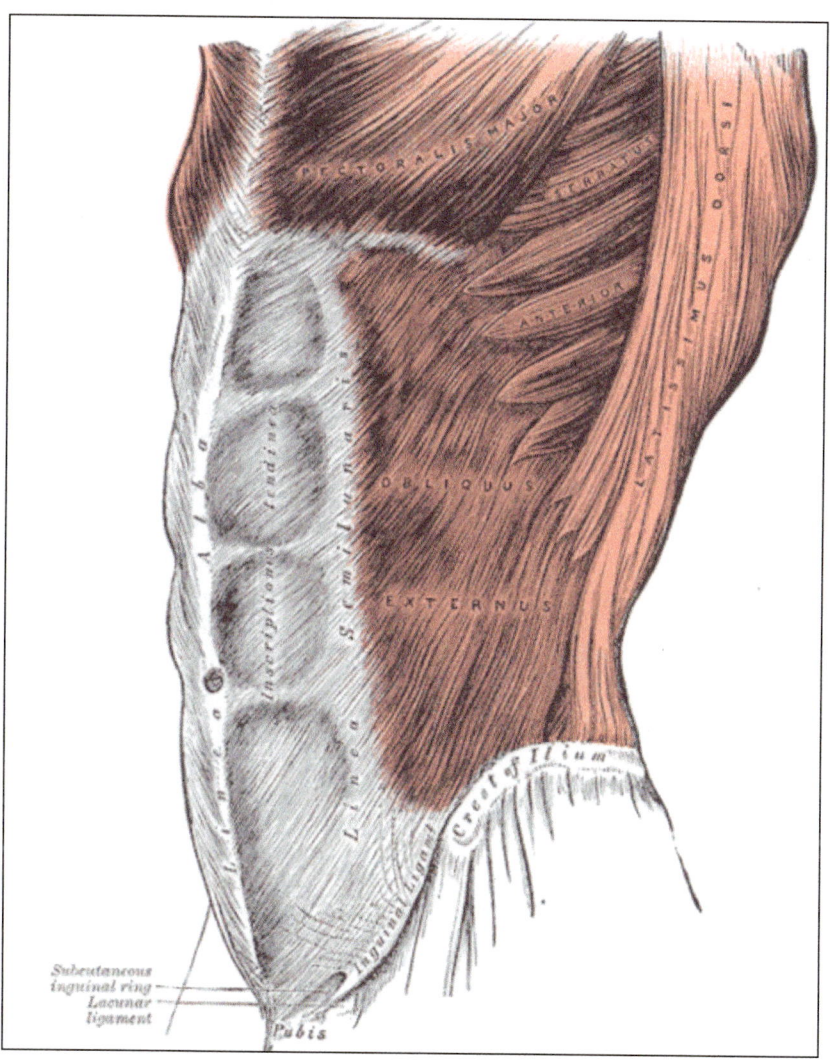

## Perineum with Pelvis - Female

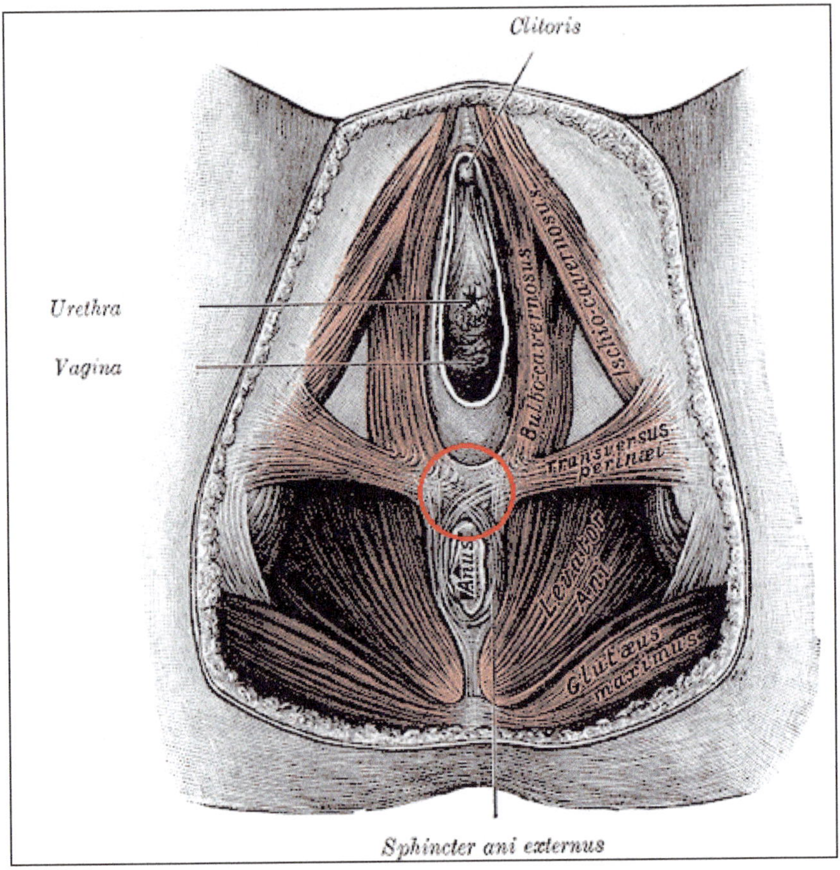

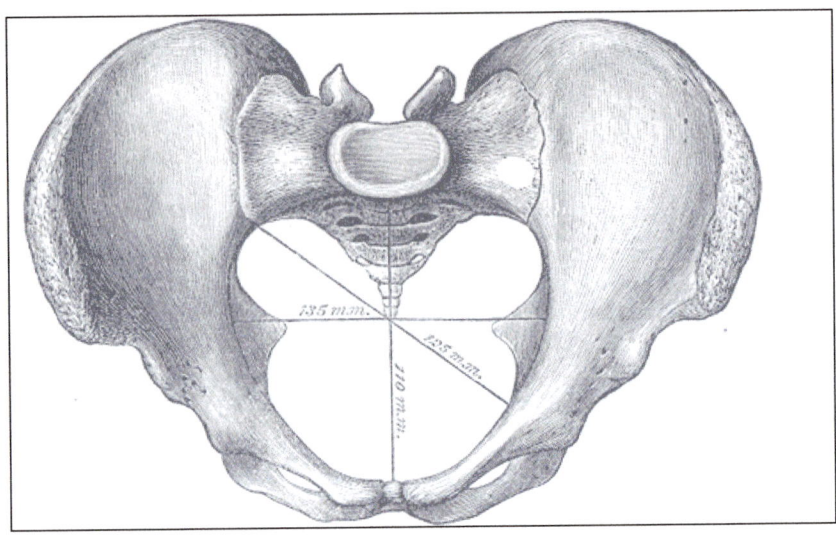

## MALE

ISCHIO-CAVERNOSUS
BULBO-CAVERNOSUS
TRANSVERSUS PERINEI
Tuber ischiad
SPHINCTER ANI EXT.
Anus
LEVATOR ANI
GLUTÆUS MAXIMUS
Coccyx

Brim of Lesser Pelvis
Pubic Arch

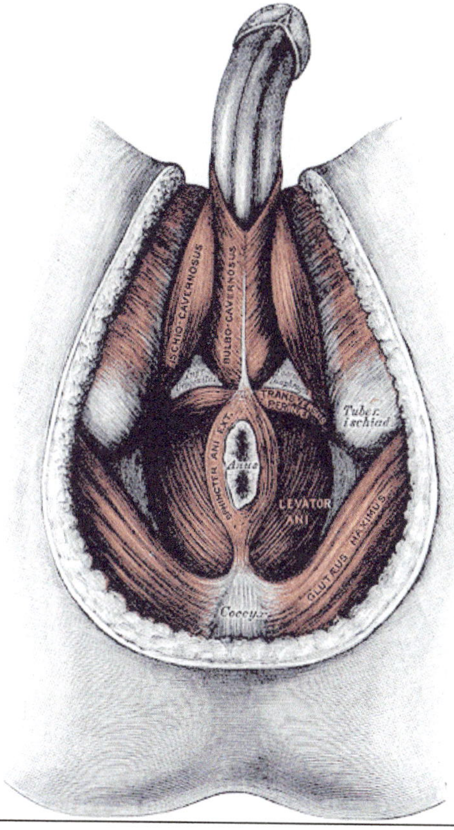

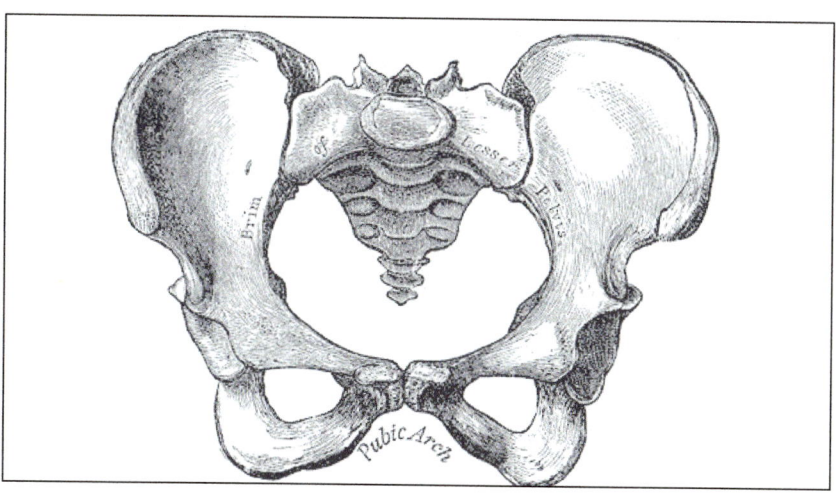

## Back

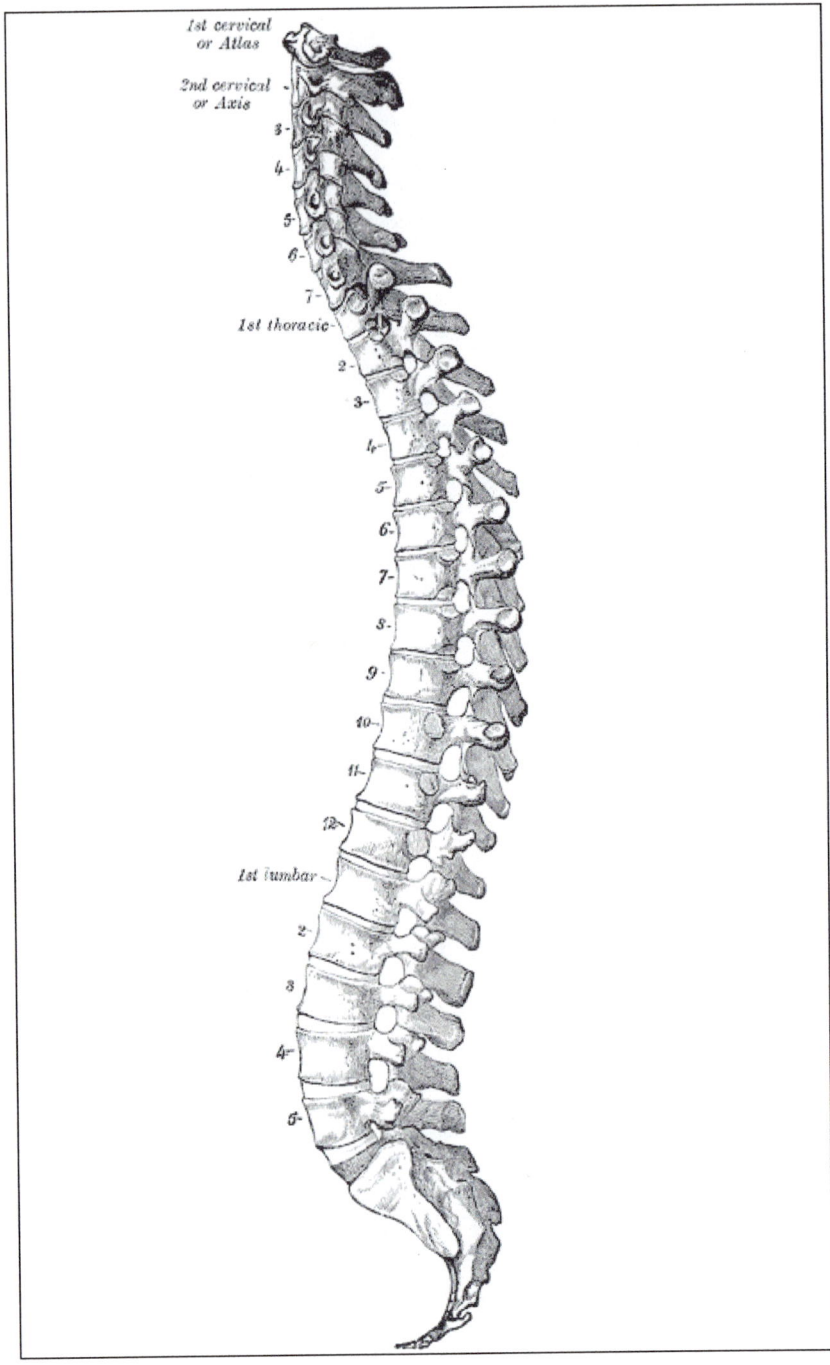

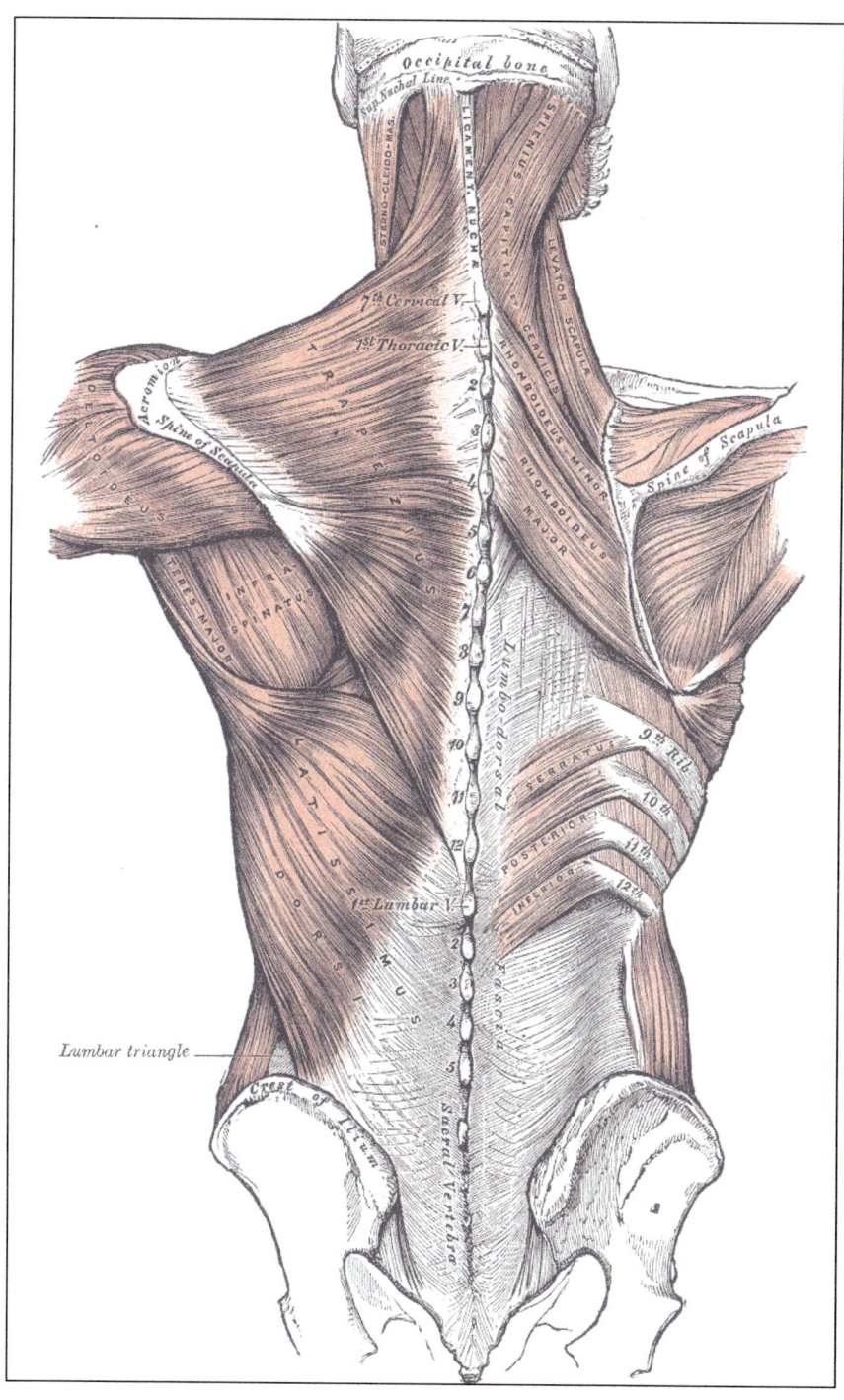

## Upper Limb

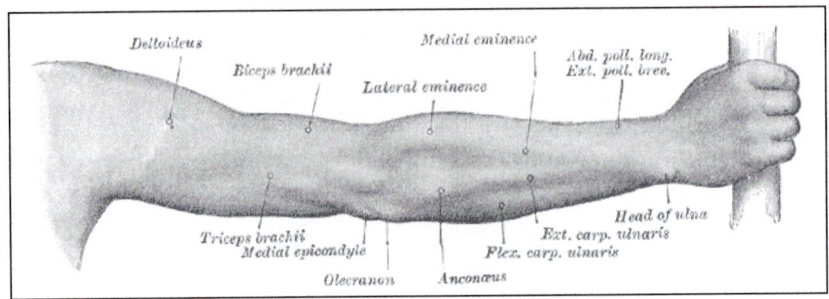

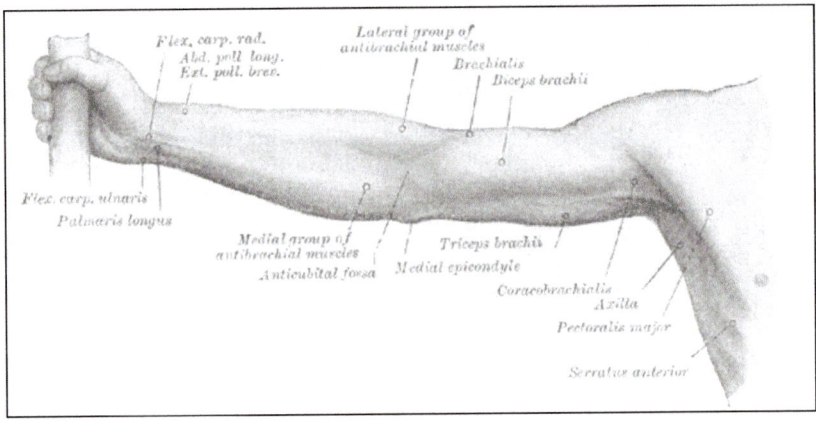

## Lower Limb

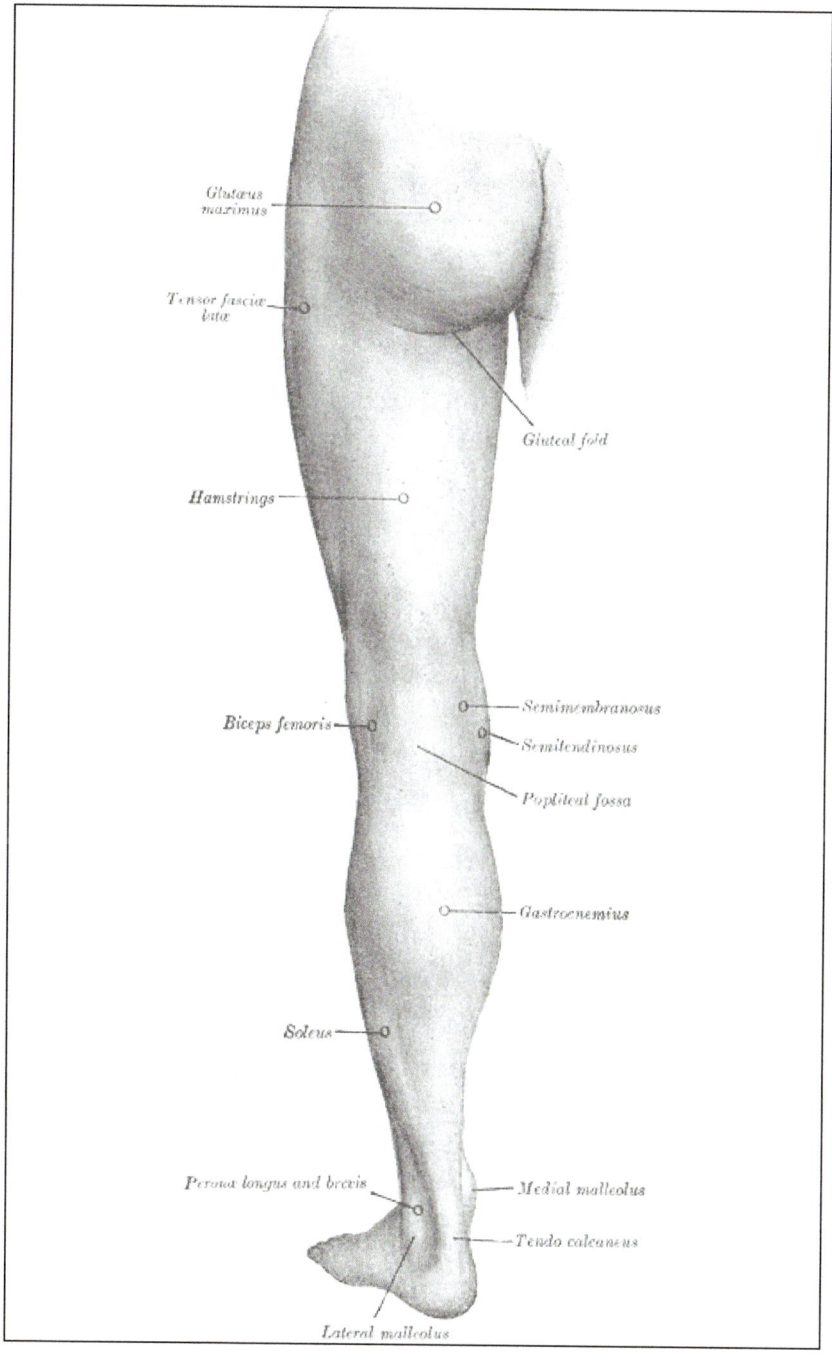

## Neck

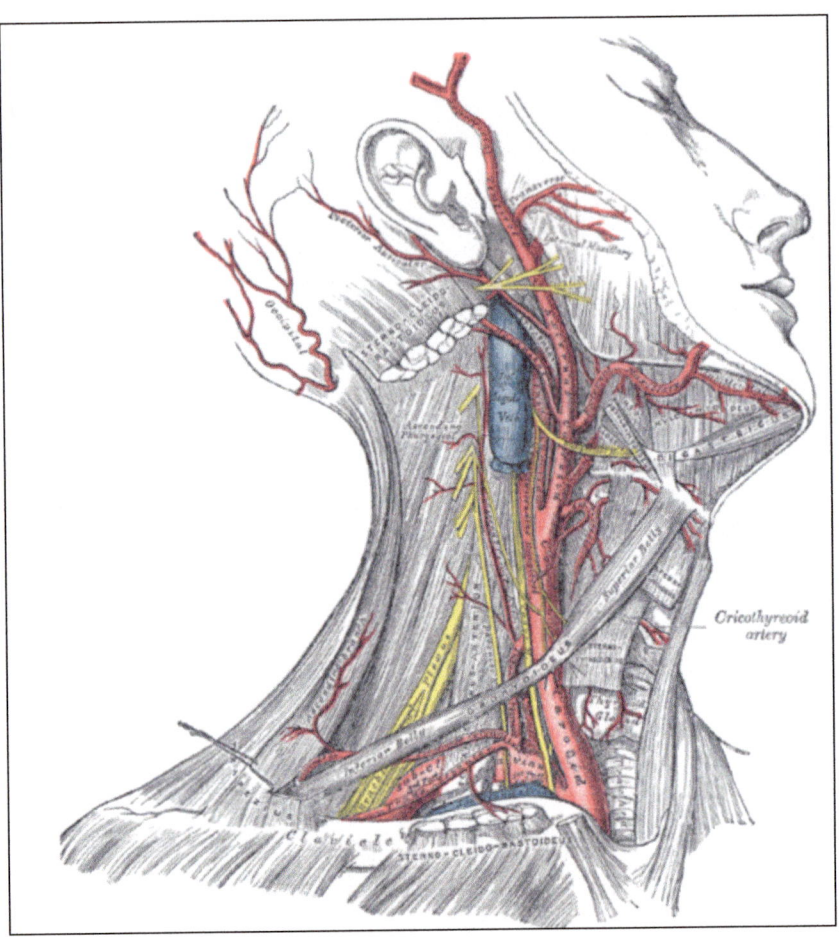

## Head

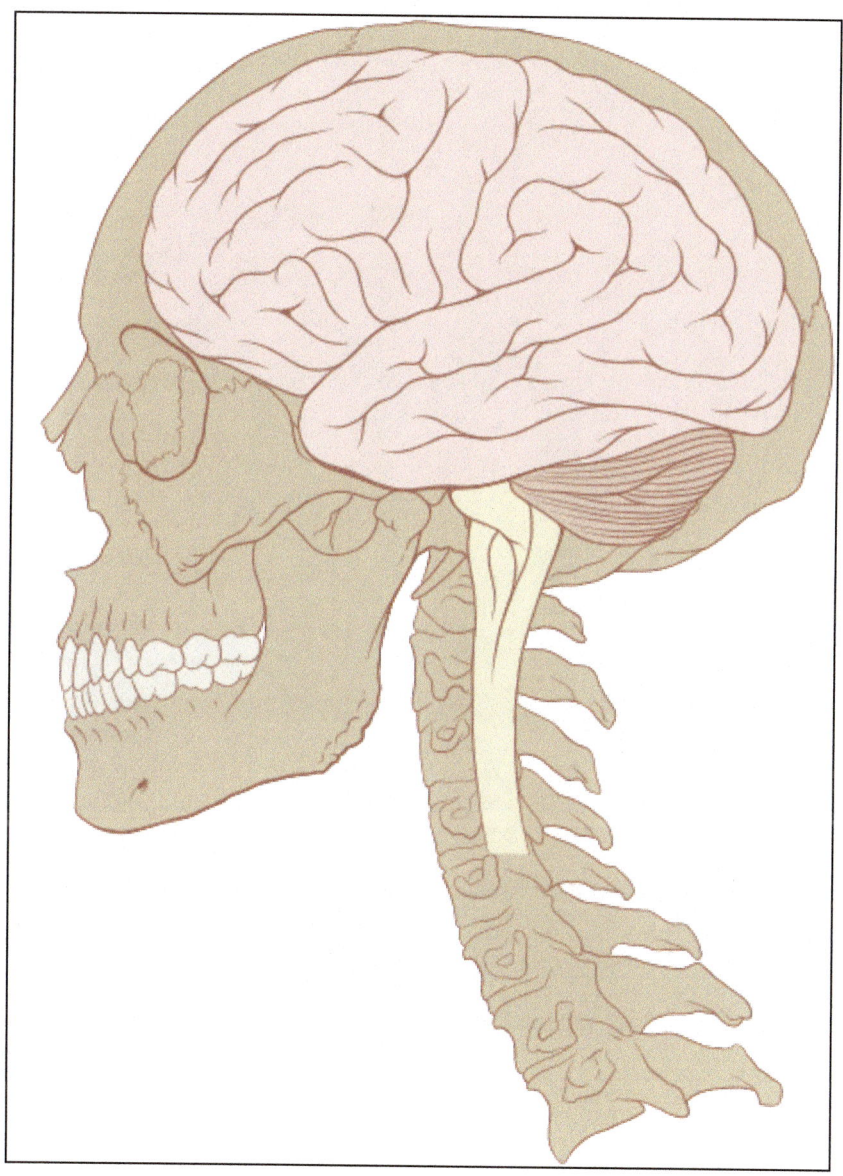

## Cranial Nerves

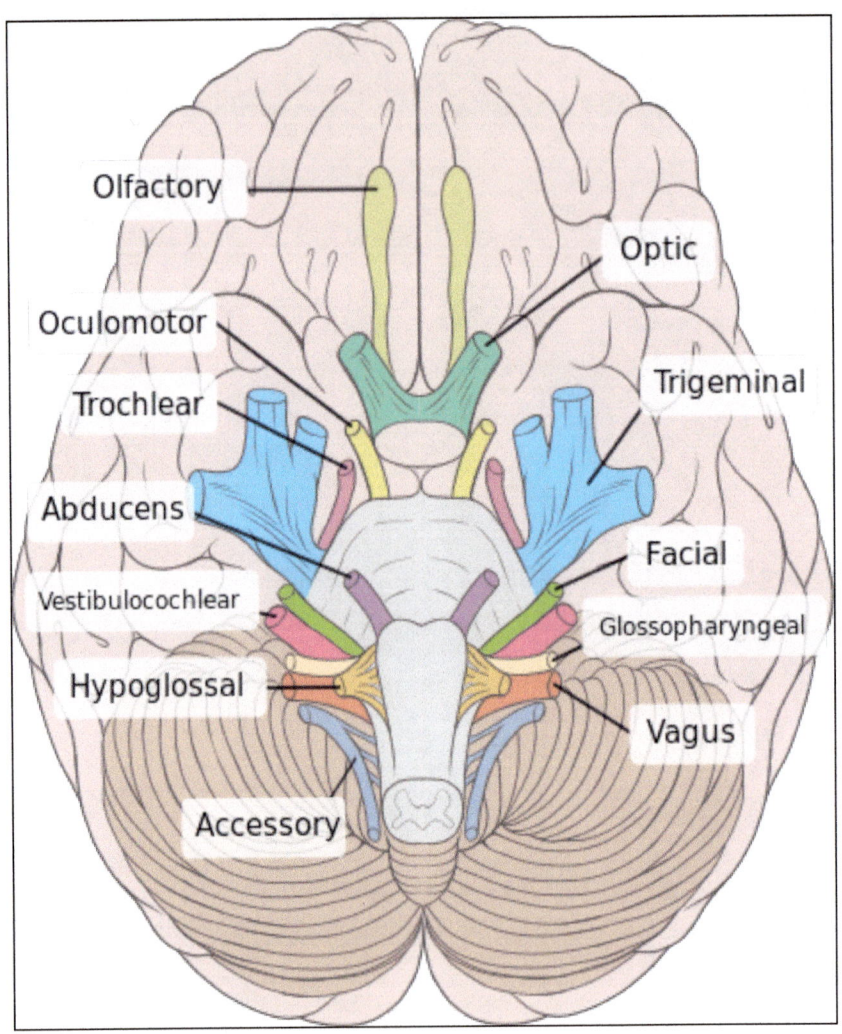

# Anatomy Chakra System Correlations

These are the basic correlations of the Regional Anatomy to the Chakra System. Standard medical charts segment the body vertically as well as horizontally.

These Chakra delineations are in comparison to standard medical terminology. When you look at standardized medical charts, the body is segmented vertically like the chakra system, not just horizontally.

The region of the human body that contains the most organs is between the neck and pubic bone in the thoracic region. The thorax is basically the chest area, correlating mostly to the heart chakra.

The abdomen correlates to the solar plexus chakra.

The perineum and pelvis correlate to the sacral and root chakras.

The lower limbs, including the legs and feet, reside within the Earth's gravitational and magnetic fields, which are Brown. These are not part of the human body Chakra System, but are important to understand for the overall health of the body.

The back correlates to the root, sacral, solar plexus, and heart chakras.

The upper limbs include the arms and hands, which correlate to several chakra areas as well.

The neck correlates to the throat/thyroid chakra.

The head correlates to the pineal gland chakra. The cranial area correlates to the crown chakra.

The circulatory system and the skin, which is the largest organ in the body, correlate throughout the entire chakra system.

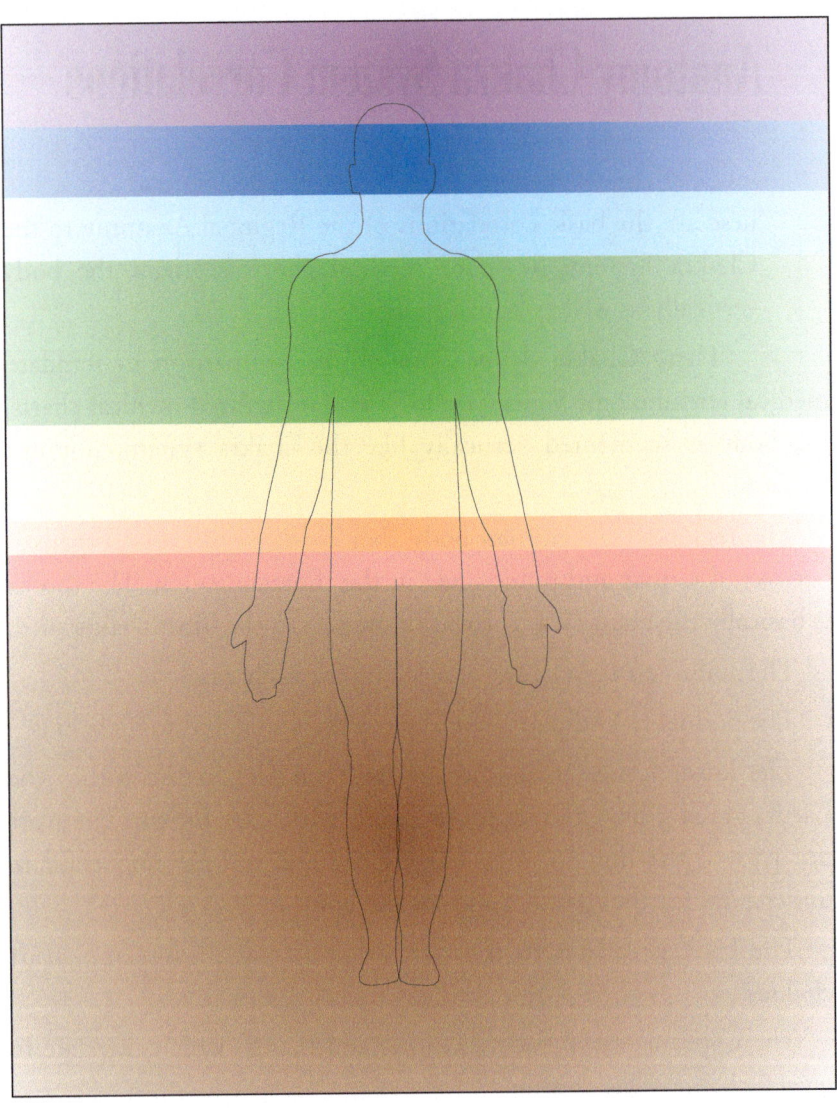

# General Chakra Mind-Pattern Correlations

Mind-patterns, or thought-bands, coalesce to manifest each chakra. As a species, humans have general thought-bands that coalesce to create specific colors in specific areas of the physical body.

Within each chakra, your individual mind-patterns delineate and refine the thought-bands into specific manifestations, whether beneficial or non-beneficial specifically to you as a unique individual.

Other species have different chakras because they have different thought-bands, especially animals, insects, plants, and so forth. Different life-forms have varying numbers of chakras due to their levels of awareness.

When we look at the Flowchart of God-Mind, level 2, level 3, and all the way down, all of the levels feed back. All of these thought-bands are projected into each one. What happens when humanity continually projects out, then projects out into animals, insect life, plant life, and into mineral life?

It lessens; it weakens and becomes less and less intense. Just like the ink in a copy machine, it gets less and less as you keep using it. That is why most species below the level of humanity have fewer chakra systems and the colors are different. The intensity is a lesser reflection of the original, yet it is still connected, it is still part of it.

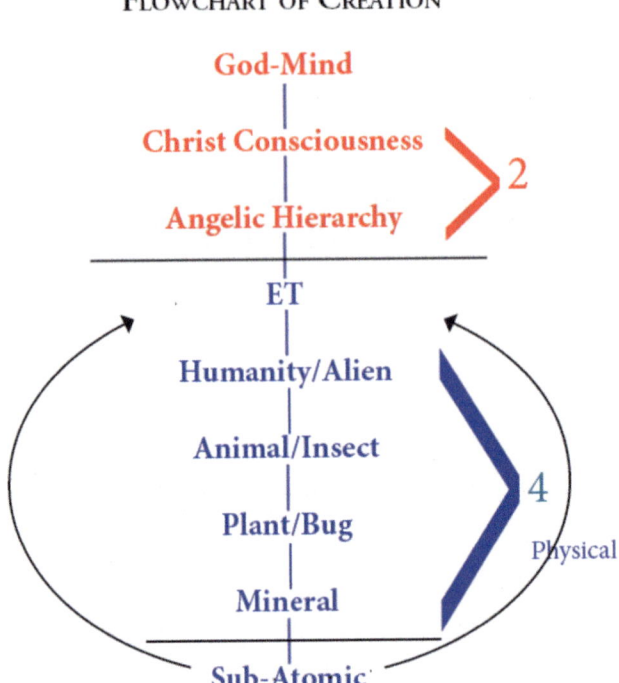

What happens to the mind-pattern when we get to a level below the level of humanity? It is more of a group mind, so there is less differentiation. It makes sense because when the energy gets less intense there is less of it to delineate, so it has to stay as a species or group mind-pattern. It makes sense then that creatures are the way they are, like animals and plant kingdoms, because the intensity is less they cannot differentiate so much.

## Chakras

### Crown Chakra/Violet

The Crown Chakra is the connection to your Oversoul and the God-Mind. The crown chakra receives information as well as provides protection.

### Pineal Chakra/Royal Blue

There are mainly two thought-bands associated with the Pineal Chakra. The first is balance. The second is the ability to create an environment and experiences within that environment.

These are general thought-bands, common to all humans.

### Thyroid Chakra/Ice Blue

The Thyroid, or Throat Chakra, correlates to communication and self-expression as well as regulates the body's support structure.

Even though these may be different thought-bands, they all correlate to each other. For example, when you create your environment or experiences, you must balance them in some way, otherwise the outpicturing will not be acceptable to you or others.

When you communicate, you must regulate the intensity of your self-expression, and you need a support structure so you can accomplish that.

All of these thought-bands are related to one another, which is why they manifest within the same chakra.

### Heart Chakra/Medium Green

The Heart Chakra correlates to feelings and processing of current emotions, and acts as a mediator between body sections.

The Flowchart of Creation/Existence represents how God-Mind rhythmically breathes out and breathes back in, over and over. This exchange of energy really represents out with the old, in with the new; as above, so below. This means that you need to eliminate and release the pieces that are no longer necessary or useful and generate new ones that are more appropriate. This also explains why release work takes place in the Heart Chakra.

## Solar Plexus Chakra/Pale Yellow

The Solar Plexus Chakra is a simple thought-band even though it has the most extensive organs in this area of the body. The mind-pattern of this region correlates to digestion. The solar plexus correlates to understanding and absorption of information and ideas.

The digestive system is extensive. If stretched out from beginning to end, your intestines would extend out for almost one mile/two kilometers.

There is a reason why you need such an extensive system. Metaphorically speaking, to translate nonphysical to physical, you need to extract as much out of an experience as possible from each moment, and then absorb all of that information before you release it and move on.

## Sacral Chakra/Pale Orange

There are several main thought-bands or mind-patterns that correspond to the Sacral Chakra: creativity, trust, truth, and reproduction. But there is something else relating to an organ in that thought-band.

Anger issues—this is why the bladder is located there. The Sacral Chakra releases anger and processes the past.

The aspects of the physical body in the sacral are creativity and reproduction. Being productive and creative in life is all related in this chakra.

The Pineal Chakra is also related to the Sacral Chakra. The pineal is heavily connected to the sacral as it provides the ability to create our experiences and environment. The sacral is essential in releasing anger associated with creations and processing them, which are either a result of the sacral or pineal thought-bands. After this realization we might want to recreate or reproduce in a different way. The pineal basically gives us the impetus to create and the sacral keeps it going. One is the source of the electricity and the other is the step-up transformer.

## Root Chakra/Pale Red

The Root Chakra correlates to survival, releasing the past, physical creation, and sexuality. The thought-band of this chakra is comprised of the connections of male/female differentiations.

The primary male characteristic correlating to creation is the sending, or projecting out, of energy.

The primary female characteristic correlating to creation is the receiving, or absorption, of energy. The creation of the physical body is only associated with the female on the sacral level and is not a male thought-band.

These are the sexual differentiations as far as the thought-bands are concerned.

## Legs and Feet/Brown
## Earth's Gravitational and Magnetic Fields

The legs and feet are not in a chakra area; however they definitely reside within a thought-band. Legs and feet represent stepping into the future, support structures in life, and movement into the future.

What if you belonged to a species that consciously realized that there was no time/space and that the past, present, and future are the same? Do you think they could float and have no need for legs or feet as humans do? What would the mind-pattern be for the support structure of these types of Beings?

# Specific Chakra Mind-Pattern Correlations

The organs located within each chakra band of the body each have a function as well as a specific mind-pattern.

## Crown Chakra

The Crown Chakra starts at the top of the head and extends to the top of the forehead. This is a very narrow chakra band in the color Violet. There is no organ that is entirely in this chakra band. Located within this Violet chakra band is the top of the cerebrum section of the brain, including both the right and left hemispheres.

The functions in this region of the brain include sensation, basic movements, skilled movements, behavior, emotion, and visual recognition. Memory is stored in this area of the brain as well as stored within cells throughout your body.

This is why when someone gets hit on the top of the head, damage can be quite extensive. Look at all the physical functions that are affected by this part of your brain.

As you know, in Hyperspace, Violet, the color of this chakra band, represents Protection. Moving your hands is a basic protective movement. You need the Violet of your brain to use your hands to direct the protective movement of your hands. You also need Violet to direct more skilled movements, such as using tools and implements, playing a musical instrument, cooking, sewing, yoga, and so forth.

Scientific research demonstrates that electrical brain stimulation (EBS) or focal brain stimulation (FBS) with an electrical probe creates movement in various body parts.

Behavior and emotion are intricately related in the same area of the brain because you physically express the emotions that you feel. These expressions need Violet to filter them because you must think before you act.

The visual cortex is the part of the brain that processes visual information, located in the occipital lobe at the back of the brain. Visual recognition is not actual sight that "sees," but rather visual recognition is about understanding what is seen.

Damage to the top of the cerebrum often impairs visual recognition. This can result in the individual seeing what is front of him/her, but not being able to recognize what he/she sees.

Damaged visual recognition is one symptom in Alzheimer's disease. The person recognizes something but he/she does not have the capacity to know how to filter the energy of what is seen or protect him/herself because visual recognition is damaged.

The brain needs visual recognition to know what kind of movement to command the body to make as a response to what it sees. Visual recognition allows the person to understand what he/she feels as well as what sensations he/she receives. In a brain that functions correctly, the responses are immediate because the brain processes more information in a split second than any computer in creation.

Heavy metals, including aluminum, can contribute to Alzheimer's disease. When a person has a build-up of heavy metals in the body over the course of a lifetime, the metals can affect the sheathing over the brain. The heavy metal can infiltrate the brain and affect this chakra area.

Energetically, Alzheimer's disease is the removal of the Soul-Personality from the body's awareness. This can be compared to a body without a brain. Alzheimer's is really disassociation; it comes from a German word that means "old home."

Dementia is different than Alzheimer's disease. In dementia, the actions of the person are not appropriate. These individuals can become violent and damaging to themselves and others. A person can have dementia and not have Alzheimer's. A person can react inappropriately but not have dementia.

In the crown chakra band, the most common issues involve Alzheimer's disease and dementia.

Mind-pattern behind someone with Alzheimer's:

*I see something I used in the past,
but now I do not know what it is.*

Some items remain recognizable; what they forget is selective. To find the specific mind-pattern for a specific person, observe the object they do not recall as well as how they now recognize it. Whatever this object meant to the person explains the mind-pattern reason for the damage to that area of the brain.

Some people with Alzheimer's do not remember family members, including their own children. This is a big clue. Why does a parent choose to forget a family member, yet recognize other people? Obviously, there is something in the relationship that the person does not want to deal with anymore.

Amnesia, which is like temporary dementia, can happen to anyone at any time for a variety of reasons, especially with a severe injury to the head. Depending upon the condition of the patient, the damaged area of the brain may regenerate and life can return back to normal.

Even in Alzheimer's patients the brain can be regenerated, especially with injections of stem cells and/or live cells that can help regenerate that section of the brain. Certain herbs and glandular products may stimulate and help regenerate the brain. Chelation therapy can also help.

## Muscular Dystrophy and Multiple Sclerosis

Muscular dystrophy and multiple sclerosis partially correspond to the crown chakra; they are also related to other systems. These conditions affect the entire body so they have multiple mind-patterns associated with them.

To determine the foundational mind-pattern to the illness, it is important to look at when the symptoms first started as well as where they first manifested in the body.

You must be very careful when delineating the mind-patterns for the diseases that are pervasive to the whole body, including such ailments as Parkinson's Disease.

## Huntington's Disease

Huntington's Disease is diagnosed when the inside of the brain starts to disintegrate and evaporate. Even with 30-40% of the brain gone, some people with this disease are still able walk around and continue functioning. This illustrates that there are other sections of the brain that compensate for the missing parts.

## PINEAL CHAKRA

The Pineal Chakra is from the top of the forehead to the tip of the nose in the color Royal Blue. This chakra band encompasses the majority of the brain. The pineal gland is also called the pineal body. Scientists say they are not certain what the pineal gland does. At one time it was considered a vestigial organ left over from long ago. It produces the hormone "melatonin" and the compound "pinoline." The pineal gland's absolute function cannot be tested and measured, according to conventional medical science. This is because the pineal gland is the liaison between the physical and the non-physical.

Melatonin is photosensitive; it regulates and modulates sleeping and waking patterns as well as seasonal adjustments. Melatonin is stimulated and activated by darkness and inhibited or suppressed by light. Melatonin also initiates the precursor or impulse for serotonin development.

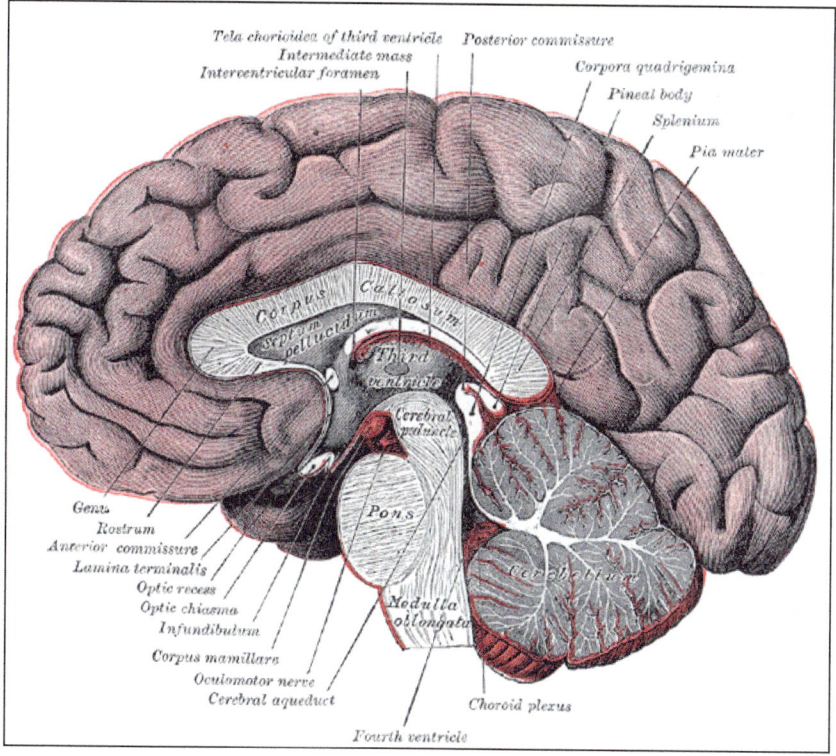

Pinoline occurs in the pineal during the metabolism of melatonin and is a component in human blood and cerebral spinal fluid. These chemicals are basically interdimensional drugs. This is why it is difficult for conventional medical science to measure or understand what the pineal does; it has several functions—both physical and non-physical. Scientists basically defer to the pituitary gland because they think they know what that does.

Mind-pattern behind the pineal:

*How I balance and create experiences.*

The pineal pulls together the energy of the right and left hemispheres of the brain to create both the logical and emotional impulses for physical manifestations. This is why visualizations are centered at the pineal.

The pituitary, hypothalamus, and thalamus are all located around and in front of the pineal; they all have very close connections. The pineal gland sends electrical impulses to these other glands instructing them to secrete and regulate hormonal levels. These then feed into other systems in the body.

Most of your five senses are located in the pineal chakra band—sight, hearing, and smell.

## Recommendations and Precautions for Optimal Pineal Gland Function

Calcification of the pineal gland is a result of the accumulation of fluoride as proven by scientific studies, which includes individuals as young as two years old. Tamarind removes fluoride from the system. Vitamin D removes calcification from the pineal gland as well as other organs of the body.

The form of tamarind is unimportant as long as it is organic; it comes in concentrate, pill, pod, and tea forms. The length of time necessary to remove fluoride depends on the extent of the contamination.

Fluoride cannot be removed via filters from water. This is known from industrial and agriculture research projects. The only way to remove fluoride is through steam distillation.

Take Dead Sea salt baths with ½ cup of organic white vinegar to remove toxins. Dead Sea salt baths will prevent absorption of all the toxins in tap water as well.

In general, most people need 2,000-5,000 IUs of Vitamin D every day. The dosage varies depending upon each person's body weight and health status, as well as sun exposure.

For pineal gland opening visualizations, use the ones outlined in these Expansions' books: ***Hyperspace Helper***, ***Hyperspace Plus, Healing Archetypes & Symbols and Healer's Handbook.***

Organic frankincense essential oil also aids in strengthening the pineal gland. The wrists have sweat glands and pores that allow for absorption of the oil. You can also use a few drops on the back of the neck, forehead, temples, small of the back, bottom of feet, palms, armpits, and groin. You can even put one or more drops in your bath water; some people put a drop in a glass of steam-distilled water to sip.

Do not use, test or experiment with psychedelic drugs or hallucinogens because they are extremely dangerous and developed for the purpose of mind-control. Too many people are left with brain damage as a result of their experimentations.

Drug use in general opens all the lower chakras so more programming can be installed and lowers the body frequencies to match the astral plane. Even marijuana with prolonged use is known to cause genetic defects, causing long-term damage to the chromosomes that in turn adversely change the aura and chakras.

Marijuana destroys brain cells and deadens the brain's ability to build nerve pathways, damages the liver, weakens organs, burns the lining of the lungs, and dulls the pineal gland. Marijuana also allows astral entities to enter your energy field and astral attachments to occur as well as open and activate programming alters and alter groups.

Mind-pattern behind all drug addictions:

*There is something about my reality that I want to blot out; there is something in my life or past that I do not want to deal with or remember.*

Using drugs to "attain enlightenment" is a dangerously rapid destructive road whose results can be achieved in a safer manner. It is not a question of right or wrong, or even legality; it is a question of safety. Through the use of Hyperspace/Oversoul tools and techniques, you can achieve much safer results. Accessing your mind in this way will bring you closer to the higher level of understanding that you seek. If you use a drug as a crutch to get you there, the results will not last, and as stated, can open the doors to an extremely long-term destructive path.

## THE PITUITARY

The pituitary gland is directly in front of the pineal. The pituitary is a master organ because it commands the orders, chemically and otherwise, to the other endocrine systems. These other endocrine glands secrete certain hormones and chemicals in the body at different levels. The pituitary gets its commands from the pineal. Electrically, the pituitary is like the CPU (central processing unit) and the distribution center of instructions.

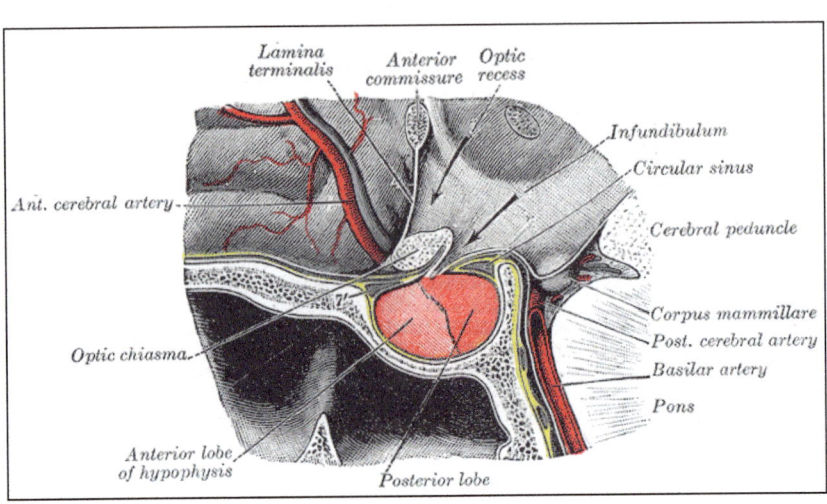

## Hypothalamus

The hypothalamus regulates sexual behavior, water intake, and the biological clock. This means all these functions are related and explains why they are located in this section of the brain. What does that tell you about these functions?

Everyone's water intake is different; it is incorrect to assume everyone needs 8-10 glasses of water a day. Most people would drown if they drank that much! Most people need much less than that.

The hypothalamus sends a signal to the thyroid, which then sends a signal to the intestinal area to regulate digestion. All these three areas are related.

In ***Healer's Handbook***, there are visualizations to change or reverse the biological clock that in turn resets the hypothalamus.

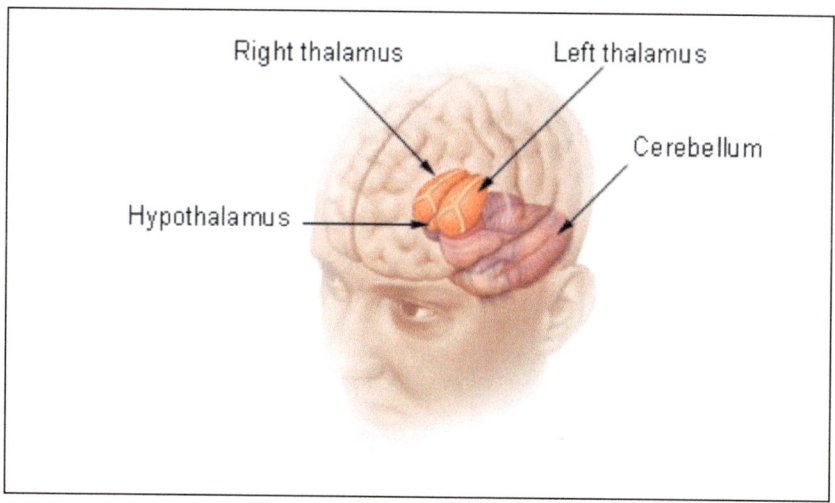

## Thalamus

The thalamus involves memory and stereotype behaviors. This refers to what you expect from others and yourself, habits and inherited mind-patterns.

Physically, memories are stored in the thalamus. Everyone has inherited ancestral memory. Some memories come from each individual's Oversoul family. However, there is also cellular memory stored in other parts of the body.

The thalamus is where people become activated when they have past-life/simultaneous regression therapies. The thalamus triggers inherited cellular memory, which will bring up an event that may or may not have actually happened to the individual's Soul-Personality. The memory that is triggered could be inherited from one of the individual's ancestors where it became genetically encoded. This indicates the experience was intense and occurred multiple times.

It takes at least three imprintings of an event or experience to become genetically encoded.

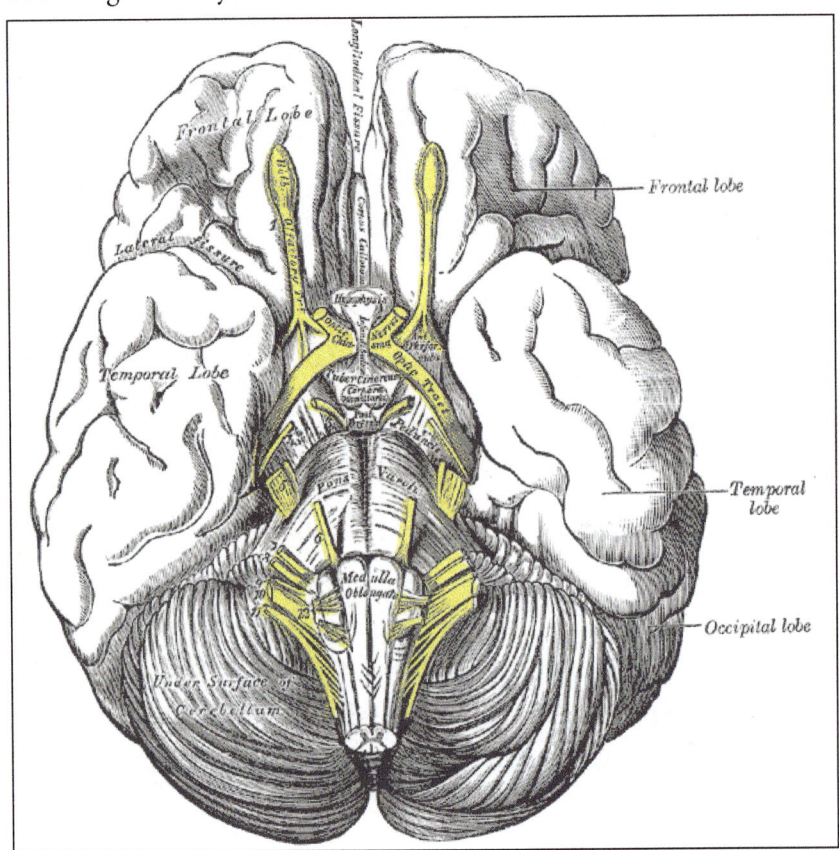

Some memories can only be triggered if a certain part of the body is stimulated in a specific way. Usually this involves current life trauma. Generally, inherited memory is stimulated in the thalamus but not always. The brain is the device and source that translates the mind-pattern.

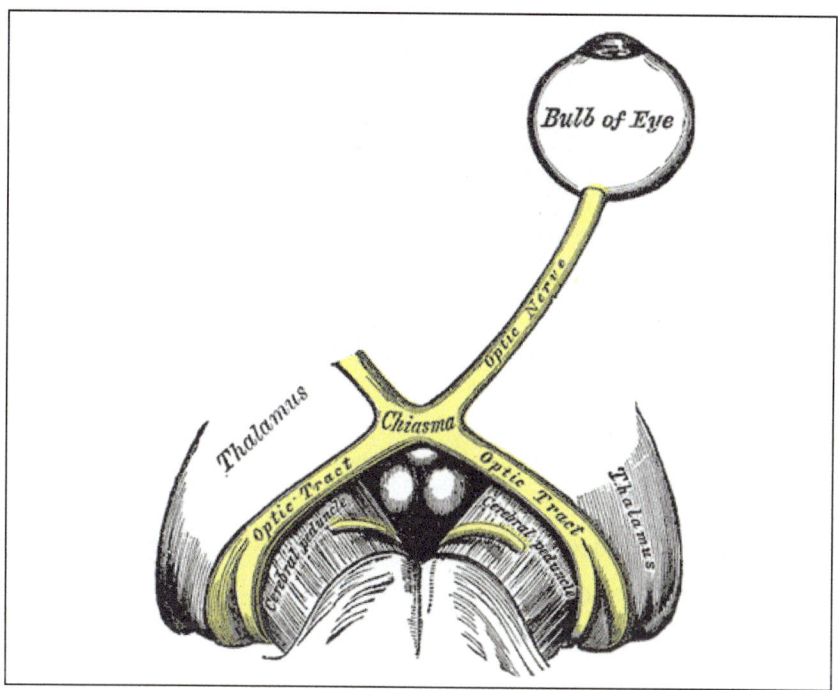

**E**YES

Mind-pattern:

*What I see and direct in my experience in physical reality.*

There are two eyes that indicate powerful vision.

The left eye correlates to female issues, logic, and physical reality.

The right eye correlates to male issues, emotion, and spirituality.

In certain circles, the pineal is considered a third eye.

Mind-pattern for the pineal:

*What I see in nonphysical reality.*

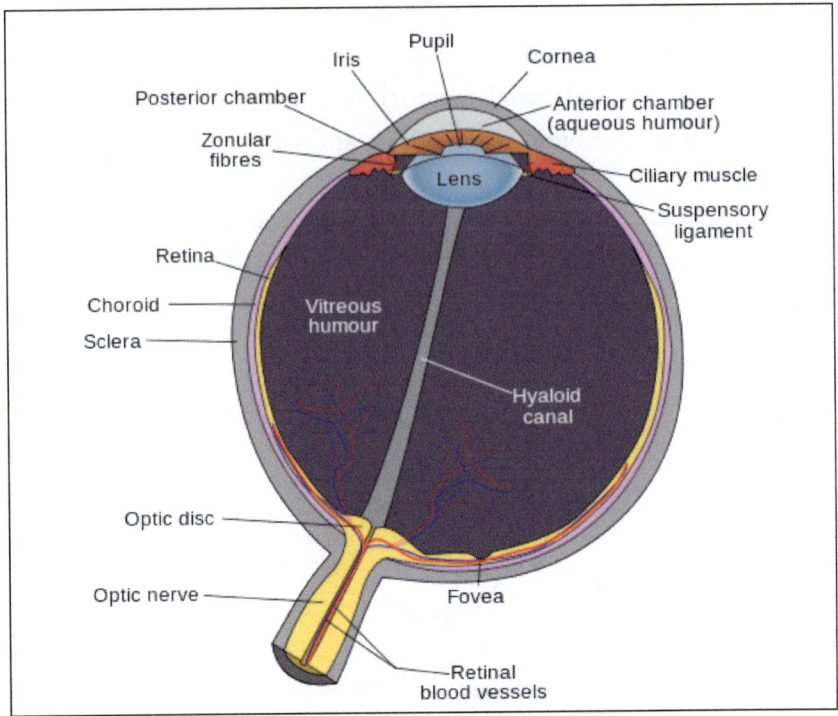

Any illness or disease that affects the eyes tells you what the specific mind-pattern is. There are several variables and conditions related to the eyes such as cataracts, macular degeneration, or irritation of the iris.

Eyes really see in reverse; the brain crosses and straightens out the visual perception. Physical reality is a reverse, or mirror image, of the non-physical/Hyperspace origins of all things.

When you see, you actually project out energy that then feeds back to you like a camera or sonar. Since everything is energetically reversed, the physical structure of the eyes and brain have to turn the image upside down and backwards so you see it correctly in a way the mind can understand.

Physically the splenium of the corpus callosum reverses everything as it crosses over this point. The right eye is controlled by the left brain, and the left eye is controlled by the right brain.

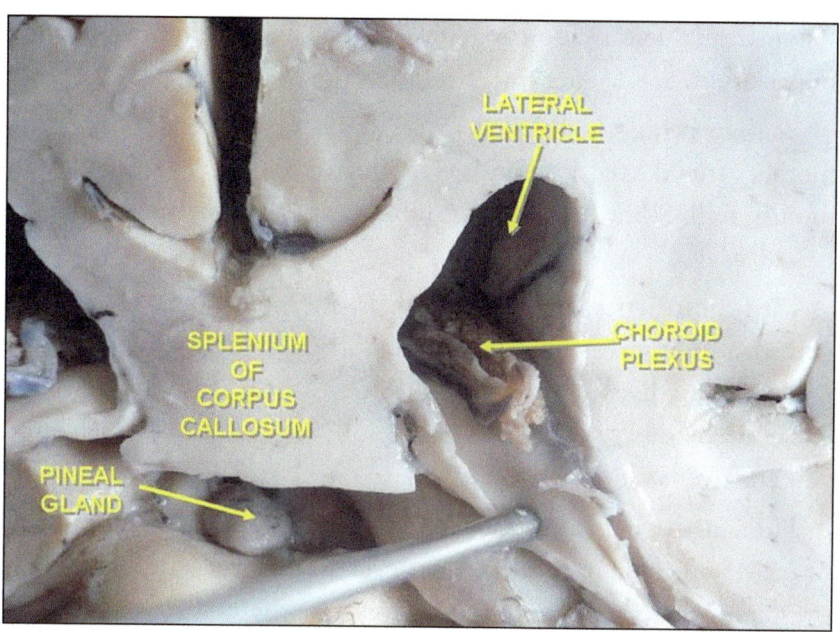

Energetically, the left half and the right half of the body are separate; this is the same principle as visual sight. The body itself is crossed over or mirroring the other side/nonphysical reality to accompany perceptions that would not be confusing. Otherwise you would see upside down and backwards, means you would not have control of your body. Everything has to be reversed because physical reality is the mirror image of nonphysical reality.

Imagine living with mirrors all the time and never knowing which side is which.

This is why the body accomplishes this; it is the physical compensation for the mirroring energy.

Mind-pattern for a person who can see far away but not close up:
*I do not want to see what is around me right now.*
*I want to go way out there.*

Society is collectively imprinted to believe that when people reach specific ages, specific physical conditions will set in, including poor vision (read "The Death Program" in *True World History* for more information).

You are being conditioned to create ill health. For example, my mother's friend lived in Florida. Her doctor told her that she had six months to live. She felt fine, but unfortunately within six months she passed away.

Medical societies, legal professionals, and political parties can kill you with their words! In school, one of the first items taught is how long humans live. Then, you continue to hear this rhetoric your entire life, so you accept these lies, adhering to the time schedule you are given.

Humans have a large ocular range, but only use a small portion of it. Most people must close their eyes and concentrate to see with the pineal instead of the physical eyes. Yet the capacity is there to see these things with your eyes open. Many people can do this, but without understanding what they are seeing, may be labeled crazy or diagnosed with eye issues, for which they are medicated.

When children tell adults they see discarnate entities, energy fields, hyperspace symbols, and so forth, they are often told it is their imagination or taken to doctors for evaluation.

People are conditioned from childhood to shut off this ability, so you must learn to reopen and strengthen the pineal. Just like a muscle that is not used, these abilities weaken, but they are still there. In addition, everyone sees everything but people have been de-focused to only see a narrower spectrum—eyes, ears, nose, mouth—and not to look at what is going on around the head—energy, symbols, shapes, pictures, and so forth.

## CRYING

The physical reason you cry is to remove toxins from the eyes.

Mind-pattern:

*I release what I see from the ocean of life;*

*I purge/cleanse what I see/experience in life.*

Your tears have salt in them. Salt cleanses, so when you cry you cleanse what you are looking at. This is why the tear ducts are around your eyes. You use them to try to cleanse the experience you see.

## SINUSES

Mind-pattern:

*How I let others affect me.*

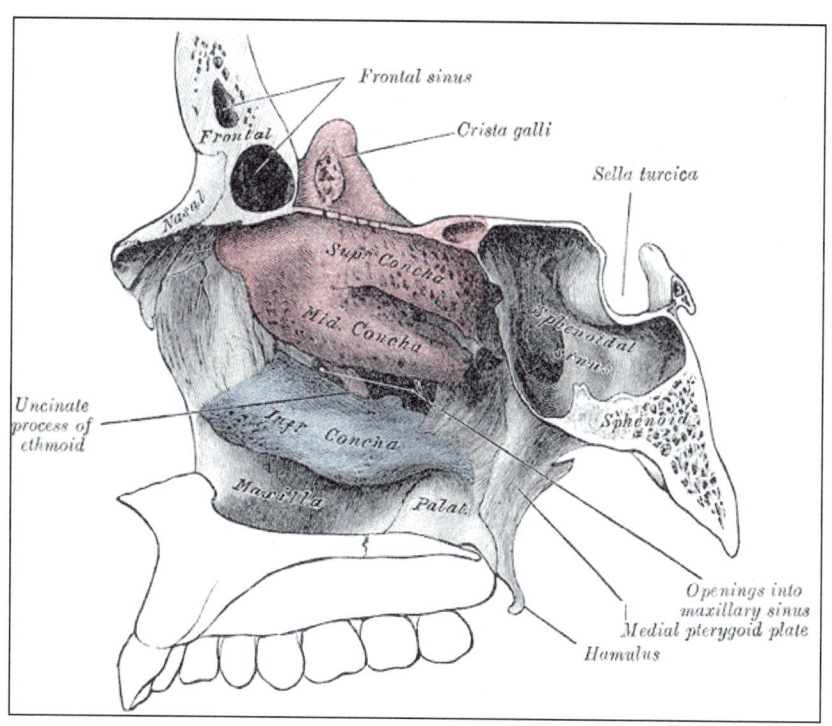

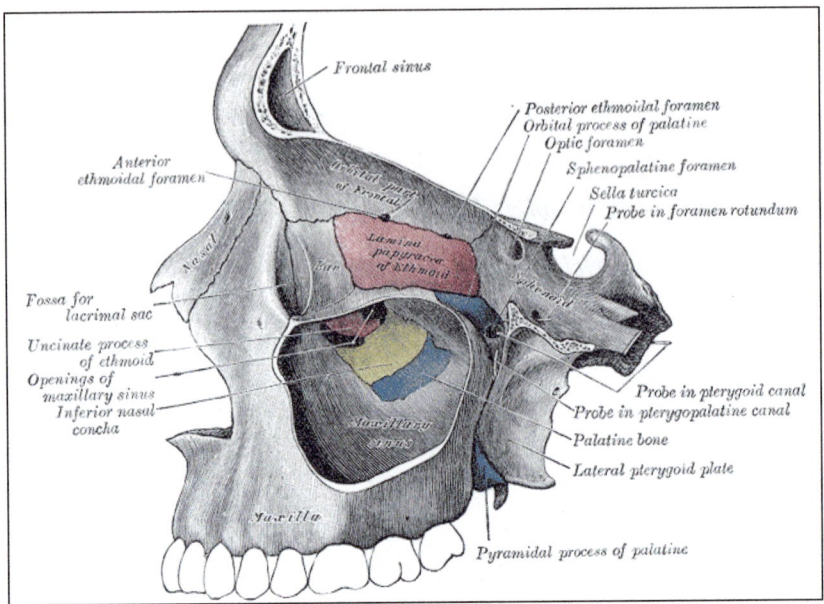

That is why you experience sinus problems whenever someone irritates or annoys you.

When this happens, look at the reflections of the irritation or annoyance to understand what you are projecting out so you can take responsibility for that aspect of your personality and mind-pattern.

Whenever you project out a mind-pattern, that mind-pattern automatically attracts those who reflect it back. This is why you find a certain person annoying. Whatever you find annoying about that person correlates to the same mind-pattern you have within yourself.

When you repeatedly meet people with the same annoying and irritating characteristics, this is only a magnified reflection of what you project out.

Even if you are only with a pet without any humans present, the pet may begin behaving in ways it never did before, such as urinating on furniture. This is because the animal picks up your mind-pattern and reflects that out. Most people look at the animal and think, "What is wrong with it?" or the other person and think, "What is wrong with him/her?"

You are highly challenged when you truly look within at yourself. The foundation of any illness is based on a mind-pattern for which you are not taking responsibility. Once you correct the mind-pattern, the illness can permanently leave.

### Nose

Do you know what the nose knows?

Mind-pattern:

*What is right in front of my face; what is obvious to me.*

*I, me, it is all about me, everything is about me.*
*The world is made for me.*

The world is made for you because what you create or reflect has to come from you. So, you must take responsibility.

Slight nose injury:

*I am not paying attention to the most obvious things in my life;*

*I need to pay attention to them.*

Breaking your nose:

*It has been a long time since you took the*
*obvious into consideration.*

The sense of smell is one of the earliest sensory modalities because it warns you if food is okay to eat or if the food may sicken you. Over the centuries, humans have eliminated their understanding of smells, because many are considered socially unacceptable.

Now, people are conditioned to ignore or totally shut off their sense of smell.

Often, smells are eliminated or masked with sprays and perfumes.

## Snoring

Snoring:

*Stubbornness.*

The connection between snoring and stubbornness involves individuals who will not change their mind-pattern and subliminally need attention. They are consciously afraid of attention, so they get it when they are asleep or unconscious.

Most people snore when they sleep on their backs. If you move the person they stop snoring, but they do not quit snoring on their own. Generally snoring is a human mind-pattern. If you have a cat or dog that snores, they reflect you.

## Auditory System

Mind-pattern:

*What I hear in my experiences.*

Severe pain in the right ear:

*What I hear hurts me from a male figure or what I hear about my emotions or creativity is hurtful to me.*

So, you need to know exactly what that is.

Fluid in the ears indicates a blockage. Fluid is liquid and liquid/water relates to emotions. Mind-pattern:

*I feel emotionally overwhelmed by what I hear.*

Pierced ears:

*What I hear can pierce me or hurt me.*

Mothers who pierce their children's ears project their own mind-pattern onto the child through pre-natal socialization. This means in the womb the child was imprinted with the frequency of the mother's nervous system.

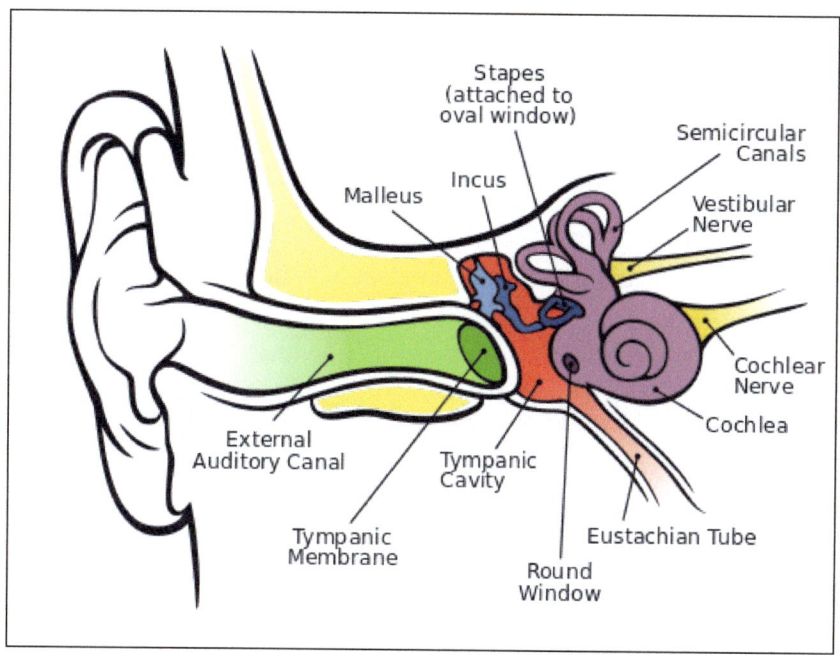

In some cases the mother does not even have pierced ears, but lives vicariously through the child. Often, the child grows up to resent the parent for doing this to him/her.

Persistent earaches in children, particularly in one ear, usually mean the child does not want to hear what the parent says. Parents who berate their children with negative comments often have children with ear issues. While the child's mind-pattern must be examined, it is the parents who must first start working on their mind-patterns to boost the mind-pattern of the child.

Earaches can be the result of a ritual. Something in the ritual hurts or angers the child, and the child does not want to hear it.

There are two reasons ears get bigger as you get older; one is physical and the other is energetic. The purpose of the ears is to hear vibrations. As you get older because of mind-pattern, the tubes, nerves, and arteries become harder. In response, the ears get bigger to compensate.

The energetic reason your ears get bigger is because as you become aware of the experiences around you, you want to hear more.

When ears close up or become deaf:

*I do not want to hear any more.*

Some people have selective hearing. My father only hears my mother when it is time to eat. He does not hear her when she says anything else.

## THROAT/THYROID CHAKRA

The Thyroid Chakra is from the tip of the nose to the collarbone in the color Ice Blue. This area includes the tongue, teeth, salivary glands (parotid), thyroid, parathyroid, larynx, and tonsils.

### TONGUE

Mind-pattern:

*Tasting life expressions of Self.*

The tongue directs the vibration of communication physically and energetically.

Piercing the tongue:

*I am clamping down on the things I need to verbalize.*

Burning the tongue:

*I am angry I said that.*

What does it mean if you have a favorite flavor or taste? Or you dislike a particular food or taste? What you like or dislike indicates a great deal about your mind-pattern.

For example, if you do not like the taste of bitter foods, this may mean you feel you have a bitter life. If you like bitter foods, this could mean that you are bitter about your life. However, sometimes bitter is the antidote to correcting and balancing your mind-pattern. If you avoid this type of food it may mean that you avoid the antidote that could be your healing.

If you crave a sweet life, you may crave sugar or sweets as you look for sweetness and pleasure. Chocolate is a mix of both bitter and sweet flavors—this might represent a more balanced perspective of life, as well as fat, which represents a craving for smoothness in life.

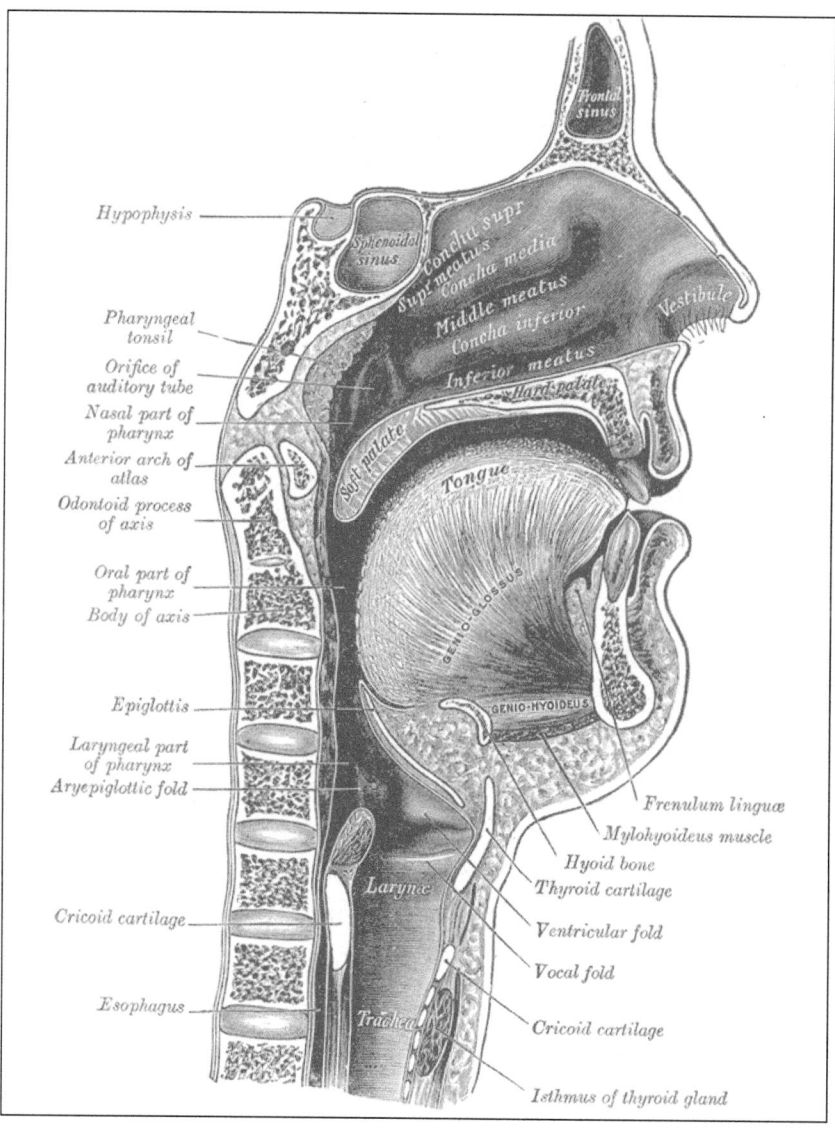

If you like smooth, creamy food, you might be looking for a smoother life. If you like food that has more texture, or even eating meat from a bone, then you may like having more rough spots or challenges in your life—something to chew on.

Some people do not like foods that are too sweet. They say, "Oh, it is too sweet" or "It is too rich." Mind-pattern behind this:

*I am restricting myself from the sweetness and richness in life.*

For example, some people see different objects in their hands when they do the Ocean of Life visualization exercise (***Healer's Handbook***). If you have small items in your hands, this represents you do not like overly rich foods; you think you do not deserve them.

People who like salty food followed by something sweet may be programmed to abruptly switch altars.

If you prefer bland food, you may prefer to stay with your status quo rather than venture beyond your well-established borders and boundaries. You prefer "safe" and like to stay with what you know.

Craving spicy foods means, "spice up your life"—you do not want "boring," you want fast, hot, and exciting activities and adventures. Hot spicy foods also promote perspiration. The people of cultures that include hot spicy foods in their diets tend to have hot temperaments that need to be cooled.

In addition, these cultures are usually found in hot climates in regions filled with instability and volatility as well as diseases such as polio, malaria, and other hot-climate illnesses. The people here are generally zesty and energetic with fast-paced lives and challenges. This is why these countries are unstable, reflecting the foods they consume, which in turn reflects the temperament of the people.

If you like bland food but are out with people who like spicy food, this means that you need to spice up your life; and those who like spicy food need to tone down their lives. There must be matching color, tone, and archetype or you could not all be together.

If you prefer dry food, you like your information "cut and dry."

Food is always a representation of what you put in your mind. Whatever food you like or do not like to consume tells you the type of information you accept or reject as well as your preference for learning. Your food choices are not "good" or "bad"; they are simply a statement of how you are in this moment. Food preferences offer another way to understand your mind-pattern that in turn affects the health of your body.

### TEETH

Mind-pattern:

*How I adjust to my life.*

The reason you go to the dentist is to physically act out a need to adjust something in your life, one or more experiences that you cannot verbalize. When the dentist works on your teeth, your mouth is "numbed" because the adjustment process is something that you do not want to talk about.

Even if you fix your teeth you must work on the mind-pattern that created the issue in the first place or you will develop a similar issue or even one that is more severe somewhere in your body.

Teeth cleaning:

*There is a layer of adjustment I need to remove in order to continue.*

Root canal:

*I do not have the nerve to make this adjustment.*

Tooth extraction:

*I am not going to deal with the issue; I am just getting rid of it.*

Crowns, implants, and veneers:

*I am artificially covering up or replacing an issue.*

Cavities and fillings:
*Victimization and needing artificial assistance to adjust to life.*

Crooked teeth:
*I am incorrectly adjusting to my current life situation.*

Severe overbite:
*What I adjust to in my future, not what is in front of me now.*

Severe underbite:
*I am only going to assimilate and adjust to my past. I am not looking at my present or my future.*

## SALIVARY/PAROTID GLANDS

The salivary, or parotid, glands break down learning experiences, making it easier for you to accept and/or assimilate the experience.

Mind-pattern:
*I need to deal with the pieces instead of the whole.*

Blockages in the salivary/parotid glands:
*I am not going to make my life easier.*
*I refuse to accept an easier way of doing this; I want it the hard way.*

## THYROID GLAND

The thyroid gland regulates metabolism and the speed at which your body digests what it intakes. The thyroid gland supports the expressions of what you learn, and helps prepare the information for use.

Mind-pattern:
*Supporting expressions of learned information.*

Some people have fast thyroid metabolism, called "hyperthyroidism," and some have slow thyroid metabolism, called "hypothyroidism."

Hyperthyroidism:

> *Talking too much and belittling Self.*

Hypothyroidism:

> *Not speaking up for Self and insulating.*

Thyroid cancer:

> *Held resentment from what you did not say or what you said that was incorrect.*

Cancer is always the result of resentment. Statistically, women have greater incidences of thyroid cancer than men.

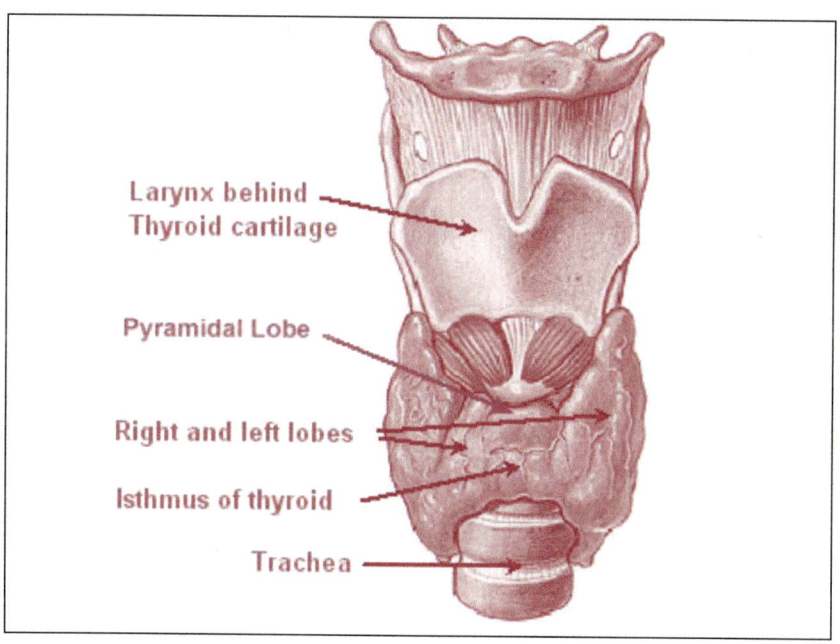

## Parathyroid

Mind-pattern:

*Supporting life structures and expressing support.
No one listens to or pays attention to me.*

There are four parathyroid glands in the human body.

Generally, when a thyroid gland is surgically removed, the parathyroid glands are also removed because they are connected.

The parathyroid glands produce Vitamin D. Vitamin D helps to absorb calcium into the bones. When you have problems with the parathyroid glands, you do not produce enough Vitamin D to help absorb calcium into your bones, which is why your bone density drops.

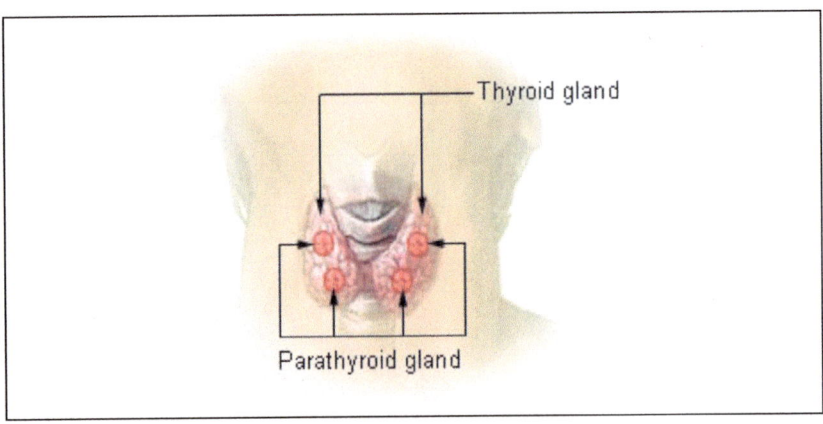

The thyroid and parathyroid glands are connected energetically as well as physically. To have a support structure in life, you need to be able to express what you are learning about life. If you cannot do one, you cannot do the other. So this is why if one organ fails, the other also fails.

Even if your thyroid and parathyroid glands are removed, you can still work on the mind-patterns because the energy of the tissue still remains. You can work on the mind-pattern of expressing what you resented having to learn.

## LARYNX

Mind-pattern:

*How I express and communicate my thoughts.*

People who do not have Hyperspace/Oversoul tools often try to ground and balance their emotions with food or smoking.

Smoking puts Brown energy into your energy field. In Hyperspace, "Brown" is the color code for grounding and balancing.

Your larynx absorbs this Brown energy, thus grounding you. Physically, your voice deepens. This happens to both males and females. Some women think that a deeper voice makes them sound more powerful and masculine, causing others to take them more seriously, especially women in business positions.

Men with a light, squeaky, or higher voice may not be taken as seriously as a man with a deeper voice. Often, males do not like other men with these types of voices.

Mind-pattern of a male or female with a light or squeaky voice:

*Do not take seriously what I am expressing.*

*Make light of my expressions (of any issue).*

*I am still a child stuck in my childhood.*

This indicates the individual is stuck in childhood. Have you ever heard a woman with a little girl voice or a 50-year-old with a voice of a 7-year-old?

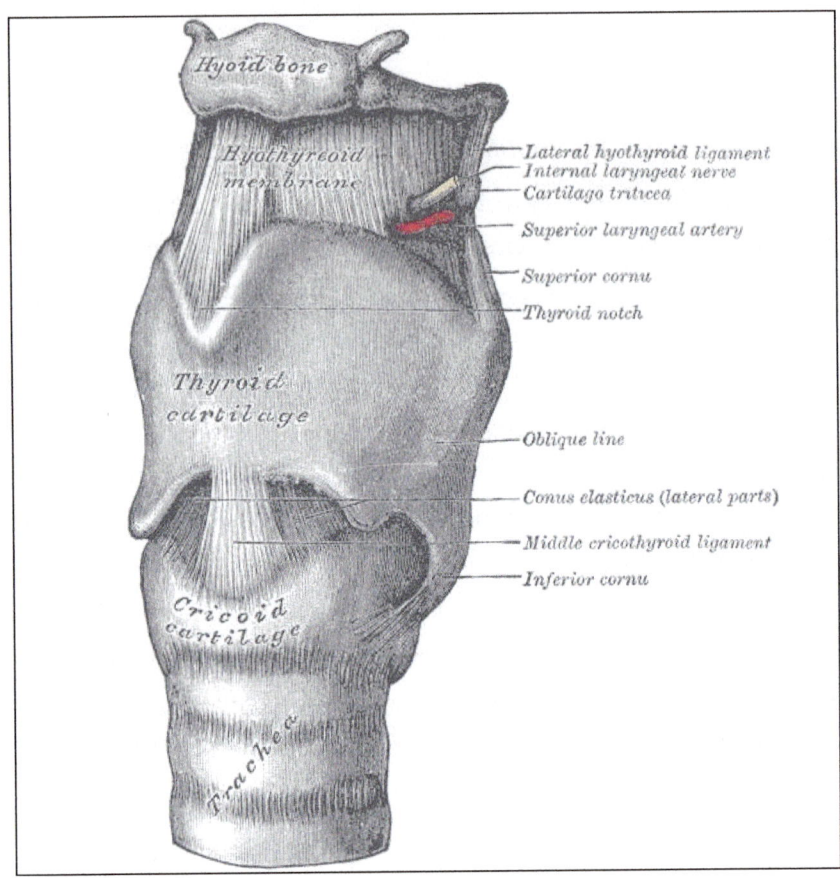

People who use child-like voices are mentally and emotionally stuck in childhood. Most likely, some type of trauma happened to them at the age of the voice that they use, which prevented them from expressing anything beyond this point in their lives.

If you have such a person in your life and his/her voice irritates you, then think about what age this person sounds like. Now, look within to determine what is irritating you from your own childhood at this age.

Women who have Monarch programming may have child-like voices because they are imprinted that this is pleasing to men.

Mind-pattern of a nasal voice:

*I have congested emotional irritations under my nose that I want to convey, but I am doing my best to block it out.*

Mind-pattern of a person's eyes that cross when he/she speaks:

*I do not want to see anything in front of me, so I mirror the translation.*

This may also be a programming function.

### ADENOIDS (PHARYNGEAL TONSILS)

The adenoids, or pharyngeal tonsils, were once believed to be vestigial organs that collected or festered germs from the lymphatic and blood system. From the 1940s through the 1960s, many people had them removed, which then increased their susceptibility to colds, flus, and strep throat, amongst other disease/illnesses.

In the 1970s, the medical profession reversed their viewpoint, only taking the adenoids out when absolutely necessary.

Mind-pattern:

*Filtering and monitoring what has already been expressed.*

Throat illnesses:

*I have anger and frustration because I am holding back what I need to say.*

Strep throat:

*What I already experienced is festering and unspoken, making me angry and hurt.*

This is why children have frequent sore throats. They are angry, hurt, and frustrated by the inability to express themselves properly, so they build up anger in the throat area.

## Heart Chakra

The Heart Chakra is from the collarbone to the sternum in Medium Green, encompassing the thymus gland, lungs, heart, liver (left upper lobe), and esophagus.

### Thymus Gland

When you experience an illness or something invasive in the body, the thymus activates and sends out T-cells to attack the pathogens.

Mind-pattern:

*Fighting for what is good or protected for me.*

Sometimes, thymus gland illness/disease is related to unresolved childhood issues.

### Lungs

The energetic reason you have two lungs is because they represent the breathing in and out of the Breath of God-Mind. Whenever you have a pair of organs, it is because the mind-pattern behind the organs is so powerful that you need to have both the physical (left) and nonphysical (right) representation. Breathing in energizes your body; breathing out expels negativity.

An energetic Soul-Personality needs two bodies, otherwise known as "twins."

Mind-pattern:

*Energizing Self and expelling negative spiritual ideas.*

Asthma:

*I am overwhelmed by my emotions.*

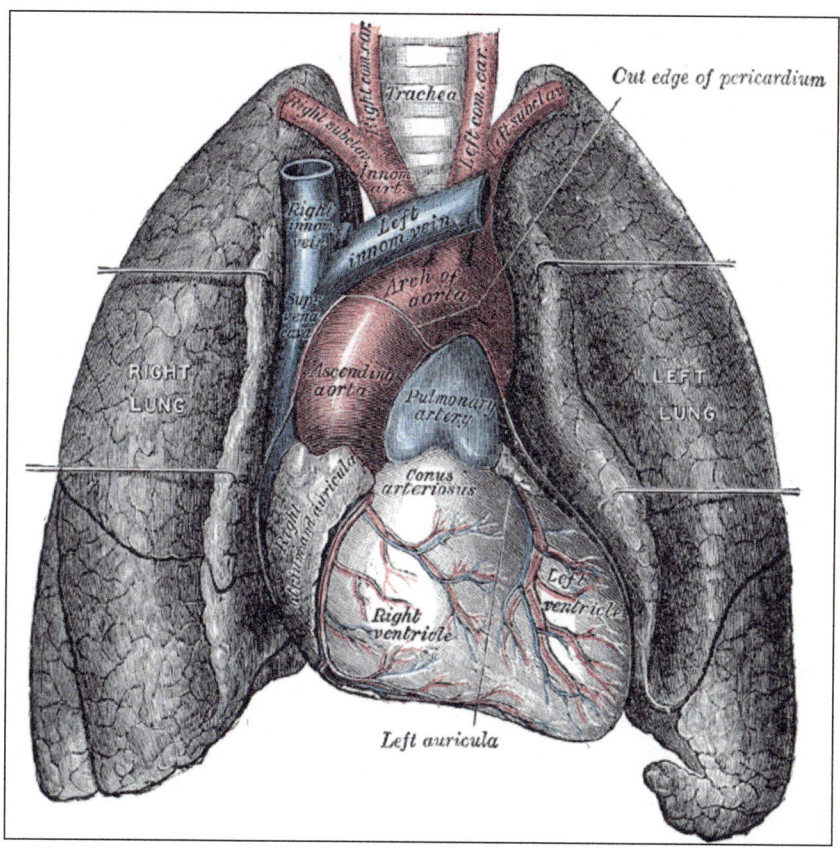

Usually, asthma develops in childhood and usually the issue is one parent in particular who overwhelms the child. Rye grass extract often eliminates the physical symptoms of asthma while you work on the mind-pattern that created the situation in the first place.

Fluid in the lungs:

*Overwhelming emotions to the point of not being able to take in or release any more ideas of self-expression. I am overwhelmed by what I've done so far.*

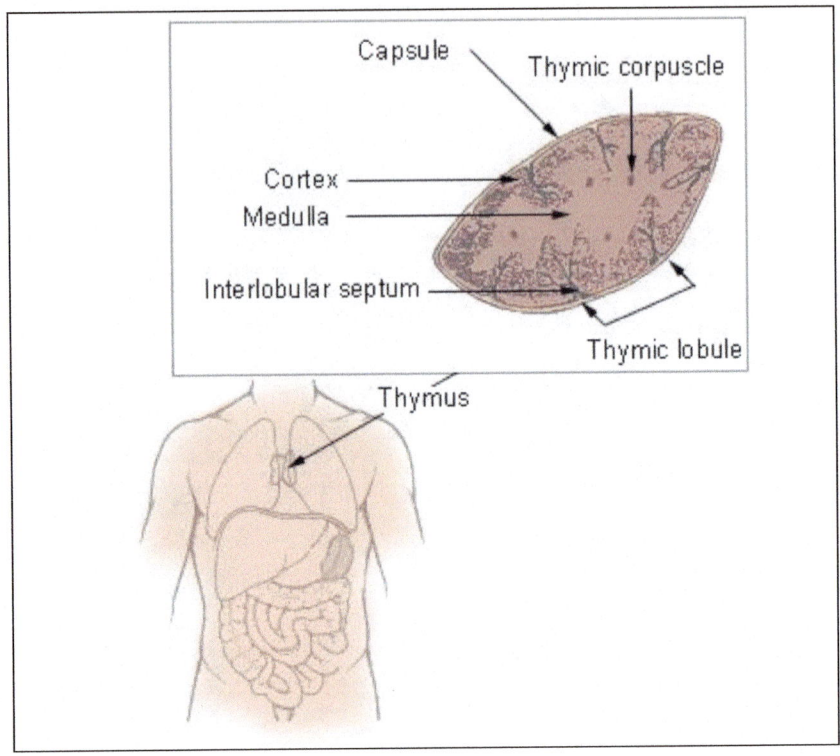

## Heart

Mind-pattern:

*Flowing joy and happiness in life.*

You only have three main arteries in the heart but four chambers. The four chambers represent physical reality. The left ventricle pushes the newly oxygenated blood to the rest of the body. Left represents physical reality; right represents nonphysical reality. Energetically, it makes sense that the left ventricle pushes the oxygenated blood out to the rest of the body.

Poor circulation:

*I do not receive any zest out of life;*
*I need something to perk me up.*

*I do not allow joy and happiness to circulate through my life.*

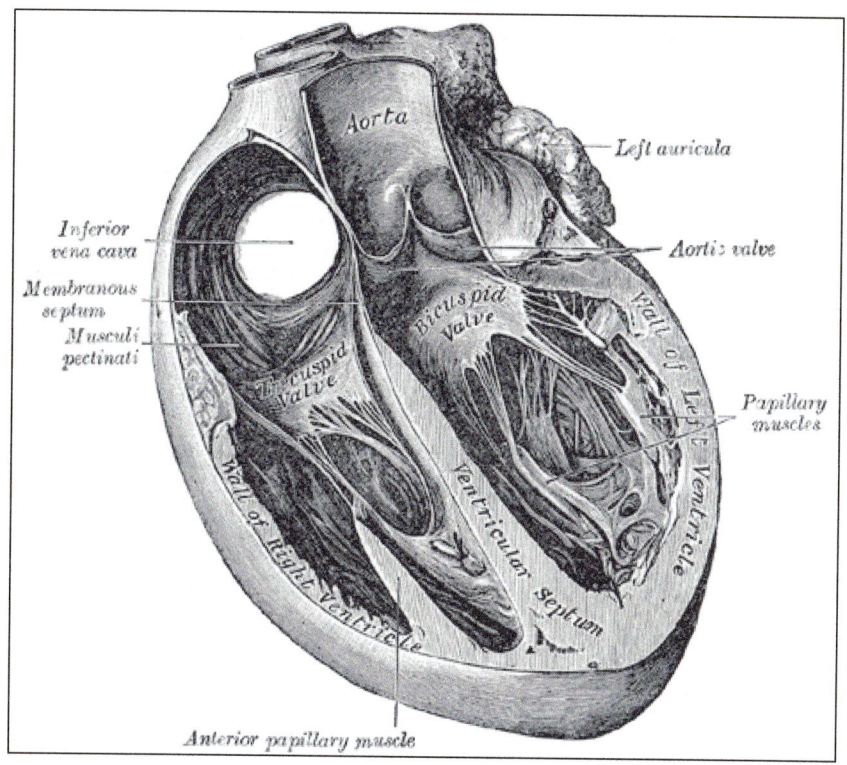

## BREASTS

Mind-pattern:

*My ability to Self-nurture.*

When a woman's nurturing ability is rejected or suppressed, the breasts are negatively affected—this can happen to males, too.

## LIVER

Mind-pattern:

*Detoxing and processing current life experiences.*

This is why the liver is full of toxins. Your liver accumulates the toxins that represent your perceptions of difficult and hurtful life experiences.

When the liver is overloaded with toxins, it releases toxins into the bloodstream. This is what causes jaundice, a yellow coloration of the skin.

That is why when something major happens to the liver, it can be fatal.

Liver disease:

*I cannot process my life past or current life experiences.*
*I cannot filter or process them;*
*I have no energy left to deal with them anymore.*

This is usually an overwhelming feeling that then means the heart chakra must be addressed as well.

The liver is treated with both Medium Green and Pale Yellow because the liver is a large organ that spans both chakra areas.

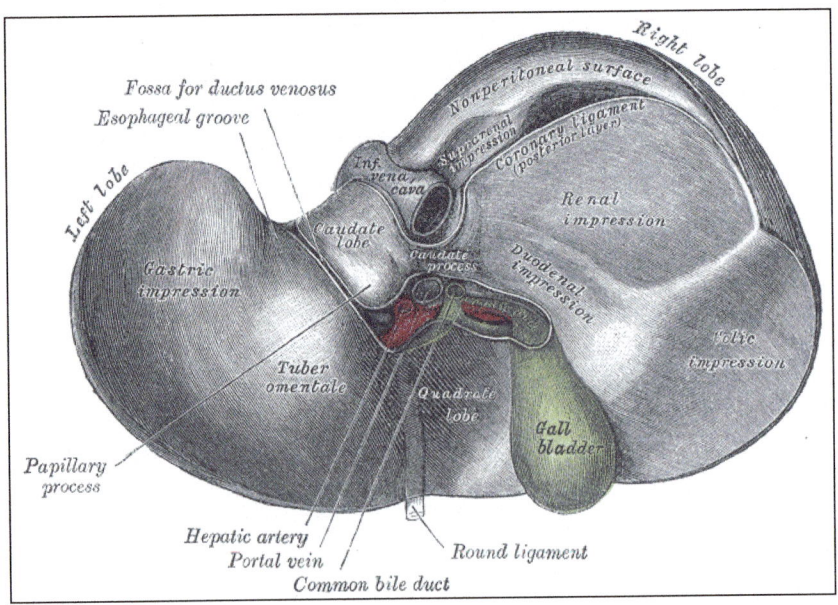

## Esophagus

Peristalsis is the contracting and relaxing of the esophagus muscles to allow food to flow into the stomach and digestive system.

Mind-pattern:

*Allowing understanding of information to flow properly.*

Blockages in the esophagus:

*I reject what I am taking in; I do not want to understand it; I want to get rid of it.*

Hiatal hernia:

*I do not want to understand this; I am not even going to let it go this far.*

Vomiting in the esophagus:

*I am losing my recent happiness; I am blocking or getting rid of it.*

Acid reflux:

*I learned something but I am not keeping it; I am not holding that information in me.*

Sometimes, people with acid reflux also have sinus issues. Both issues deal with irritations and annoyances relating to what is in front of you.

This combined mind-pattern says:

*I am not holding that information inside me. I see people and things that annoy and anger me, therefore I am getting mad at it.*

Inflammation of the esophagus, called esophagitis:

*Held resentment.*

Esophagitis is an inflammation of the esophagus from acid reflux that can lead to cancer.

## Solar Plexus Chakra

The Solar Plexus Chakra is from the sternum to the navel in Pale Yellow. Located in this chakra band are the stomach, large and small intestines (which are connected), the liver (right lower lobe), spleen, pancreas, and gallbladder.

### Stomach

Mind-pattern:

*Holding onto information until it is ready to be understood.*

Not absorbing food due to bleeding or ulcerative conditions and may include diarrhea:

*I cannot retain information. The information is painful and hurtful to me. I do not want to hold onto anything.*

Ruptured stomach:

*I do not want to store information for understanding later; I do not even want to be here.*

Gastric bypass surgery or stomach stapling:

*I cannot handle any more information; just a little bit of information at a time.*

People who have gastric bypass surgery or stomach stapling can only eat a few ounces of food at a time. These people have significantly insulated throughout their lives, storing too much information throughout their bodies and cannot handle it anymore.

This surgery is only performed on extremely obese people who have many layers of fat. The operation has a high hemorrhage death rate. The stomach can stretch, rupture the staples, and cause death.

There is another method to control obesity via limited food intake using an inflatable and adjustable gastric band that is placed around the top portion of the stomach. The mortality rate is significantly less than the gastric bypass surgery. The mind-pattern must be changed for any surgery to be effective. Otherwise, you can gain back the weight you lost, plus more.

Obesity:

*I am insulating and putting up walls between me and the outside world.*

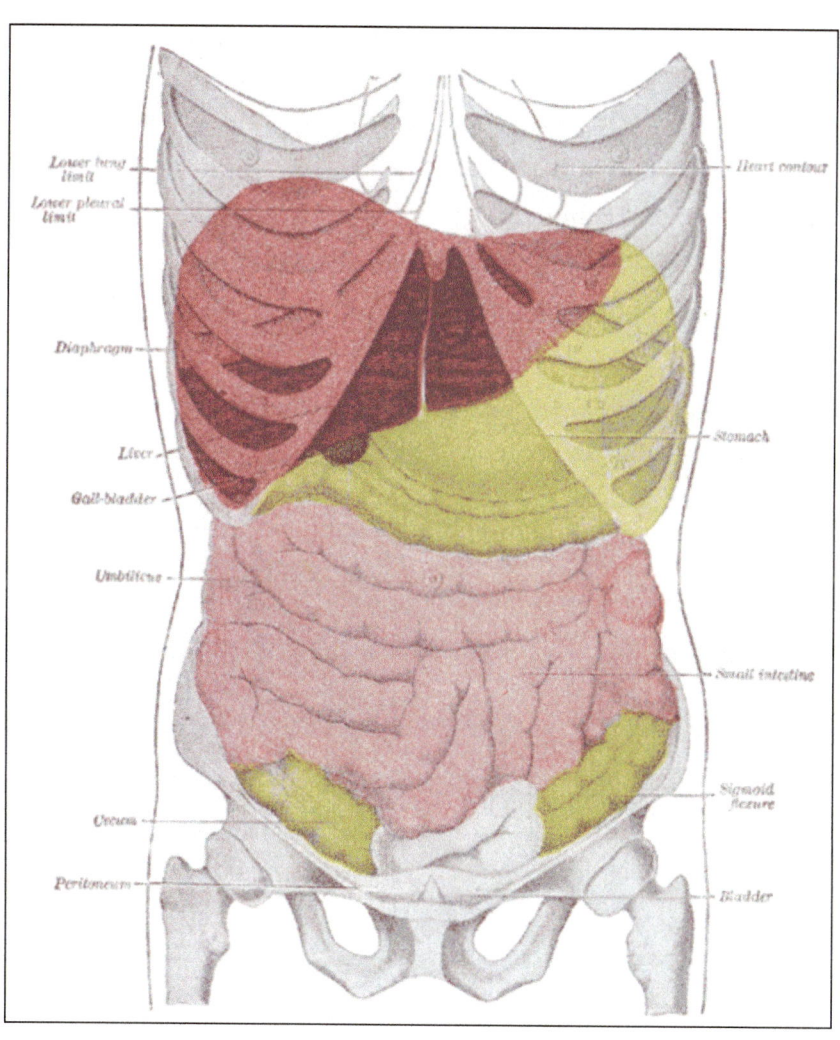

The majority of extremely obese people were sexually abused in childhood. These people retaliate by gaining weight so they are no longer attractive, plus the sheer physical weight of these people makes them feel powerful when mentally and emotionally, they feel powerless.

## Digestion Begins in the Mind

Your thought to eat begins in the mind.

Your mind uses your brain as a central device to order electrical current to the various body systems so the body is maintained.

This is a schematic of the how food becomes energy in the body. We start with thought or mind-pattern as it enters the brain. The brain is a device the mind uses.

What you think about when you eat affects your body.

If you do not like the food you are eating, how can you expect your body to utilize it?

If you like the food, your body follows your thoughts and much more easily assimilates the food.

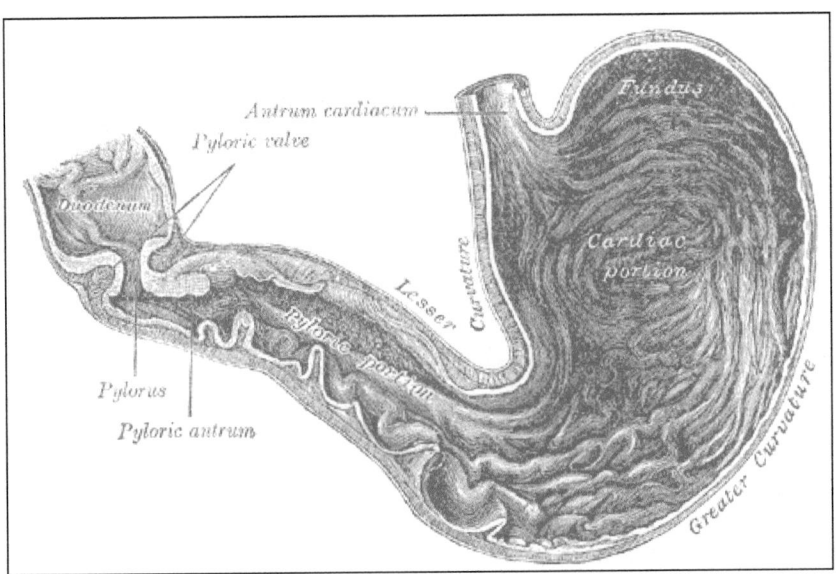

When you eat, you can mentally direct the food to the cellular structure with instructions on what do with the food. Body intelligence generally wants to store all food as fat in case of starvation.

People who are fast learners generally tend to eat quickly, symbolically trying to digest and download information. However, they may eat so fast that they are not able to absorb all that they learn.

People who are slow eaters need to take time to absorb, assimilate, and digest what they are learning.

A person who eats one food and then another is usually highly focused and structured. This type of person is generally not a multi-tasker.

What a person chooses to eat first, and the order of types of food eaten, gives you clues to the types of information they are able to assimilate before moving on to the next type of information.

Drinking too much liquid while you are eating:

*I am diluting information, washing it out and getting rid of it because it is too much for me to absorb.*

These kinds of people may be prone to constipation issues. It is better for your digestive track to eat your food first so it can be absorbed and drink the majority of liquid after your meal.

### LARGE INTESTINE/COLON

Mind-pattern:

*Getting every opportunity to absorb and understand the main points of an experience.*

Ulcerative colitis:

*I do not want to accept, hold onto, or assimilate my experiences.*

I was once diagnosed with ulcerative colitis, but it is now completely cured. There was a time in my life where I was going through severe physical, mental, and emotional trauma as well as financial distress. This caused me to develop ulcerative colitis.

I used this affirmation to help reverse my condition:

*I now accept all that I learn about myself and others.*

I also extensively used Pale Yellow in my intestinal system. Then I used Violet to seal in and protect the Pale Yellow. Whatever you eat passes through the protected Pale Yellow so the food can be more easily absorbed while the intestines are healing.

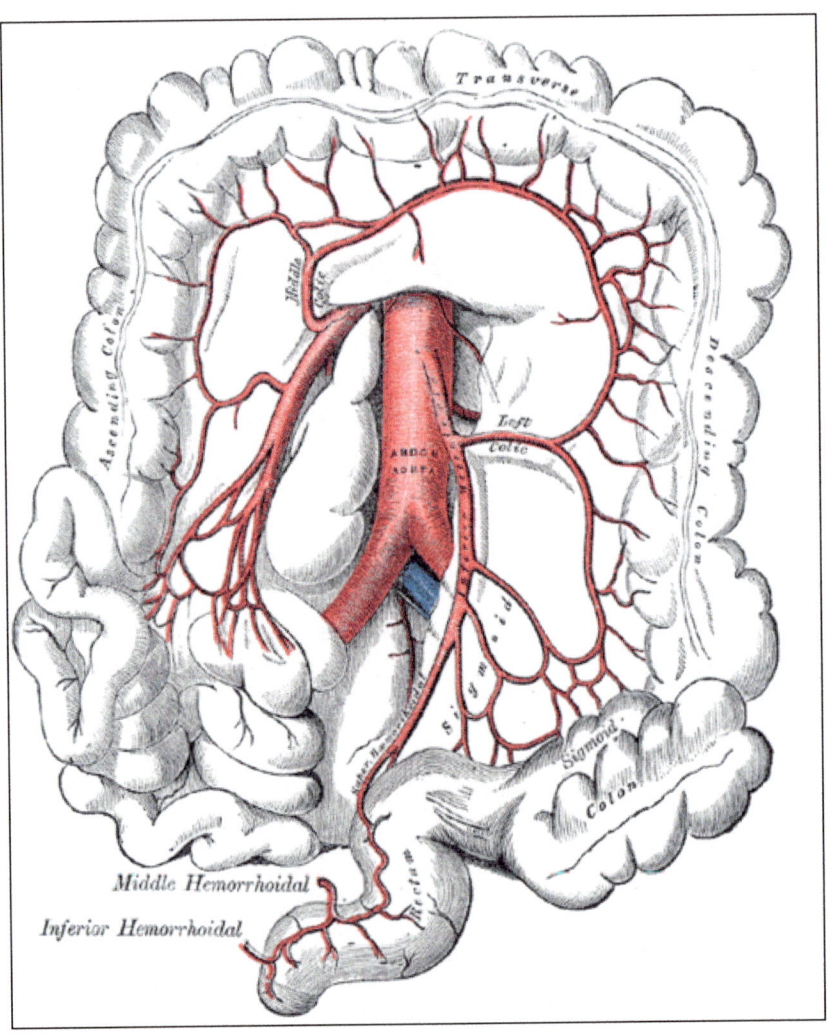

A doctor in Los Angeles advised me to take Tienchi tea, which is also available in pill and tablet form. While I worked on my mind-pattern, the tea helped to heal the intestines. I have not had an episode now for many, many years.

### SMALL INTESTINE

Mind-pattern:

*Digesting the smaller details of an experience.*

When you have issues with larger experiences, you have issues in the large intestine. When you have issues with the smaller details of experiences, you have issues in the small intestines.

The absorption process is assisted by the cilia, which help absorb and direct the distribution of nutrients.

### LIVER (RIGHT LOWER LOBE)

The liver has four lobes because it needs to process many experiences in the present.

Mind-pattern:

*Processing of non-emotional life experiences.*

### PANCREAS

Mind-pattern:

*Understanding and accepting the happiness or sweetness in life.*

Insulin overproduction:

*I cannot hold onto happiness in life;
happiness is slipping away from me.*

When insulin is overproduced, your blood sugar drops below what is healthy.

Insulin underproduction:

*I can see the happiness in life, but I cannot feel it;*
*I know that it is there but I cannot appreciate it.*

When not enough insulin is produced, the blood sugar cannot be fully absorbed, and cells are not fed the energy that is needed.

Normal insulin production but still not being able to absorb blood sugar:

*I do not accept happiness; I can get and have happiness but I do not accept it. I have low self-worth, low self-esteem; I self-punish and self-sabotage; I feel guilty.*

Stevia helps regulate insulin production. Peppermint tea aids blood sugar absorption. Pancreatic glandulars can help support overall pancreas health.

Insulin production is related to the heart chakra with issues of emotional isolation and abandonment. Even though not many major organs are in this area, it is the most emotionally important because all your emotional absorption and release takes place here.

### Gallbladder

Mind-pattern:

*I feel bitterness in my life; I am bitter about my life.*

The gallbladder produces bile, a digestive aid. Gallstones develop and calcify as a result of your mind-pattern, preventing the bile from releasing and your food from digesting.

## SPLEEN

The spleen is located next to the stomach, on the left side. The spleen is the size of your fist. It purifies and makes white blood cells, which are part of your immune system.

Mind-pattern:

*Keeping Self protected.*

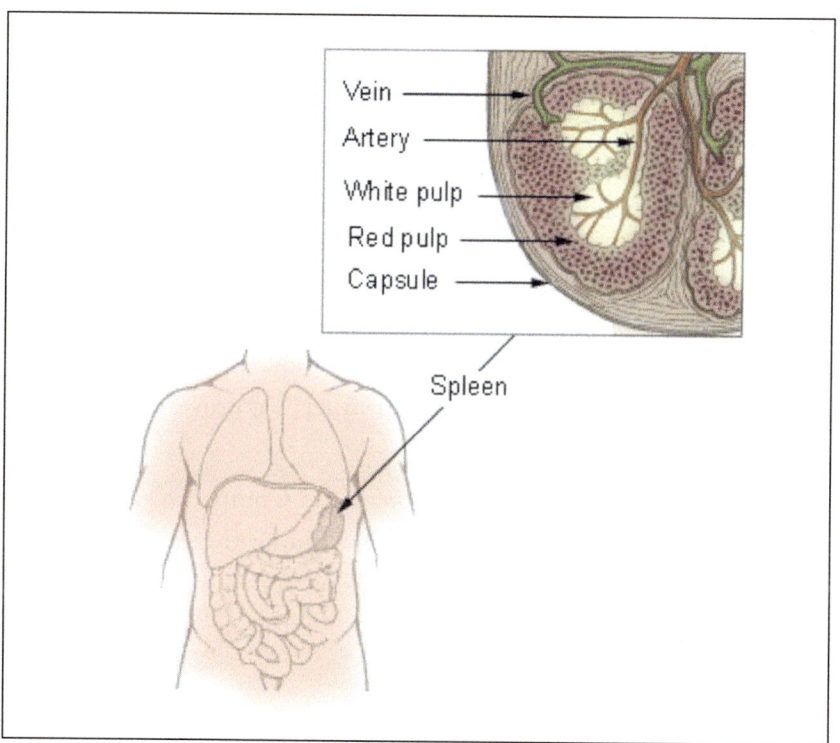

The spleen is specific about what it protects; it protects your happiness and joy in life of the stored information in your stomach, so you can deal with and understand it. White blood cells balance red blood cells for the flow of life.

Leukemia:

*A resentment of not having happiness in the flow of life.*

Leukemia is a blood cancer where the white blood cells eat the red blood cells, which results in death due to no more available food or oxygen for the body.

The opposite can happen where you produce too many red blood cells, resulting in blood clots that can cause aneurisms or strokes.

Blood:

*The flow of happiness and joy in life.*

Blood clots:

*Something is blocking my happiness.*

Where the blood clot forms is the clue to the blockage of your happiness. Many people have blood clots in their legs.

Legs:

*Your support structure and stepping into the future.*

A blood clot in the leg means you are blocking the happiness in your future. Whether it is in the right or left leg provides more clues to the specific issue.

Many doctors prescribe the medication "Coumadin" to thin the blood. This is also used as a rat poison, killing the rats by internal hemorrhaging. This can be the same result for humans. Other side effects are seizures and memory loss. Aspirin is now sometimes prescribed instead of Coumadin.

## SACRAL CHAKRA

The Sacral Chakra starts at the navel and extends to the pubic bone. The color is Pale Orange. This chakra band contains the kidneys, adrenal glands, ovaries and uterus (female), urinary bladder, appendix, and the lower portions of the small and large intestines/colon.

### KIDNEYS

Mind-pattern:

*Processing past experiences.*

There are two kidneys because you have many past experiences.

Kidney stones:

*I am unable to process my past experiences.*

### ADRENAL GLANDS

Mind-pattern:

*Your ability to cope with all life experiences.*

This is why they activate when you are under stress. They are located just above the kidneys because they help you process past experiences.

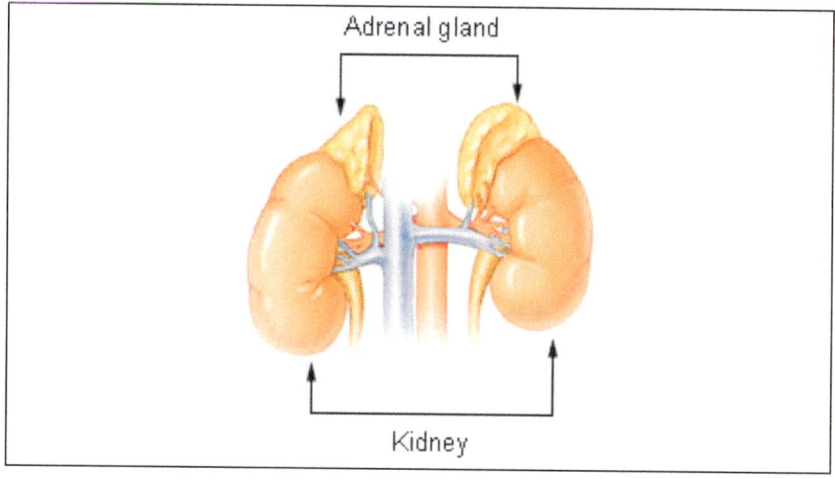

Sometimes, the adrenal glands are located within the Solar Plexus/Pale Yellow Chakra Band.

Adrenal failure in females due to the production cessation of specific uterine hormones:

*My creative support and development has stopped;*
*I cannot cope with my life experiences.*

Sometimes the thyroid and larynx are also affected, so this additional mind-pattern must be addressed:

*I cannot speak about how I feel.*

## Ovaries

Mind-pattern:

*Creative energy or power for physical and nonphysical experience.*

## Uterus

Mind-pattern:

*Creative support and development.*

Hysterectomy:

*I am noncreative with low self-worth. I have issues of creative support and development, so I am useless and rejected by others.*

## Urinary Tract/Bladder

Mind-pattern:

*Releasing anger.*

This is why as people chronologically age they have more bladder issues. Angers build up and are expressed negatively in the bladder and urinary tract. People who do not care what or how they express anger as well as those who suppress anger have bladder/urinary issues.

### SMALL AND LARGE INTESTINES/COLON

The Small and Large Intestines/Colon are also partially located in the Sacral Chakra.

Small Intestines in the Sacral Chakra:

*To take new and learned ideas, keep what is necessary and eliminate the rest. This is my last chance to get the final bit of understanding from what I have taken in.*

Large Intestines/Colon:

*Releasing unnecessary past experiences.*

Colon Cancer:

*I resent my past experiences; I do not want to release my past experiences because I am angry about them and I cannot deal with them.*

Constipated Colon:

*I hold onto wasteful experiences that are unnecessary but I still want to look at them repeatedly.*

Indigestion Bloating:

*I have fear about what I am learning so I insulate against it.*

Hormonal Bloating (usually in females):

*I am fearful about creative issues so I insulate against this.*

### APPENDIX

Mind-pattern:

*A need to purge ancient genetic past.*

Ruptured/Infected Appendix:

*The information I learned about my ancient genetic past is hurtful to me.*

Ancient genetic past means not just humanity in general, but your specific family ancestral history that is genetically stored and active within you. This means that you have learned information about your ancient past that was hurtful and disruptive.

This can outpicture in the eruption of your appendix, confirming that you cannot process or digest the information.

This is old cellular memory that you inherited that needs to be released, centered in the appendix because the appendix is considered a vestigial organ that is no longer necessary. The appendix was used to digest food that is no longer eaten, such as shells and bark.

## Root Chakra

The Root Chakra starts at the pubic bone and extends to the top of the thighs.

The color here is Pale Red. The main organs present in this Charka Band are the genitalia for both male and female, and the prostate for males.

Male Genitalia:

*Creative power and energy for physical and nonphysical.*

Female Genitalia:

*Receiving energy for creative power for physical and nonphysical.*

When you have issues with creativity and personal power, these issues physically outpicture in these areas of the body. This happens to anyone who feels their creativity and productivity is ending and/or diminishing to the point where they cannot envision a future.

### Prostate

Mind-pattern:

*To create support and development.*

The male prostate correlates to the uterus of the female.

## LEGS AND FEET

The Legs and Feet are not part of the Chakra System, but resonate with the Earth's magnetic field. From the top of the thighs to the bottom of the feet the color here is Brown. There are no organs in this region of the body, which only includes muscle, connective tissue, skin, lymph, and sweat glands.

Mind-pattern:

*Stepping into the future and support structure.*

Heels of the Feet:

*Vulnerability in the present that affects the future.*

In Hyperspace, Brown is the color code for now/present.

People often ask about their connection to the Earth. Remember that humans are not native to this planet, so you do not have an energetic connection. This is why you need to keep Brown in the lower part of your body—the color Brown grounds you into this reality.

Brown begins to fade in the energetic field of anyone who is getting ready to pass on, or even those people who do not want to be here.

Some people think that putting energetic roots into the ground helps them. In reality, this can result in pulling up into your Self all kinds of dangerous energies such as electromagnetic energy, magma, underground bases, and so forth.

In the same way, some people think they can dump their energetic waste into the Earth. The Earth is not your garbage can—your energetic waste goes back to your Oversoul, not into the Earth.

When you work with Hyperspace energy, you stop right beneath your feet. Do not pull anything up from the Earth and do not dump anything into the Earth.

# Body Energy & Exercise

The major nutrients your body needs are:

Protein

Fat

Sugar

Water

Minerals/Vitamins

Not everybody needs the same amount. For example, the body of a 400-pound sumo wrestler has different nutritional requirements than the body of a 90-pound woman.

In the same way, not everybody needs 8 to 10 glasses of water every day. When you drink too much water, you wash away digestive enzymes as well as other important nutrients that your body needs. Over-hydration can be as dangerous as under-hydration.

Over-hydration prevents oxygen and nutrients from entering your cells. This means that you can actually drown from the inside out. Women with high estrogen levels retain water. Even men can have estrogen levels that are too high, causing water retention.

The amount of water your body needs not only depends on size, but also on your level of physical activity, climate, and if you are indoors or outdoors. Learn your body's needs and then take care of it in the way that is unique to you, depending upon each day's variables.

Lactic acid can build up when you over-exercise to the point where you have used up all available sugar and water in your system. When sugar and water cannot break down any more, they become lactic acid, a waste product. This is toxic to your muscles, causing them hurt, feel tired, and even cramp. Stretching your muscles when they cramp helps the built-up lactic acid to drain out.

Twenty-five percent of lactic acid that builds up in the body gets flushed out through the kidneys and the bladder. The rest gets oxidized and used as other types of energy. That is why it is important you keep your kidneys flushed.

Sugar is stored in the muscles and is the first thing to be utilized when you exercise. This is because sugar is the easiest, most convenient source of energy for the body.

When you exercise, the sugar breaks down into pyruvic acid and from there into carbon dioxide and water. From here, your body needs oxygen to complete the exercise. This is called the "Krebs Cycle."

Mind-pattern for craving sugar:

*Trying to fill mental/emotional holes with sweetness.*

Physically, you may crave sugar due to a hormonal imbalance, parasites, and/or your system lacks sugar.

Fat covers the viscera, or internal organs, of the body as a protective coating. Your body does need a layer of fat to maintain optimal health.

Fat is not stored in the muscles, making it more difficult to access when you exercise because fat needs to be broken down. You need fat for energy.

Under normal conditions, the fat layers of the body are almost inexhaustible. As a general rule, athletes and people with anorexia are the only people who exhaust most of their storehouses of fat. The menstrual cycle in females can be disrupted and even stop as a side effect of losing necessary body fat.

Women require 20-30% body fat. Men need between 10-16%. Having less than this amount is a dangerous situation because without fat reserves, people can actually die. Some people have only 3-4% body fat.

Because the body needs fat for energy, to survive, the person must eventually gain body fat back, or the person could actually die. The body has cellular memory, so the body must re-set its capacity to store fat. The body must protect itself, so when the person starts eating again, the food is stored as fat as a protective/survival mode. So starvation really just puts you in a loop that accomplishes nothing other than harming the body.

## CELLULITE

Cellulite is really toxins between the fat layers.

Mind-pattern:

*I have some deep fears I will not release.*

Cellulite on the hips:

*I always feel out of balance, especially with thoughts of my future.*

Cellulite on the buttocks:

*I carry the weight of my past with me.*

Cellulite on the thighs:

*I have childhood trauma and abuse issues that I carry with me.*

Cellulite in the abdominal/stomach area:

*I am anxious and worrying about what I am learning, digesting, and assimilating.*

## EXERCISE

It is important that you exercise in a way that optimizes the benefits for you and your lifestyle.

Jogging and running, as well as trampolines and impact sports, cause the brain to jolt against the skull, resulting in small concussions and even hematomas on the brain. In addition, these activities can eventually lead to joint, muscle, and bone issues.

Mind-pattern for jogging or running:

*Running away from your life.*

Walking or speed walking is healthier. Burning the fat takes longer, but the results are the same. For example, if you jog 10 miles in three hours or walk 10 miles in six hours, your body receives the same benefits, but the results take longer.

Weight training builds bone density and muscle mass. Weight training is actually more aerobic than what is commonly termed as aerobic activity because weight training requires more oxygen and therefore the benefits are longer lasting.

Weight training causes minute tears in the muscles, so only do your weight training every other day. This gives the body time to recuperate. Resting allows the muscles to grow back together, thus gradually enlarging. Simply put, weight training is gently ripping the muscle and then repairing it.

At some point, your muscles reach the maximum enlargement for your genetics. When this happens, maintain your weight training and exercising.

Bodybuilders often take steroids to increase muscle mass, however steroids add to cancer and other health issues. Physically, it is best to reduce carbohydrates and sugar levels while increasing protein intake. You may need a digestive aid and of course, drink steam-distilled water as appropriate for your specific body needs.

Muscle burns more calories than fat. Even if you only exercise intermittently, simply by having a more active muscular system your body burns more calories.

# Body Movement

Here are some terms that are helpful for you to know:

**ABDUCTION**
An action that means away from the body.

**ADDUCTION**
An action that means toward the body.

**CIRCUMDUCTION**
Moving in a circular motion.

**DEPRESSION**
Pushing part of your body down.

**ELEVATION**
Moving a part of the body in a straight upward motion; for example shrugging your shoulders.

**EXTENSION**
Increasing the angle of what you are doing.

**EXTERNAL ROTATION**
   Turning away from the body.

**FLEXION**
   Decreasing the angle of what you are doing.

**FUSCIFORM**
   Bowing in the middle.

**INTERNAL ROTATION**
   Moving toward the body.

**LONGITUDINAL**
   Stretching the muscle forward, making it longer rather than wider.

**PRONATION**
   In a position with palms down.

**PROTRACTION**
   Shoulders forward.

**RADIATE**
   Expanding the muscle.

**RETRACTION**
   Shoulder back.

**SUPINATION**
   In a position with palms up.

# Muscular Movement

Radiate means the muscle expands. Longitudinal is the muscle stretching forward, making it longer instead of wider. Fusciform is when it bows in the middle.

Doctors make you take a grip test; I was told mine did not match my age. Who determines what age determines what number on a device? I question it. You cannot compare yourself to someone else. Everyone is individual. Maybe your grip is right for your genetics and predisposition.

Just like those weight charts, they do not take into account bone density, exercise level, or other factors. I have seen fat people who were heavier because of muscle mass but they were told they were falling into the obese category and they were not.

There are people considered overweight by the charts, but that is normal for them. If they were to lose weight, their bodies would weaken. You have to go by the mindset. What is normal for one is not normal for another. And I understand they are looking at a wide range to get these numbers, but you still cannot apply it to everyone. You have to look at the person and the mind-pattern.

# Blood Pressure

Systolic represents the left ventricle pressure that propels your blood. Diastolic pressure measures after the heart relaxes and is the 'in-between' beats of the heart. Systolic is the high number and diastolic is the low number. You do not need to check your blood pressure all the time unless you have a problem.

Hypertension or high blood pressure is considered 140/90 or higher. Doctors look at the bottom number more because if your pressure is high even when your heart is relaxed, that means there is too much pressure in your arteries and capillaries. It can cause a stroke or aneurism where the blood vessel bubbles and pops. You can also have a stroke in areas other than the head. Some people have purple spots on their legs that are basically a mini stroke in their blood vessels.

Most of the heart calibration machines available in health clubs may not be accurate or maintained well. Those are not reliable calibrations. Just like blood pressure machines, you do not know who calibrated it, how long it has been there, etc. Your blood pressure can elevate from being in a doctor's office and becoming anxious.

What is normal for one person is not normal for another. For example, Janet's normal blood pressure is 80/40; they think she is dead. A measurement of 20/70 would be high for her, even though that is considered 'normal.' You have to go by the person.

Someone says the new borderline for blood pressure is 120/80. That is ridiculous. That means more people will fall into the high blood pressure category so doctors can prescribe more drugs.

What happens when you put someone on medication to regulate blood pressure? Your body becomes dependent on it, so the body's intelligence says it does not have to regulate anymore because something else is doing its job. The same problem occurs when doctors give women 'Synthyroid'; the thyroid stops functioning naturally because it picks up the artificial hormones in the system and reduces its own production. So the doctor raises your medication because your thyroid production is lower. This is for the rest of your life.

This is the same with female hormone replacement; thank goodness studies now say women should not take estrogen. Maybe they killed everyone they wanted to kill by giving them breast cancer or uterine cancer. Stay away from all soy products because it causes more estrogen to develop.

There is a new blood pressure monitor that you put around your wrist like a band and it gives you a quick digital reading by picking up the impulses from the blood vessels in the skin. It takes readings over a long time, day and night. Then you can see what is normal for you.

If you have consistently high blood pressure, the mind-pattern is:

### *I feel constantly pressured in my life.*

Your body translates this into a condition where cholesterol builds up in your arteries. This creates more pressure, which can create a heart attack or stroke. Then doctors give you medications. They all have toxins in them that cause liver damage, which gets into your lymphatic system and then the kidneys and before you know it you are a big mess.

The mind-pattern "I feel pressured in my life" makes the body accumulate plaque in the arteries and veins because it is an insulation—I need to protect myself in life.

To herbally treat blood pressure, use red yeast rice, garlic, red wine (Pinot Noir has the highest capacity to reduce plaque), and wild rice (a grass seed that grows in the Great Lakes area). Studies show that if you eat ½ cup of wild rice every day for 90 days, the cholesterol level drops and the plaque leaves the body. Wild rice is not genetically altered, yet. Many people do not like its nutty taste. Remember to also flush the arteries with Purple, which will pull the plaque out of the body.

Also, Vitamin B-3/niacin, calcium and Vitamin D pull plaque out of the system and actually put calcium back in the bones and makes your bones stronger. It is helpful for women with fibroids, cysts in their breasts, kidney stones, and gallstones. Niacin will loosen the plaque from your arterial walls and literally lets it slide out of the veins and arteries. When you feel the niacin flush, stop taking it! That is the sensation you feel when it slides out of your circulatory system. It means you took too much too fast. Generally, where someone has a plaque issue, I recommend 100 mg of niacin for two weeks. If no flush, go to 200 mg. Stop after the flush or you will collapse the vascular walls. Maintain it with garlic. Odorless garlic scrubs the arteries and keeps them clean.

Another very good method of removing plaque and lowering blood pressure is black cayenne pepper. Get it in capsule form.

# Healing Archetypes for Mind/Body Correlations

Three complex archetypes related to healing are as follows: The 'N' archetype in Medium Green, the triangle in Brown, and the square in Royal Blue.

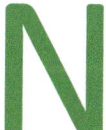 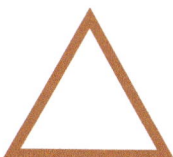 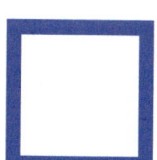

Brown represents physical reality; Medium Green relates to the Heart Chakra and creation, Royal Blue corresponds to Hyperspace and the mind-pattern. The three archetypes represent: "Creation within physical reality in relation to the mind-pattern."

## Color Codes for Optimal Body Function

Correlate the chakra colors with the organs and general theme or function of the area as it relates to them. For example, the heart is energetically Medium Green and the mind-pattern deals with emotions. The bladder, Pale Orange, concerns releasing anger and is focused in the creative area.

Thyroid is Ice Blue, dealing with communication and expression.

Medical science says it does not know how to regenerate nerves if the spinal cord becomes severed. But this can be done; nerves can regenerate.

Copper is a conductor of electrical energy and enhances the electrical flow in the body. Visualize and use Shiny Copper in the spine and skeletal system, Royal Blue in the brain, and Pale Yellow from the neck down in the spinal cord and nervous system to regenerate nerve tissue as well as maintain optimal nerve function.

Flush the arteries and veins with Purple, which will pull the plaque out of the body.

What about sensitive teeth? What will you do for that? Use Shiny Copper for strengthening the teeth. Put Ice Blue around that to prevent sensitivity. Inside the Shiny Copper put Pale Yellow for the nerves. Strengthen the bone so you no longer feel sensitivity.

# Flowchart of the Human Body and Digestive System

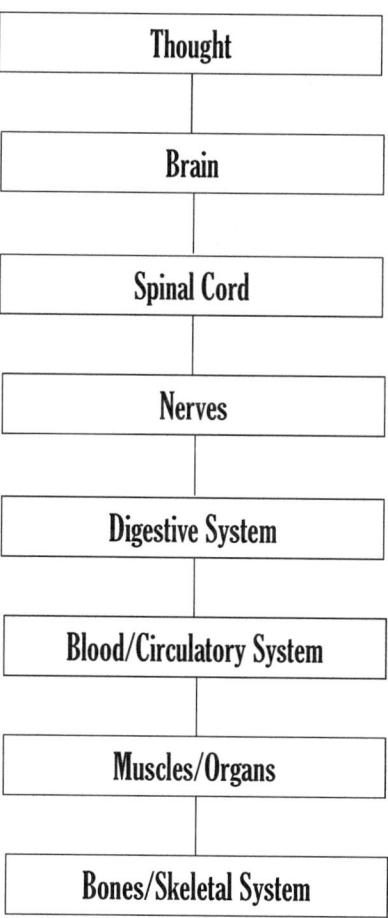

This is a schematic of how food becomes energy in the body. We start with thought or mind-pattern as it enters the brain. The brain is a device the mind uses.

The brain is the central device that orders electrical current to the various body systems in order to maintain the body. If you look at it multi-dimensionally, thought is around the body feeding into it.

Let us examine how the brain and body interact when you ingest food.

What you think about as you are eating affects the body. As you eat, drink, or ingest anything, you should mentally direct where the cellular structure of that intake should go. Otherwise, if you do not specifically direct it, the body intelligence will tell it where to go and will tell it to add extra fat storage in case of starvation mode. That is just what the body does genetically.

I had a client once who binged and swallowed quickly; as he ate he condemned himself. I have come across people who lived in countries where they never knew when they would have to flee or run. They would gorge themselves as fast as they could, even if they were not hungry. They were brought up believing at any minute soldiers would come and they would have to leave quickly. There was another client who had to eat quickly because everyone else in his family would take all the food.

People who are fast learners tend to eat quickly because they are symbolically trying to digest and download the information. People who are slow eaters need to take time in what they are learning. They need to absorb information slowly. Then they can go onto the next piece of data.

A section eater eats one thing on the plate, then they eat the next thing on the plate. These non-mixers of food are structured or focused. They are not multi-tasking people. They can only focus on one task at a time until it is finished, then they move on to the next.

We can break it down even further. Look at what order they choose to eat first, then last. This gives you a clue to the type of information they are able to assimilate before they can absorb another type of information.

Drinking too much liquid while eating is also detrimental. You should really drink after you eat.

Mind-pattern:

*Diluting information, washing it out and getting rid of it.*
*It is too much for me to take, let me dilute it.*

It is better for your digestion to drink after you eat because your intestinal track is absorbing the liquid and not the food. Usually, those people have constipation problems.

## CELLULITE

Cellulite is really toxins between the fat.

Mind-pattern:

*I have some deep fears I won't release.*

Cellulite is really a question of doing release work.

Women require 20-30% body fat. Men are normally between 10-16%.

Having 3-4% body fat is dangerous; you will eventually die because there is no energy. Here is what happens. There is no way anyone who reduces their body fat so low can survive; eventually they will gain back fat to sustain their bodily functions. The body has cellular memory; it knows you tried to kill it and goes into starvation mode. So it resets the capacity to store fat; when you start eating again, your body stores it as fat. Your body says, "You aren't going to kill me again, I'll store even more fat." So, you defeat the purpose by starvation.

Especially for men, most weight is in the abdominal or stomach area. The mind-pattern is about what you are learning, digesting, and assimilating in life. If you are not happy about your life or what you are learning about yourself or others scares or worries you, then you gain weight to cushion or insulate against the outside world.

Women carry most of their weight on the hips, backside, and the thighs. Cellulite on the hips indicates you are always feeling out of balance, especially towards the future. Weight on the backside represents carrying around weight from the past. It is past issues you are carrying around and not releasing. Women often tend to externalize if they do not verbalize and release, so they carry their baggage around with them. Cellulite on the thighs is related to childhood traumas. Many women have abuse issues. These are not necessarily sexual, but something that happened in childhood that they still carry around with them.

# Spine and Nervous System

The spinal column relates to the nervous system. At the top of the spine, right below the base of the skull, is the atlas C1 vertebra. Some chiropractors believe that by manipulating the atlas only, all spinal conditions can be corrected. Because it is the first part of the spinal column, some chiropractors believe if that atlas is misaligned it will automatically affect the rest of the spine. This school of thought says that by adjusting the atlas, a chain reaction begins, aligning all the other discs and vertebrae.

The C2 vertebra is called the "axis." Some people report by adjusting the atlas and axis their vision has improved.

The atlas C1 and axis C2 lead down to the coccyx, or tailbone, which is misaligned in most people. The cervical region has seven vertebrae; some people have eight. After that is the thoracic region with twelve vertebrae. The lumbar region has five vertebrae. The sacral region has five vertebrae fused together and the coccyx region has four vertebrae fused together. The total number of vertebrae equals 33. In Hyperspace, "33" means an end of a series of cycles. Generally, the lower you go down on the spine, the thicker the bones become. The upper bones are thinner, therefore more prone to injury.

Intervertebral discs have several outer layers called fibrocartilage. The internal nucleus pulpous is a gel-like substance that absorbs shock and impact from the body's movement. Herniated discs develop when the fibrocartilage is damaged or degenerates and the nucleus pulpous bulges out the side of the disc. This then puts pressure on the nerves. That is when you start having back pain.

Mind-pattern for a herniated disc:

*I feel fractured in my support structure.*

A common issue as people age is the shrinking of their spine due to disc degeneration, actually reducing their height.

Shrinkage due to disc degeneration:

*I am not important anymore. I am less than I used to be.*

*My perspective is not as high-powered as it used to be.*
*I feel put down.*

Vertebral subluxations in the cervical region C1-C7:

*I am stubborn.*

Vertebral subluxations in the thoracic region:

*I am shouldering burdens from childhood that I have not released.*

Vertebral subluxations in the lumbar region:

*I do not feel unsupported in life.*

Vertebral subluxations in the sacral and coccyx region:

*I am concerned with financial and material things.*

Scoliosis, a curvature of the spine:

*I feel completely overwhelmed in my support structure in life. I am weighed down and cannot support anything.*

The more you are concerned about a specific issue, the more it outpictures into your life. For example, when you worry about the future, the nerves and capillaries that feed into the legs and feet are also affected.

You could get adjusted by a chiropractor five times a day, but if you do not change the mind-pattern, your chiropractic adjustments will not hold.

Stretching and occasional chiropractic adjustments are beneficial to separate the vertebrae and align the spine. This allows optimal energy flow through the spinal cord, nervous system, and body.

To rebuild cartilage and maintain disc, spinal cord, and nervous system health, these supplements are helpful: Omega-3, horsetail herb, olive oil, and calcium citrate with Vitamin D. A massage with a combination of peanut oil, castor oil, and olive oil will also build and regenerate the cellular tissue in this area.

The following diagram details each vertebra with the corresponding nerves that control each part of the body.

This is what a nerve cell looks like. You can see the coating around each nerve cell, called "myelin sheath." The fingers that feed out from the nerve cells are called dendrites.

When a person is nervous, jumpy, and jittery, there is a reduction of the myelin sheath around the nerves so that the electrical impulses seem to scatter in a way that is not part of the system or network.

Degenerated myelin sheath:

*I feel short-circuited in life.*

The spaces between the dendrites are called synapses. Many problems are located in this area. Sometimes there is a lack of connection from the synapses between the dendrites of the nerve cells and the electrical flow between the cells.

Sometimes, instructions coming from one nerve to another nerve are distorted. This may cause muscular contractions or muscular atrophy, depending on the specific condition.

Not much can be done with the spaces, so the best you can do is rebuild the nerves to improve the health of the dendrites. If two dendrites touch each other, it is like touching two live wires together.

This can be very painful, causing the area to swell.

Where the myelin sheath is distorted, an electrical storm can build up to such an extent that seizures can result. When this happens in the brain, the storms become overwhelming to the Nervous System. The Nervous System cannot contain the electricity passing through, so the Nervous System shuts down, resulting in a seizure.

Fats, such as butter, olive oil, and Omega-3 can help to build up and maintain the myelin sheath. This helps stabilize and maintain the flow of electricity so it does not misfire. This is another reason why you need fats in your diet and why you must maintain the correct layer of fat for your body type and lifestyle.

People who are too thin are more apt to have the improper coating of their myelin sheath, causing them to be jumpy and nervous.

# Skeletal System

There are 206 bones in your body.

Mind-pattern for the skeletal system:

*My general support structure in life.*

There are different types of joints that help bones move in different directions:

## Synarthrosis

Synarthrotic joints have no movement; they are fibrous joints that are tied together with collagenous fibers like the suture joints in the cranium.

## Amphiarthrosis

Amphiarthrotic joints are slightly moveable cartilagenous joints. They are bones connected by cartilage like the joints between the vertebrae, ribs attached to the sternum, the pubic symphysis, and the tibia and fibula.

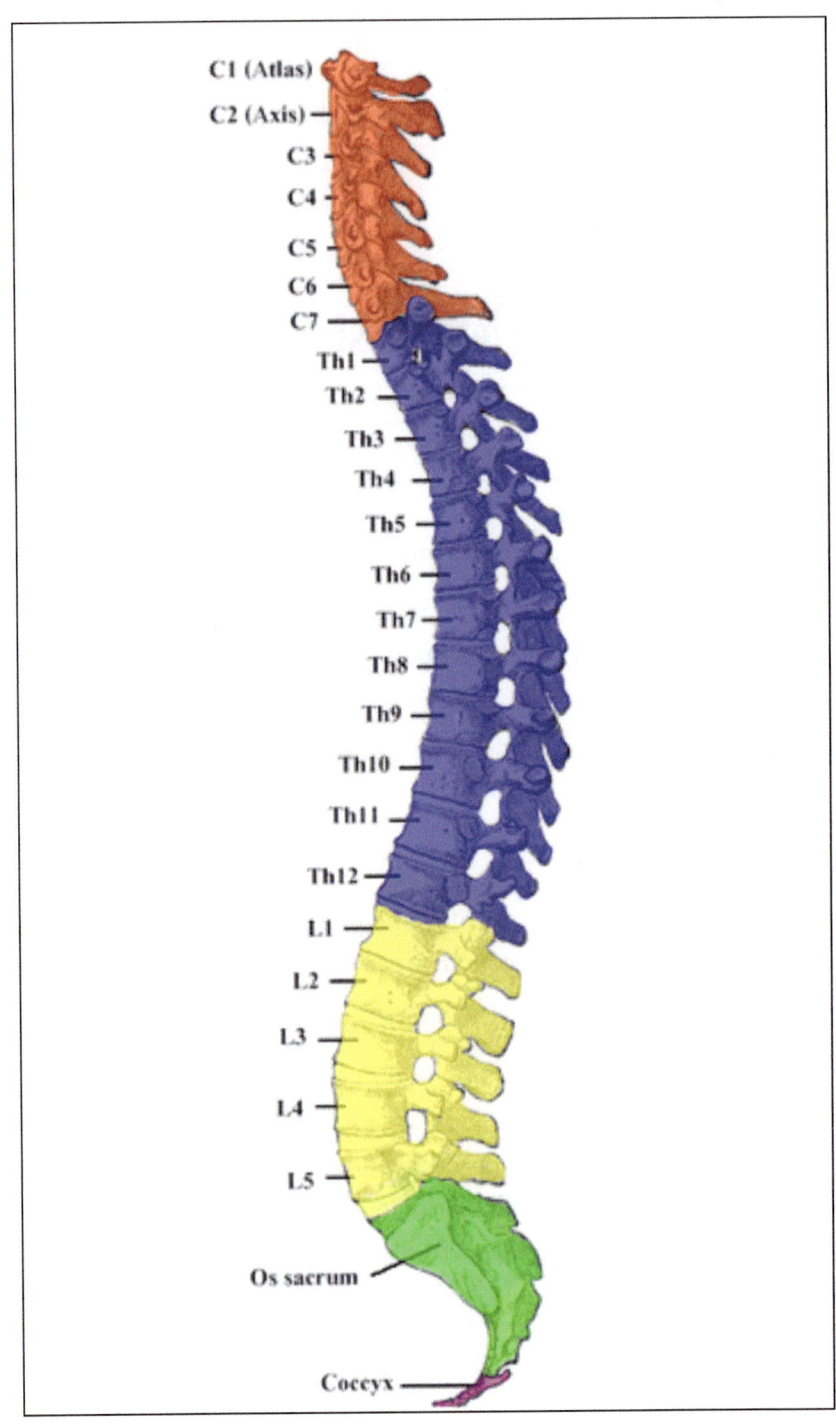

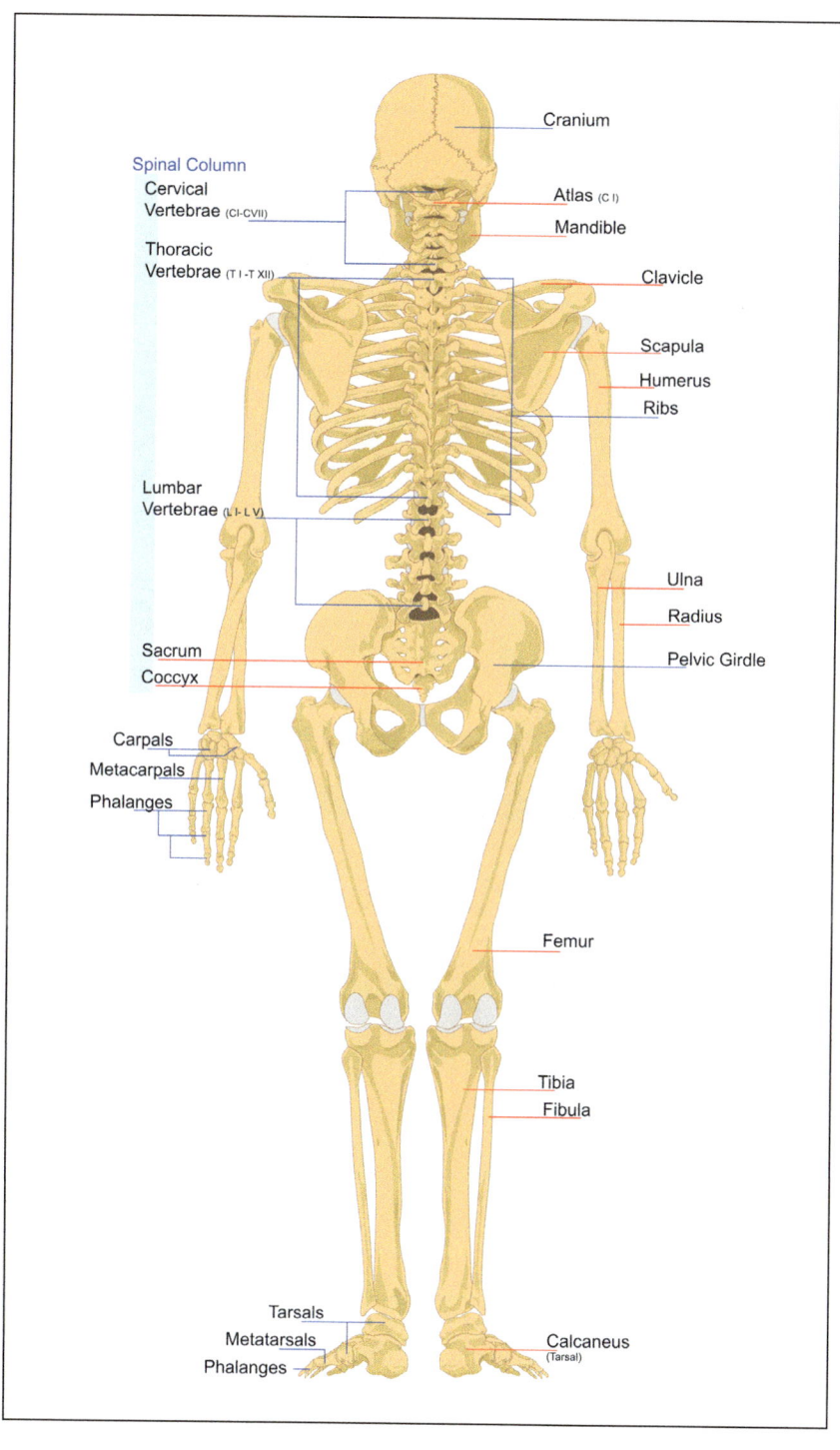

132 • Alternative Medical Apocrypha: Body-Mind Correlations

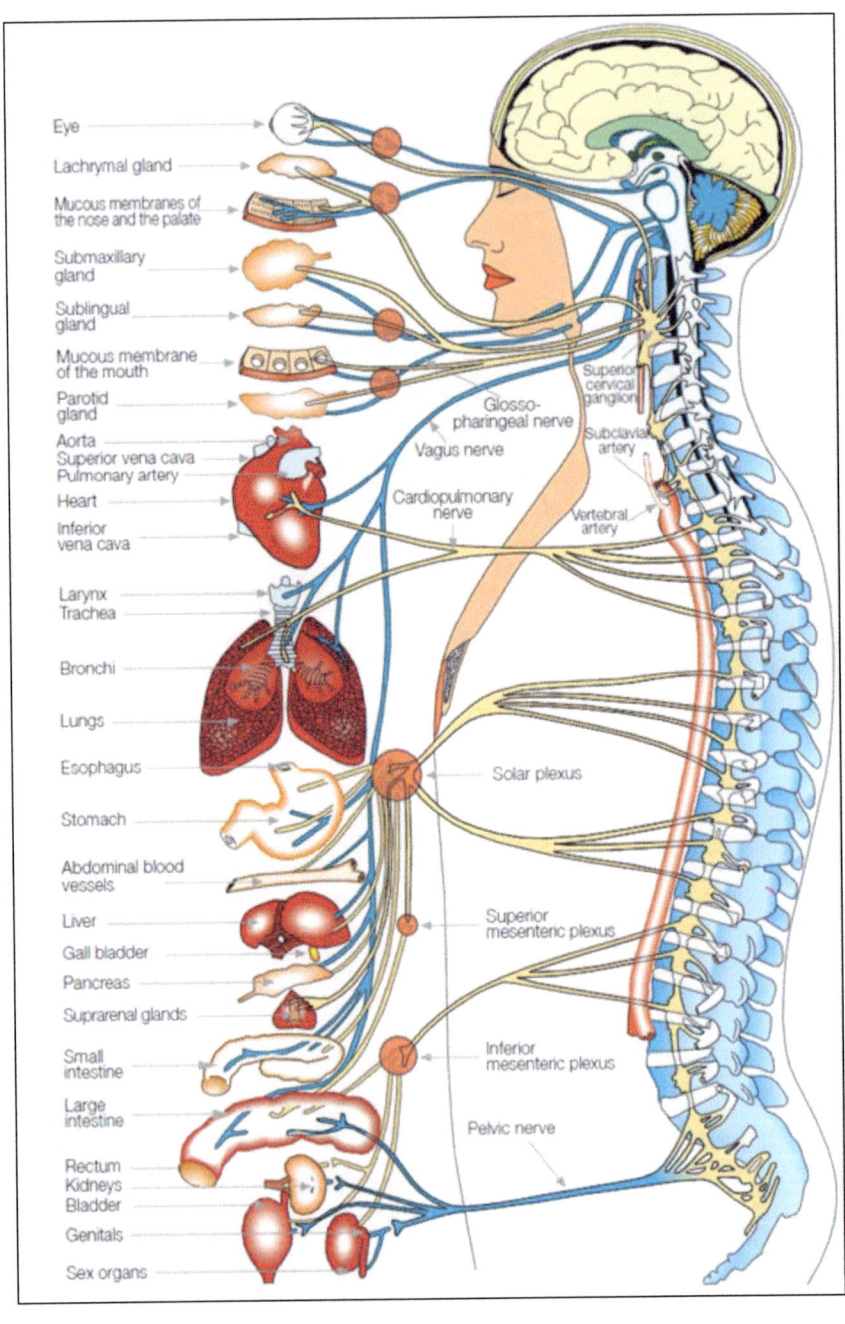

| VERTEBRAE | AREAS AND PARTS OF THE BODY | POSSIBLE SYMPTOMS |
|---|---|---|
| **CERVICAL** | | |
| C 1 | • Back of the head | Headaches (including migraines, aches or pain at the back of the head, behind the eyes or in the temples, tension across the forehead, throbbing or pulsating discomfort at the top or back of head) |
| C 2 | • Various areas of the head | |
| C 3 | • Side and front of the neck | |
| C 4 | • Upper back of the neck | |
| C 5 | • Middle of neck and upper part of arms | Jaw muscle, or joint aches or pains |
| C 6 | • Lower part of neck, arms and elbows | Dizziness, nervousness, vertigo |
| C 7 | • Lower part of arms, shoulders | Soreness, tension and tightness felt in back of neck and throat area |
| **DORSAL** | | |
| D 1 | • Hands, wrists, fingers, thyroid | Pain, soreness, and restriction in the shoulder area |
| D 2 | • Heart, its valves and coronary arteries | Bursitis, tendonitis |
| D 3 | • Lungs, bronchial tubes, pleura, chest | Pain and soreness in arms, hands, elbows and /or fingers |
| D 4 | • Gall bladder, common duct | |
| D 5 | • Liver, solar plexus | Chest pains, tightness or constriction, asthma, difficulty breathing |
| D 6 | • Stomach, mid-back area | Middle or lower mid-back pain, discomfort and soreness |
| D 7 | • Pancreas, duodenum | Various and numerous symptoms from trouble or malfunctioning of: <br>– Thyroid <br>– Heart <br>– Lungs <br>– Gall bladder <br>– Liver <br>– Stomach <br>– Pancreas <br>– Spleen <br>– Adrenal glands <br>– Kidneys <br>– Small and large intestines <br>– Sex organs <br>– Uterus <br>– Bladder <br>– Prostate glands |
| D 8 | • Spleen, lower mid-back | |
| D 9 | • Adrenal glands | |
| D 10 | • Kidneys | |
| D 11 | • Ureters | |
| D 12 | • Small intestine, upper/lower back | |
| **LUMBAR** | | |
| L 1 | • Illocecal valve, large intestine | |
| L 2 | • Appendix, abdomen, upper leg | |
| L 3 | • Sex organs, uterus, bladder, knees | Low back pain, aches and soreness |
| L 4 | • Prostate gland, lower back | Trouble walking |
| L 5 | • Sciatic nerve, lower legs, ankles, feet | Leg, knee, ankle and foot soreness and pain |
| **SACRO** | • Hip bones, buttocks | Sciatica, pain or soreness in the hip and buttocks |
| **COXIS** | • Rectum, anus | Rectal trouble |

134 • Alternative Medical Apocrypha: Body-Mind Correlations

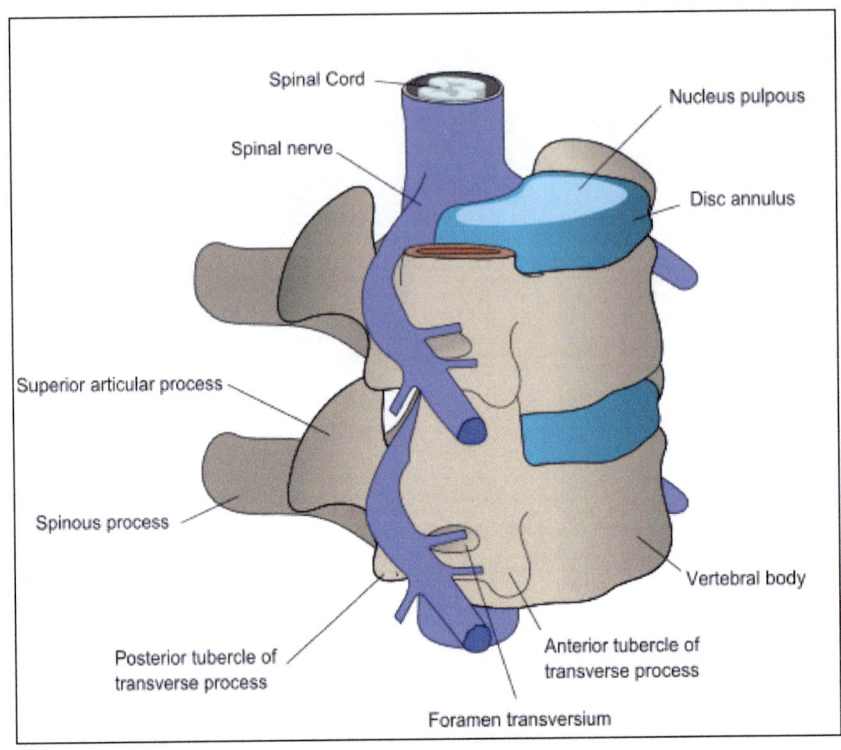

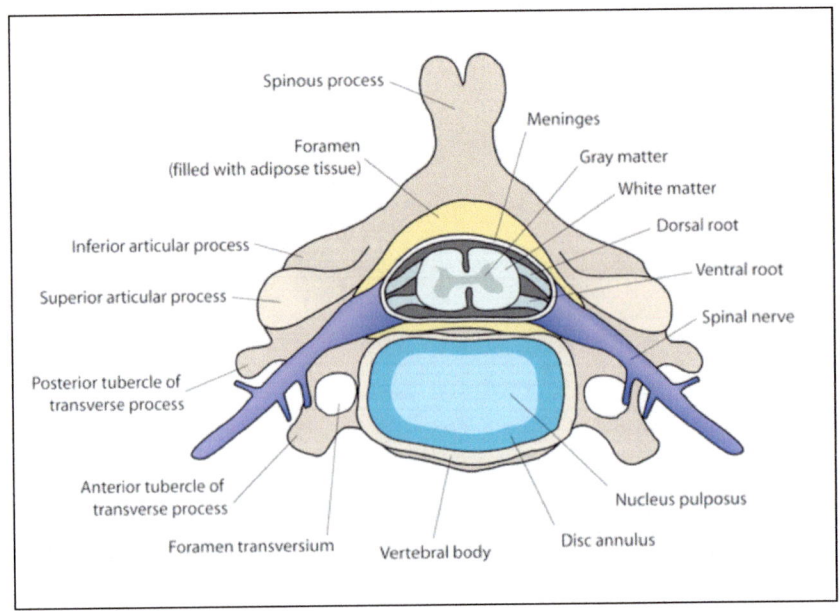

## DIATHRODIAL

Diathrotic joints are freely moveable joints surrounded by a joint capsule filled with synovial fluid like the shoulders, elbows, hips, and knees.

There are three subcategories of the joints:

## UNIAXIAL

Only moves in one direction (elbow, knee)

## BIAXIAL

Moves in two directions (in the foot)

## MULTIAXIAL

Ball and socket (shoulders, hips)

If you have arthritis, osteoporosis, or any other bone condition, visualize the entire skeletal structure as if made out of a Shiny Copper tube or pipe. Use a Shiny Copper penny as a visual aid if necessary.

Visualize and hold the color of Shiny Copper for 45 seconds in and around the bones. This color strengthens the bones, increases bone density, and realigns any subluxations in the vertebrae of your spinal column.

If you break or fracture a bone, visualize and hold the color of Shiny Copper in and around that bone for 45 seconds two or three times each day. This speeds the time of the healing.

Do the same with arthritis. Mentally visualize the shape of the bone while at the same time hold the color of Shiny Copper in it. To reduce pain, also visualize a layer of Ice Blue over the Shiny Copper.

Mind-pattern for arthritis:

*I feel hurt by my support structures in life.*

Osteoporosis:

*My support structure in life is weak.*

Broken/fractured bones:

*My support structure is broken/fractured.*

There are biaxial joints in the foot. Most injuries are caused in the toe area. The bones cannot move themselves; the ligaments, tendons, and muscles move them. They can only move when an electrical impulse from the nervous system is generated by the brain, all originating in the mind.

Vitamin D is essential to the skeletal structure; each person's need of calcium and Vitamin D is specific to that person. The bones can fuse together if there exists too much calcium in the body. Calcification can occur when there is not enough Vitamin D to absorb the calcium into the bones.

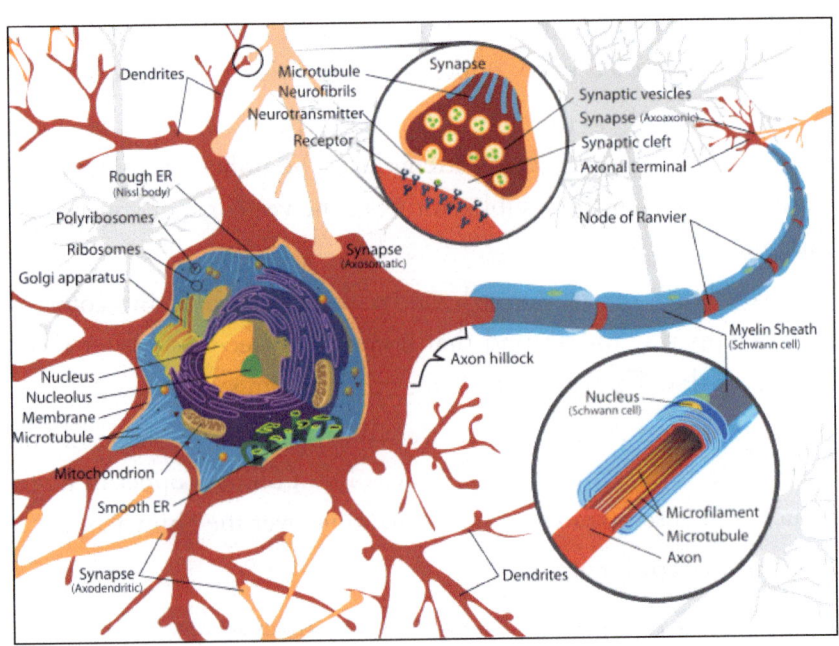

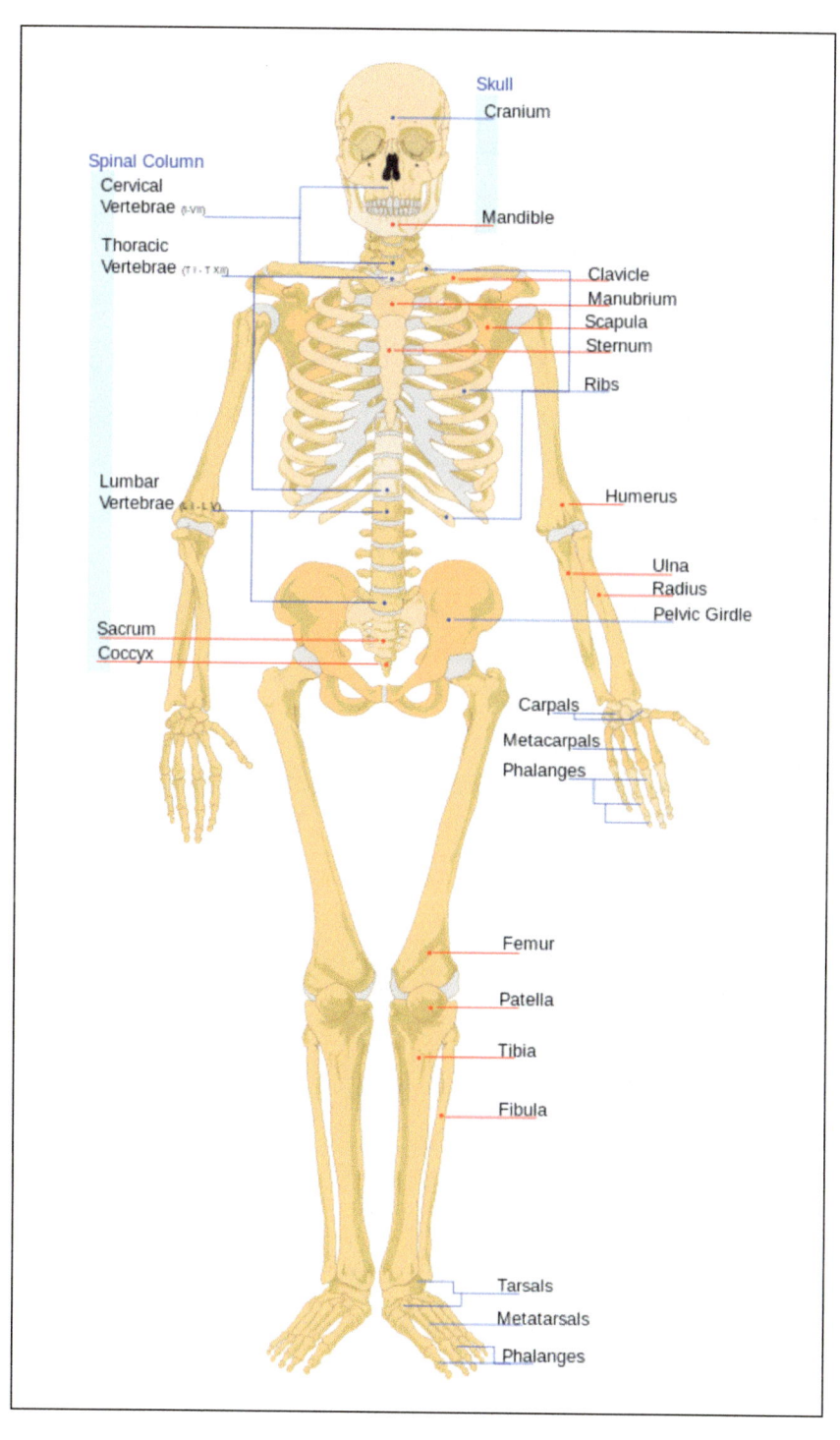

## Pelvis

### Female

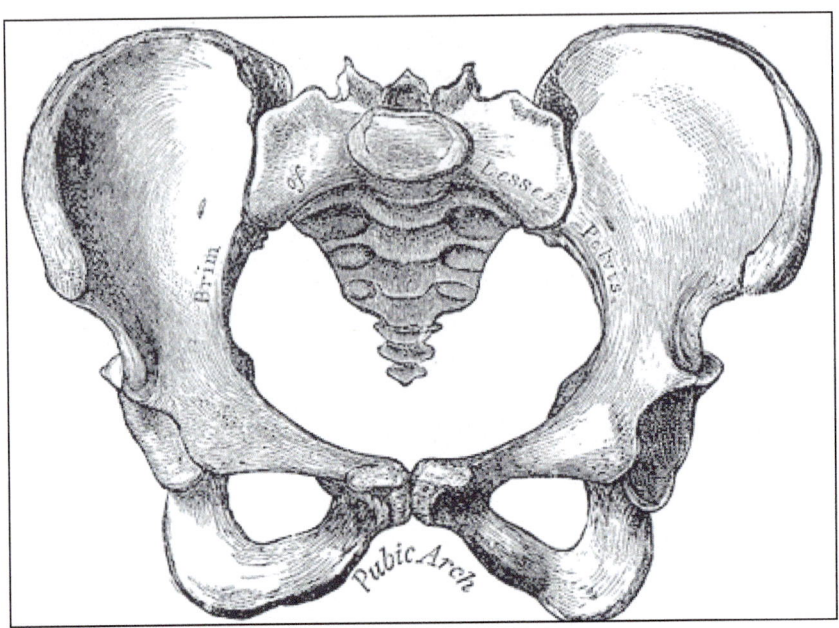

### Male

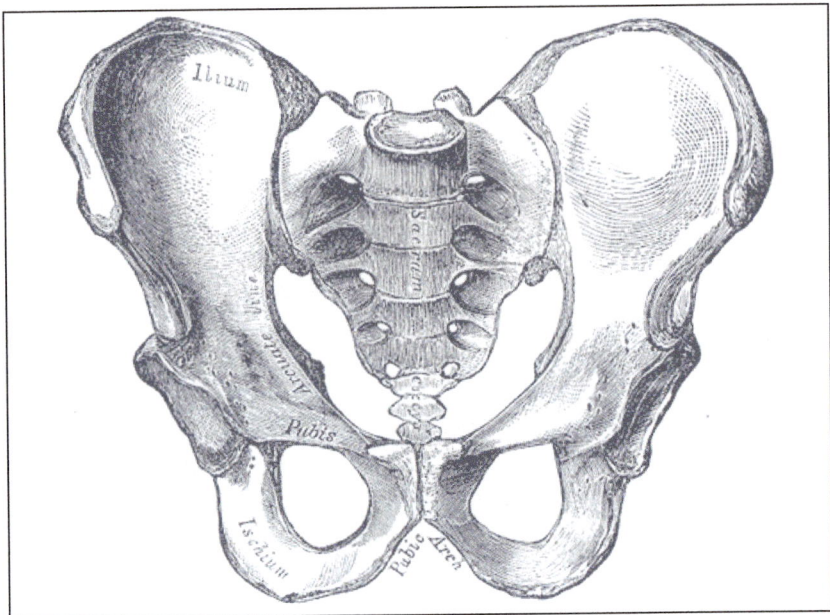

Mind-pattern:

*Balancing into the future.*

Issues with hips:

*I am worried that I cannot move forward with balance into my future.*

There are the three bones of the pelvic girdle that come together at the acectabulum joint:

Illium

Pubic

Ischium

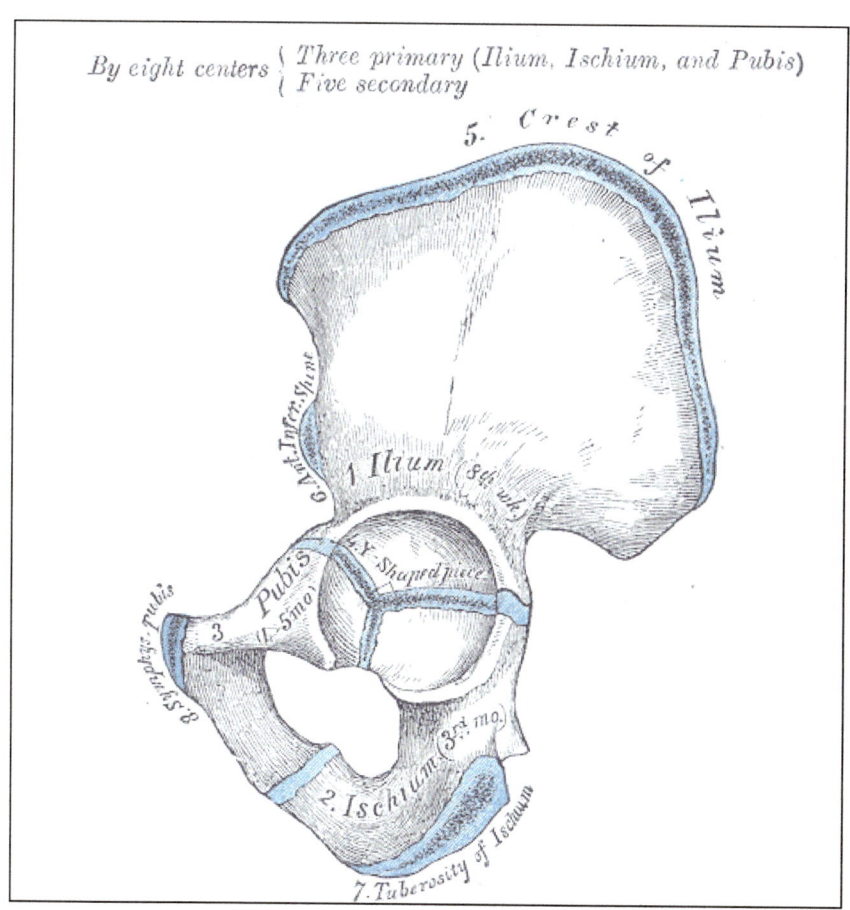

## Legs

Mind-pattern of the patella:

*Being flexible in the future.*

Right leg:

*Male figure (including Self if male), creativity, and spirituality.*

Left leg:

*Female figure (including Self if female), logic, and physical reality.*

The tibia is actually inside the leg and the fibula is on the outside. The ankle bones are called the talus, the bones in feet are the metatarsals, and the toes are the phalanges.

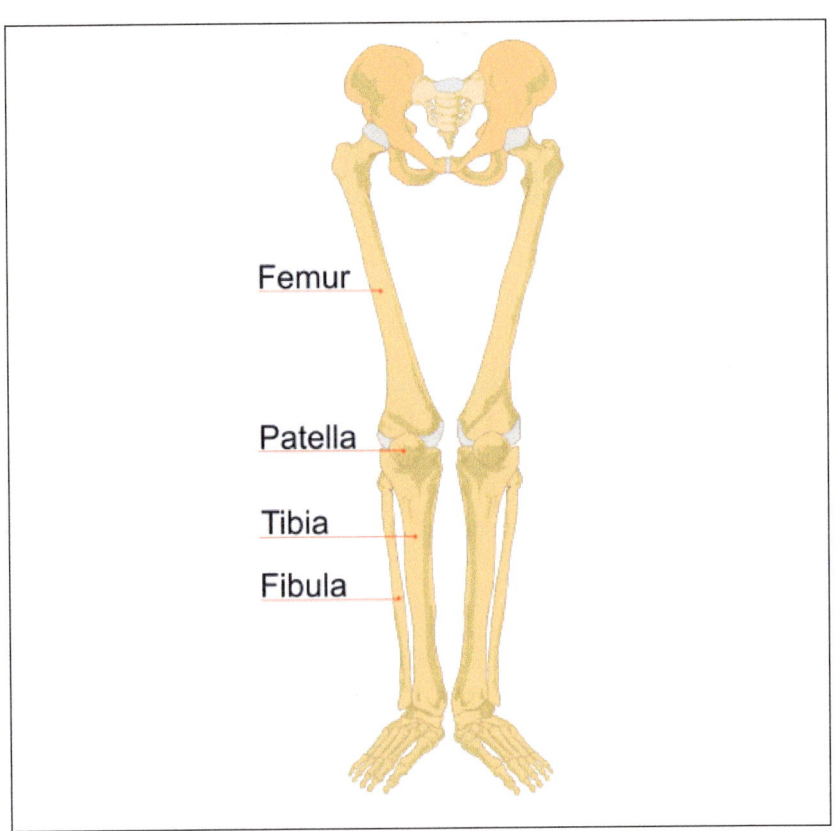

Kneecap deterioration from the back side is a common health issue. Mind-pattern:

*Issues of flexibility about the future.*

There are ways to regenerate this area and avoid invasive procedures. Take Glucosamine and Chondroitin as well as Vitamin D and calcium citrate.

In addition, rub castor oil on the kneecaps every day, letting it soak in to regenerate cellular tissues. Mentally, visualize the legs in the color Brown. Gentle weight training exercises with the legs helps to strengthen the bones as well as increase bone density.

The first corrective measure necessary when you have a problem with one or both of the kneecaps is to stay off of them. To promote healing, keep the knee wrapped tightly so you remember to not bend it too intensely or frequently.

Whenever you want to heal a part of the body, especially a moveable part of the body, do not move it. Keep it stationery or supported so it has time to build energy and density.

Many people have water on the knee.

Water on the knee:

*Inflexibility and feeling pressured with the thought of being flexible.*

*The thought of being flexible is too much for me to handle.*

Bunions are really a misshaping of the bones in the foot where it bows out. With this condition you must visualize the bone's shape as well. You are strengthening the bone as well as reshaping it. For pain, always surround the area with a layer of Ice Blue.

Bunions:

*I am not focusing properly on my future support structures.*

## Arms

The bones of the arms are similar to the bones of the legs, but with different names. The femur in the leg correlates to the humerus in the arm.

The two bones in the forearm are the ulna and radius, leading into the bones of the wrist called the carpus or carpals.

The hand has the metacarpus or metacarpals while the fingers are called phalanges like the toes.

The clavicle bone leads into the sternum, ribcage, and spinal column.

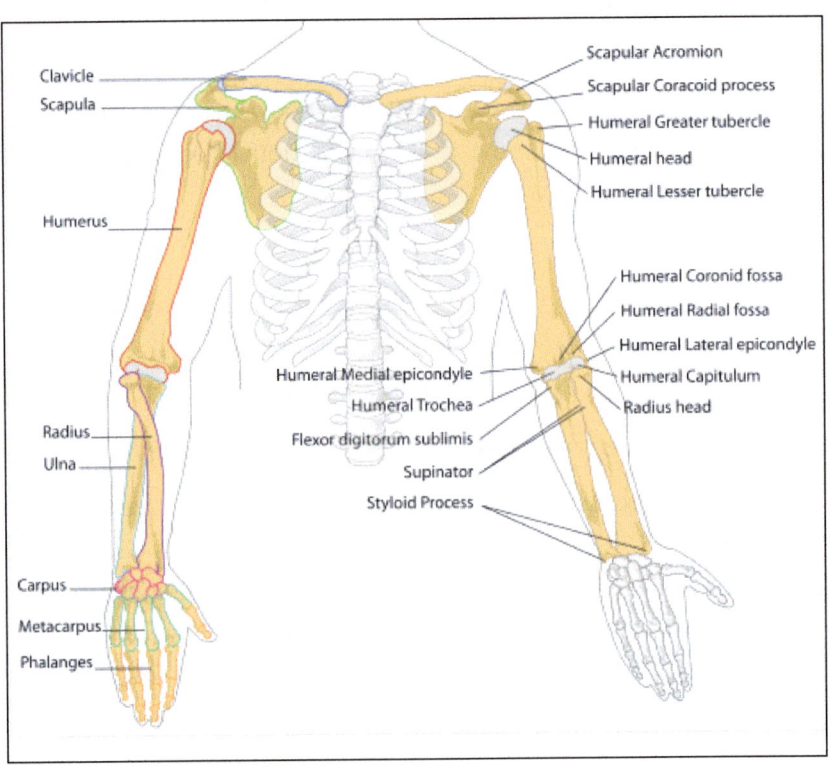

## Skull

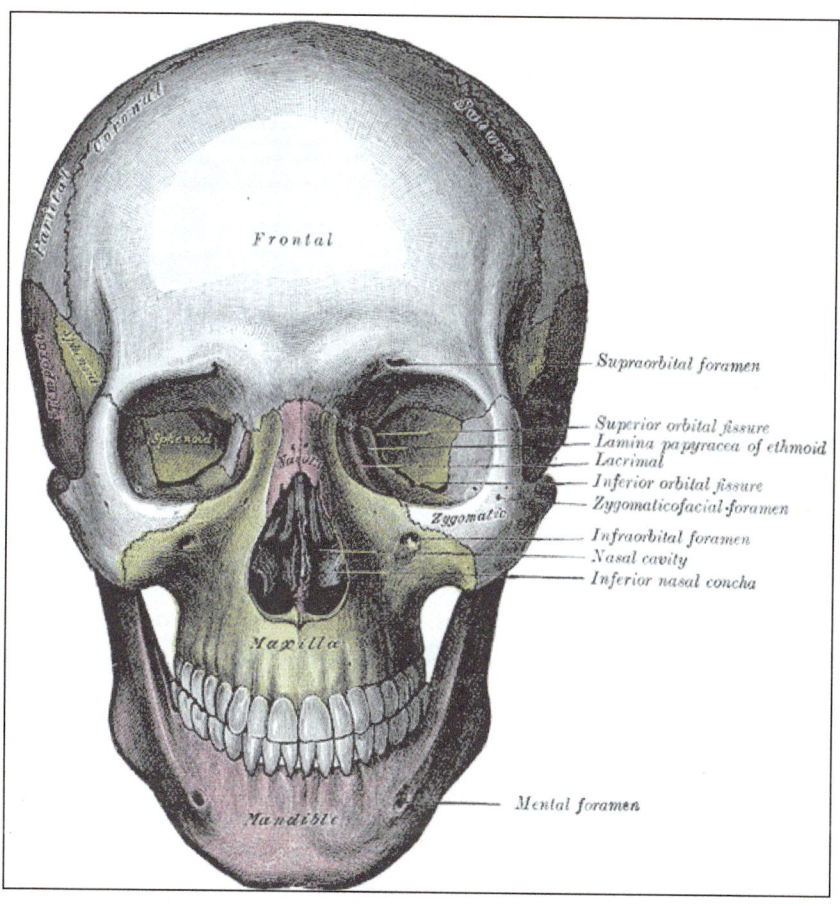

This diagram shows the human skull with the frontal bones and how the teeth and jaw fit together.

Mind-pattern for teeth:

> *How I adjust to life.*

Bottom teeth:

> *How I adjust to past and present situations.*

Top teeth:

> *How I adjust to future situations.*

Teeth on the left side:

> *How I adjust to female issues.*

Teeth on the right side:

> *How I adjust to male issues.*

Teeth in the front:

> *How I relate to the present.*

Teeth in the back:

> *How I relate to the past.*

Brushing your teeth is a form of reflexology.

Mercury fillings are a toxic heavy metal. Most dentists say mercury damage is done within the first few years of being in the mouth and has potentially leaked out.

If your bones are strong, the mercury is contained within the tooth unless it cracks or has other issues. Some dentists prefer not to remove the mercury fillings, saying that removing them may cause a toxic situation for your body. It is best to not have mercury fillings in the first place, but if you do have them, consult with your dentist before removing them to determine the best scenario for you.

Pure gold or silver fillings become electrical conductors, making electrical currents more active on the side of the mouth with the filling. You may also feel more muscular contractions and you will become an increased beacon for electromagnetic energies.

Fluoride treatments deaden brain tissue and actually weaken the skeletal structure, including the teeth. Fluoride was developed by German scientists to make populations docile. Fluoride in water is banned in Europe. In France they aerate the water and do not add any chemicals into the water.

## Mandible/Jaw

Mind-pattern:

*How I communicate my strength of character.*

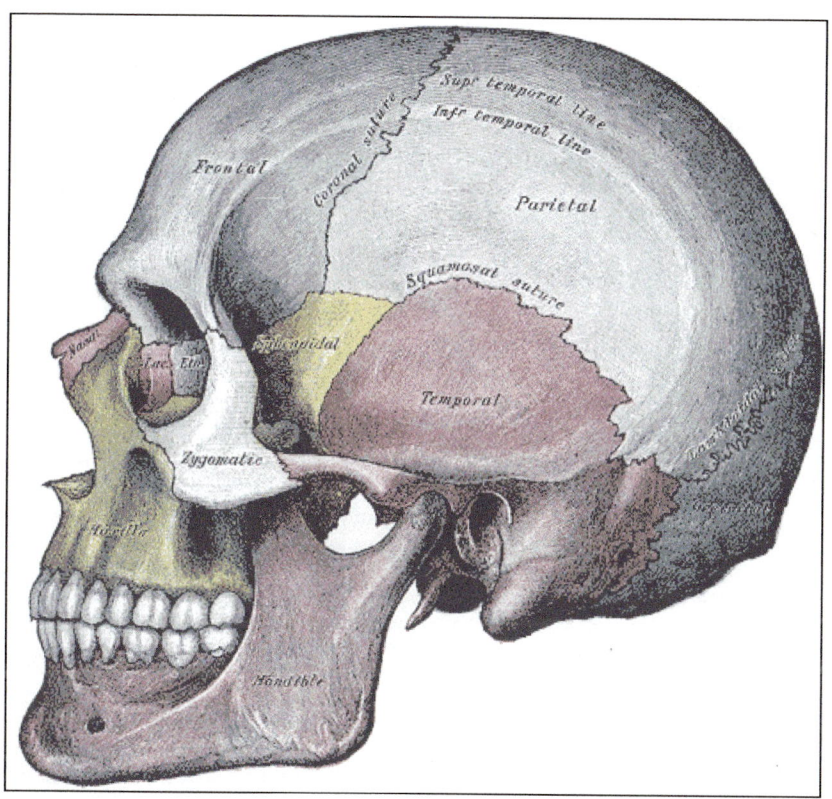

# Muscular System

Motion is always present in all body systems in groups of three. For example, in the muscular system there are muscles, ligaments, and tendons.

Ligaments connect bone to bone.

If you rip a ligament, usually it requires surgery to reattach it.

Tendons connect muscles to bone.

Many people have difficulty with tendons. For example, tendonitis is an inflammation that occurs from repetitive motion. Lifting weights can cause tendons to tear; you might mistakenly think it is a muscle.

Muscles connect to each other.

Mind-pattern of little muscular development:

*I am weak in my life and I have no way of moving through it.*

A lot of muscular development:

*I have power and strength to move through life.*

Muscular illnesses like atrophy and dystrophy:

*The way I am moving through my life is hurting me.*

The heart muscle is the most important muscular structure of the body.

Muscles are made up of fiber and they move in special ways:

## Concentric

A concentric muscle contraction happens when the muscle shortens while lifting. For example, your muscle shortens when it contracts during a bicep curl.

## Isometric

An isometric contraction occurs when there is no lengthening or shortening of the muscle. For example, when you push against an object or you grip and hold an object, your muscle does not lengthen or shorten.

## Isotonic

An isotonic contraction happens when the tension in the muscle stays constant even if the muscle is lengthened or shortened. For example, during weight lifting or pushups, the tension in the muscle stays constant.

## Isokinetic

An isokinetic or isovelocity contraction occurs when the muscle contraction and motion stays consistent but the resistance varies. This usually involves workout equipment that allows the resistance to be changed and controlled while the motion stays at a fixed speed.

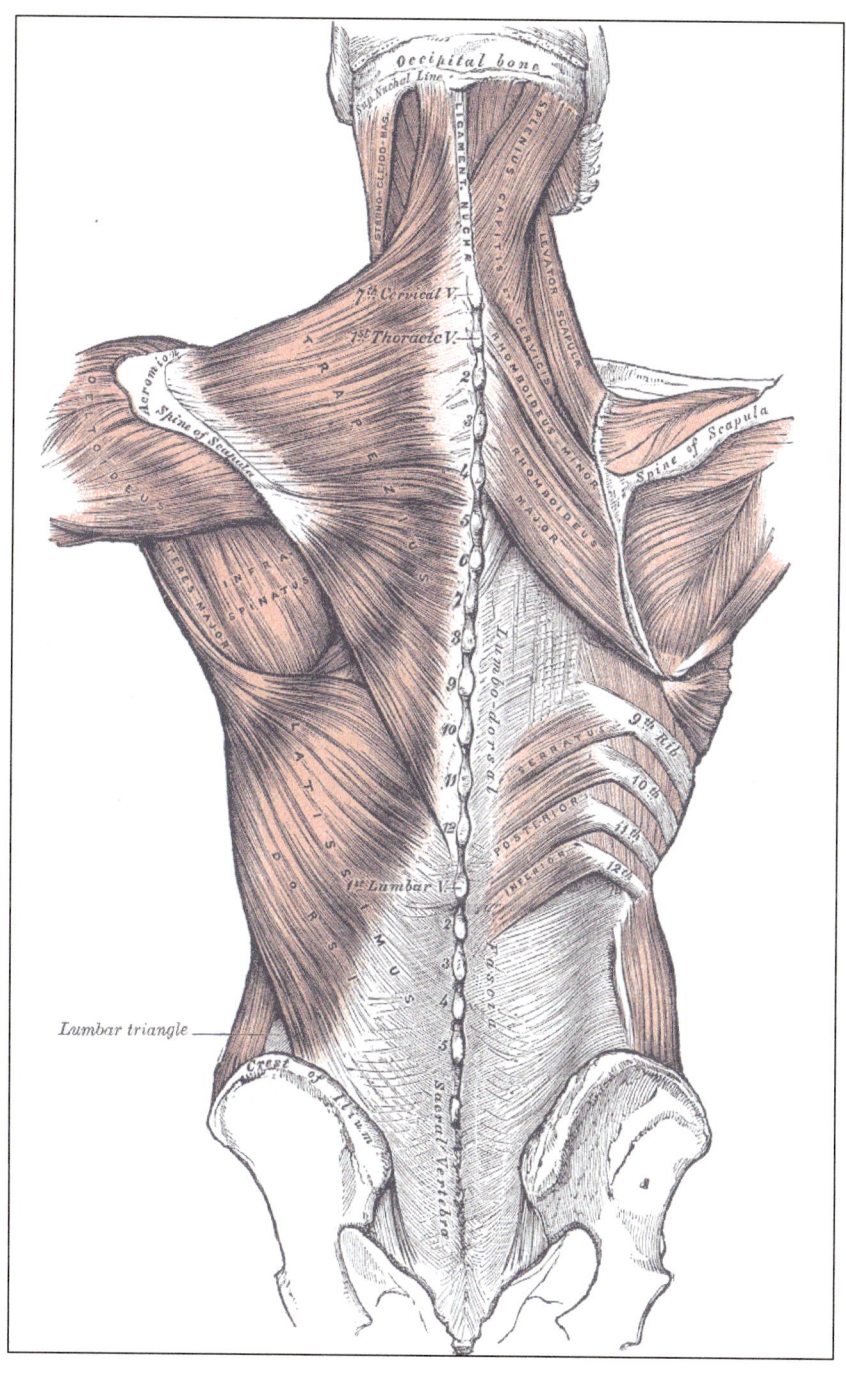

## Muscle Groups

### Trapezius

The trapezius is located in the back from the occipital bone to the lower thoracic area and laterally to the shoulder blades or scapula.

### Latissimus Dorsi

The broadest muscle of the back, also known as the "lats."

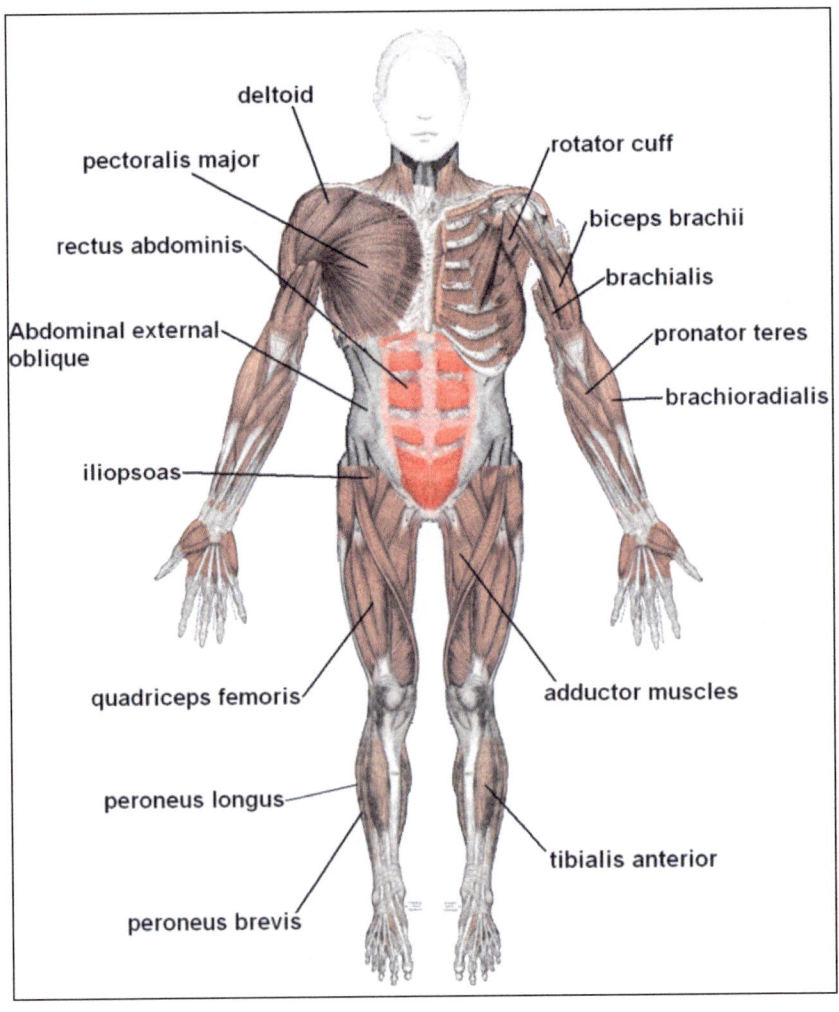

## Deltoids

The deltoids are the shoulder muscles. There are three kinds: the anterior, lateral, and posterior.

## Pectorals

The major and minor pectoralis muscles are located in the chest area.

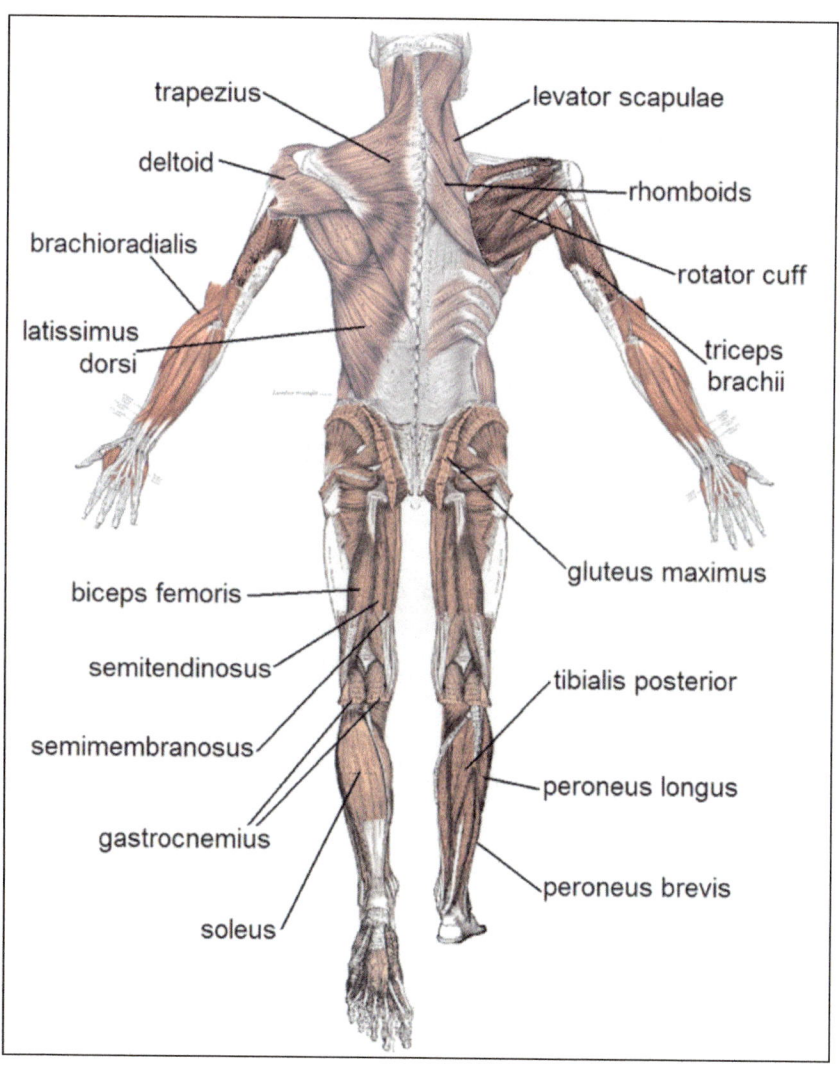

## Biceps

The biceps are located in the front of the arm between the shoulders and elbows.

## Triceps

The triceps are the muscle group located on the back of the arm.

## Brachiali

The brachialis is behind the biceps and flexes the elbow.

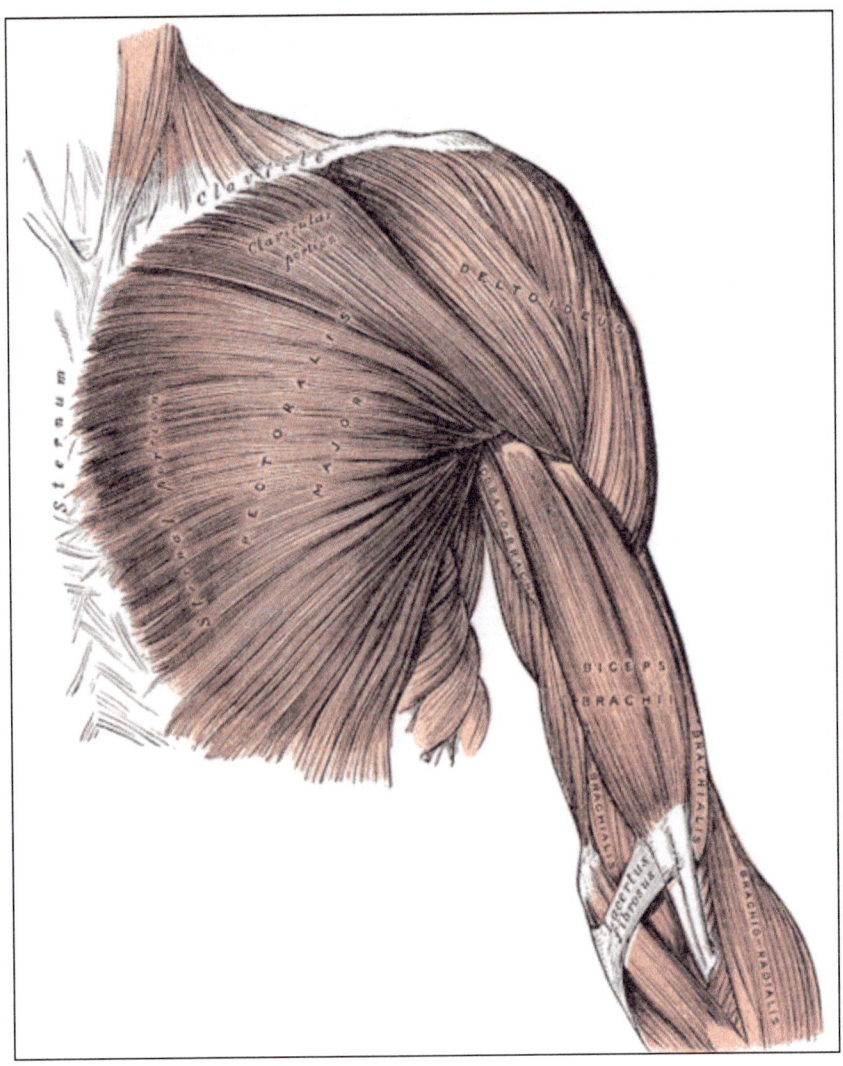

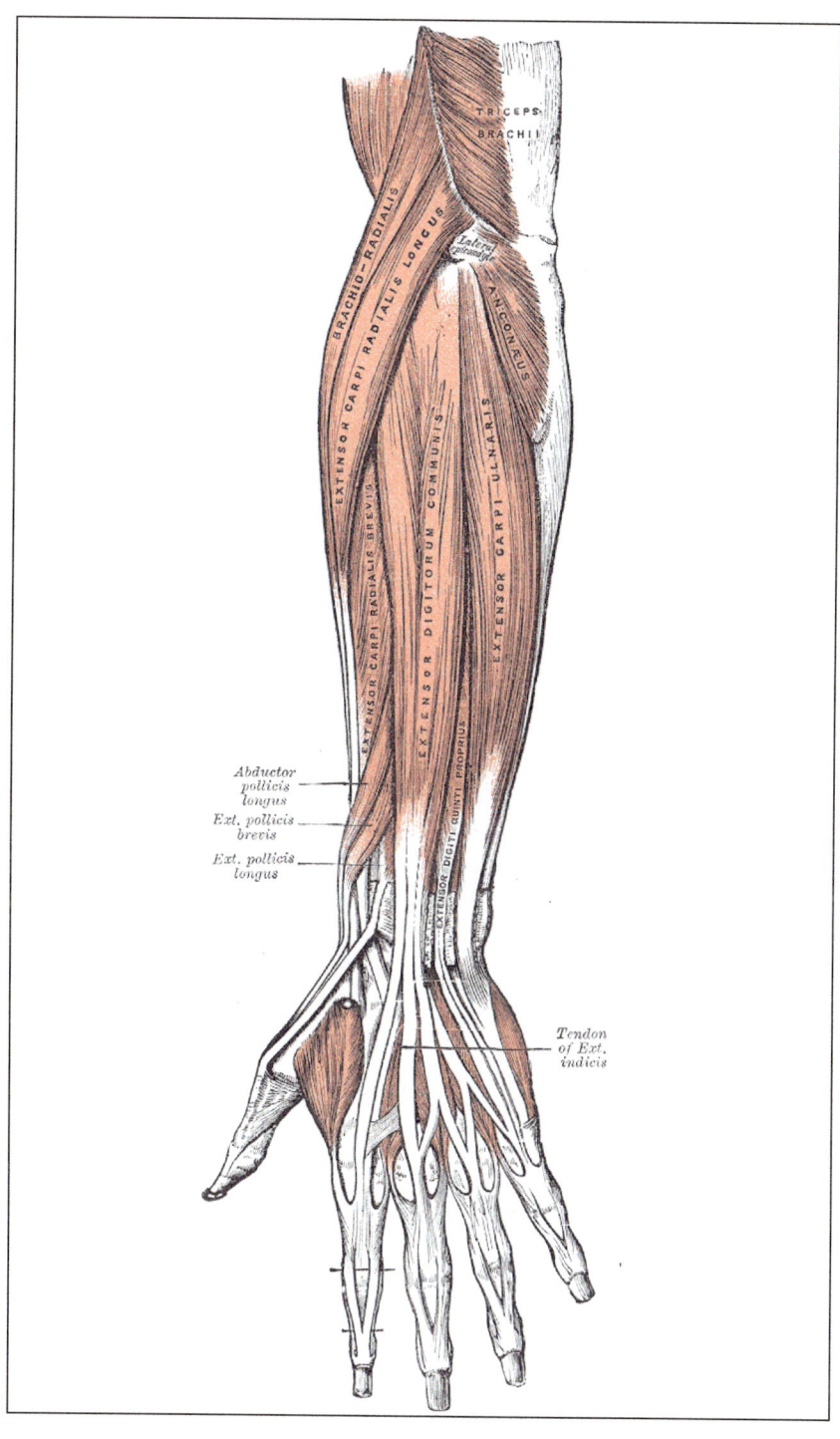

## BRACHIORADIALS
The brachioradials are located in the forearms.

## FLEXORS
The muscles that move the fingers.

## SERRATUS ANTERIOR
Located over the ribs on the sides of the chest.

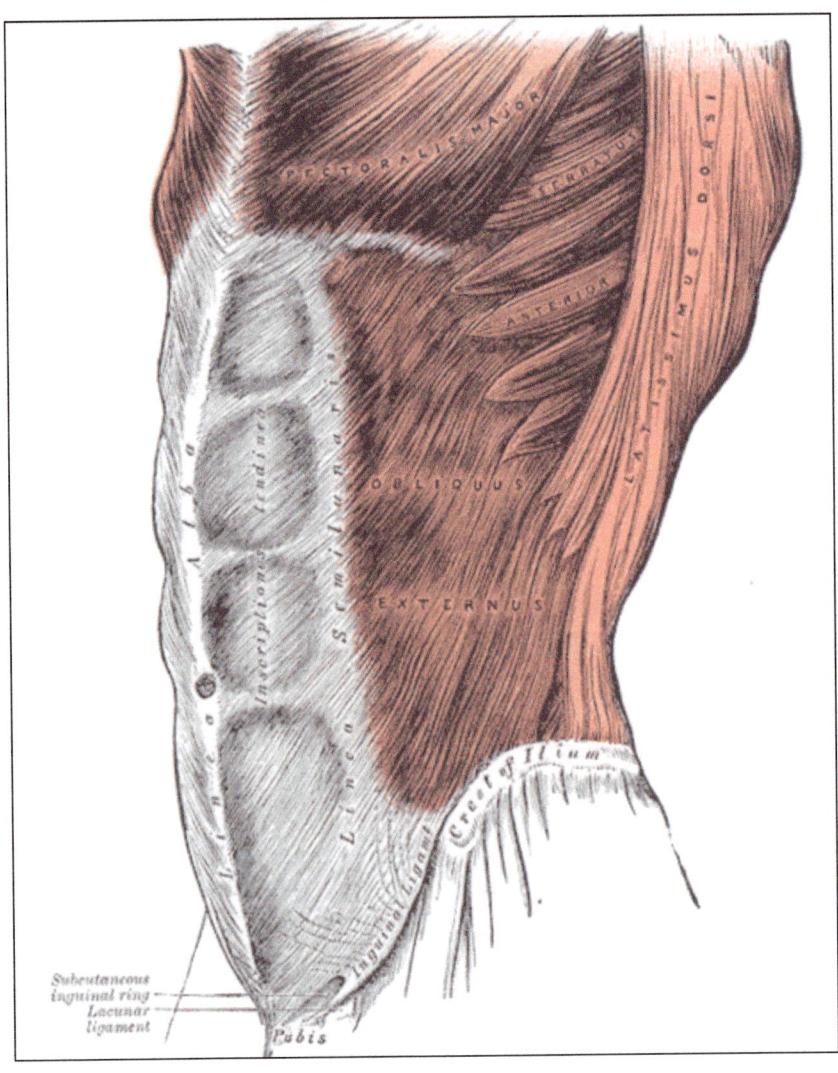

## Rectus Abdominis

Located in the abdomen, commonly known as the "abs." Depending on your genetics you could have either a six- or an eight-pack.

## Obliques

The muscles on the sides of the abdominals.

## Psoas and Iliacus

The interior hip muscles; they help with the rectus abdominis, so if you want a six-pack you will have to work together with these.

## Gluteal

There are three gluteal muscles: the minimus, medius, and maximus. These are also known as the triplets.

## Quadriceps Femoris

The quadriceps have four muscle groups that include the rectus femoris in the middle area of the thigh, the vastus lateralis on the outer side of the thigh, the vastus intermedius in the middle of the thigh underneath the rectus femoris, and the vastus medialis on the inner part of the thigh.

## Sartorius

The longest muscle in the body, which goes across the quadriceps from the hip to the knee.

## Tensor Fasciae Latae

The thigh muscle on the outside of the thigh that connects from the iliac crest of the hip to the knee. It balances the hip and works with the gluteus maximus to support the knee.

## Gracilis

The thin flat muscle located on the inner thigh.

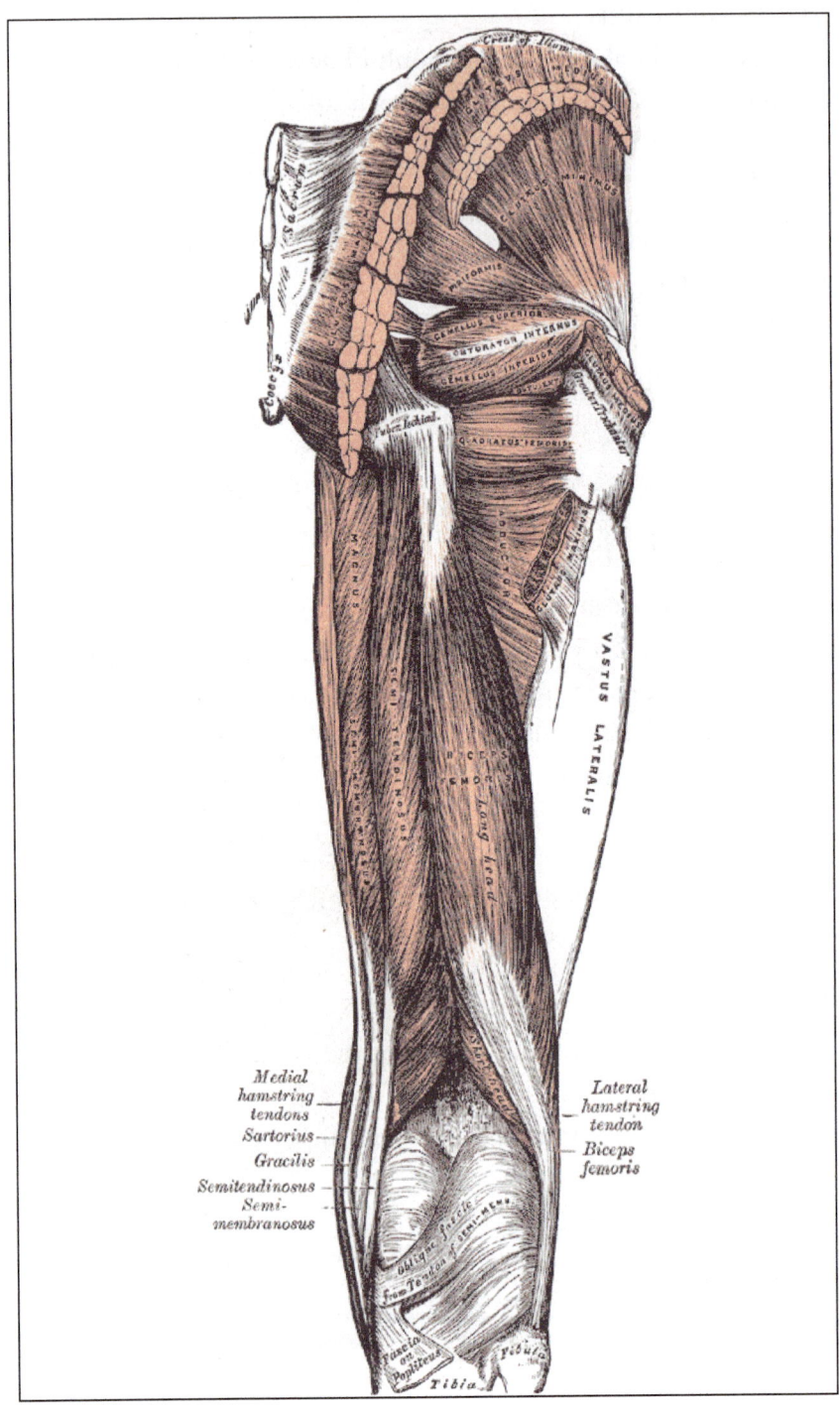

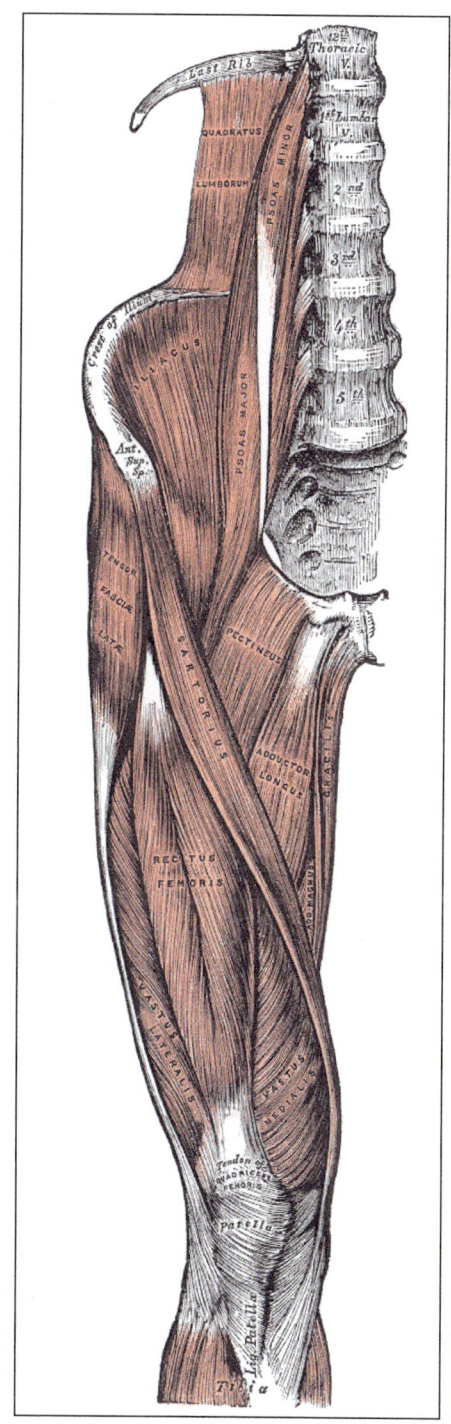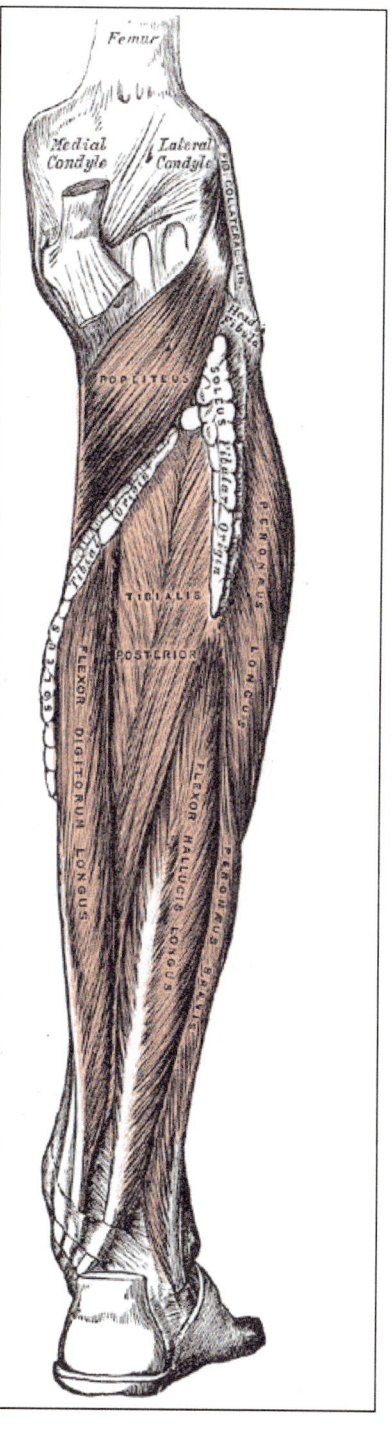

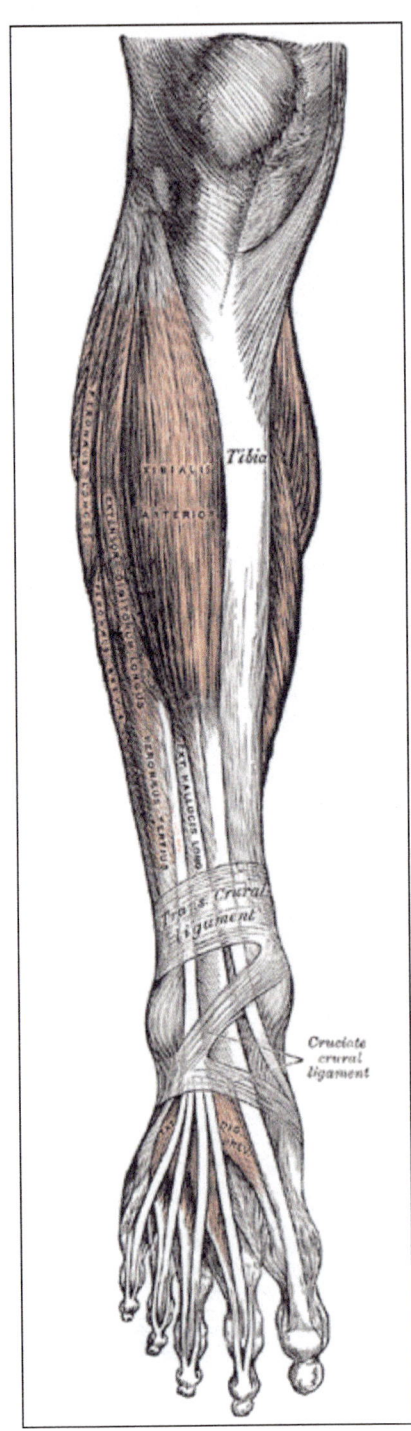
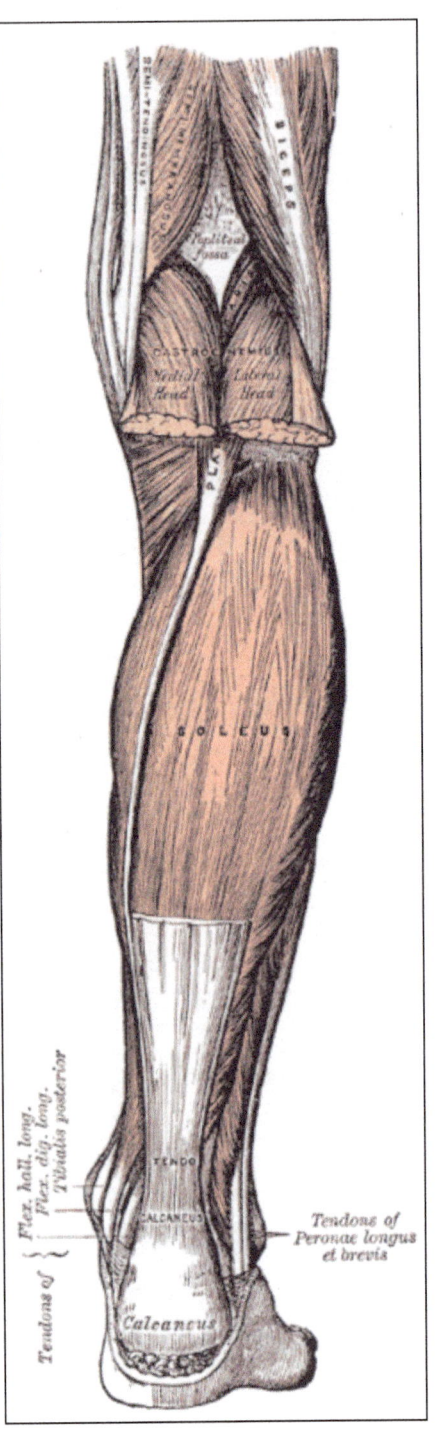

## Hamstrings

The hamstrings include the bicep femoris (long and short head), the semitendinosus, and semimebranosus.

## Soleus and Gastrocnemius

Together these form the calf muscles.

## Tibialis Anterior

The shin muscle.

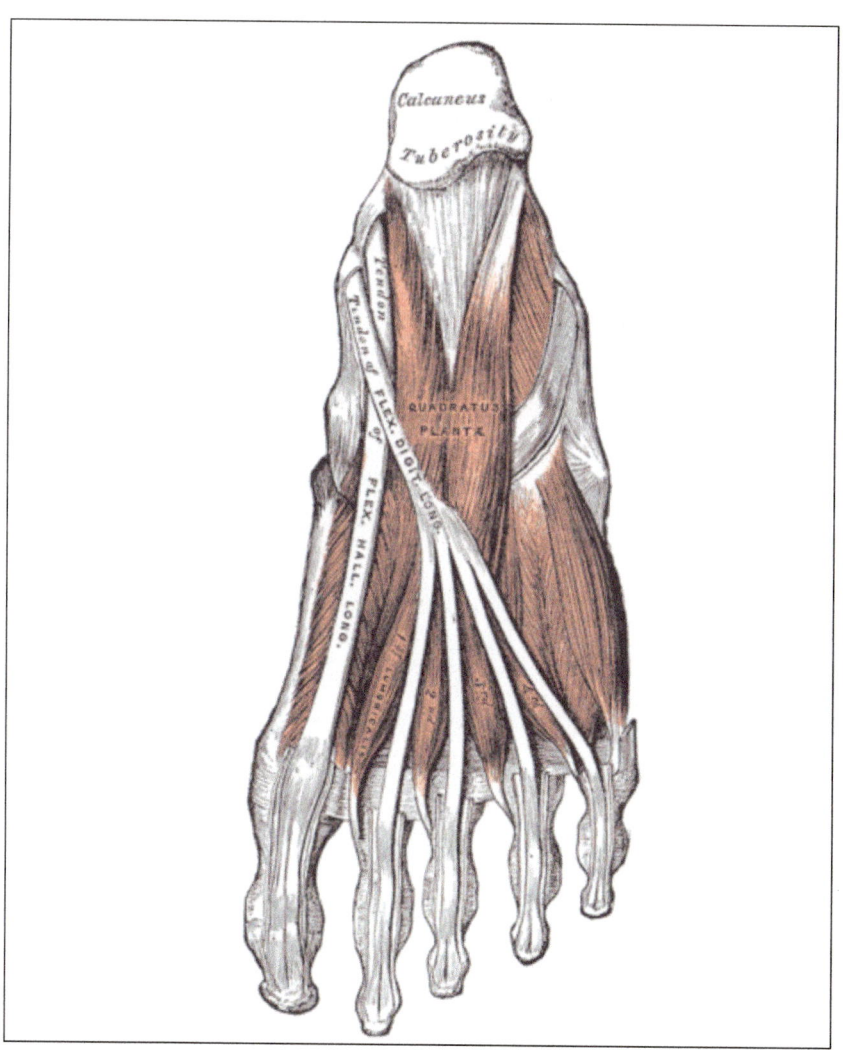

# Cancer

All cancer is caused by a virus. There are environmental conditions that enable the virus to achieve what it does in the cells.

The initial tumor is like a "master tumor" that sends out the cells that form the metastatic tumors elsewhere. There is a sympathetic and energetic connection from the initial or master tumor to those tumors that metastasize from it. Doctors must focus on this "master tumor" to stop the cancer from spreading.

Cancer metastasizes by draining from the organs or sections of the body that have the cancer. The cells drain into the lymphatic and circulatory system and from here flow through the body until they find another appropriate spot conducive to growth.

The lymphatic system does not have its own pumping system. You have to do exercise to get the lymphatic system to move. Deep tissue massage can help as well.

This is why whenever cancer is diagnosed, lymph glands in that area are examined for cancer cells. If cancer is found in the lymph glands, these glands are removed so traveling cancer cells cannot be deposited in this area.

From a surgical perspective, this makes sense, but from a holistic view it does not. Without drainage, you most likely will still have a problem in that area. Plus, once you are cut open, it is easier for the cancer to spread throughout the lymphatic and circulatory system. So even if it is removed from one area, there is a high chance that it will settle elsewhere in the body.

Most people who are diagnosed with cancer are afraid to get the surgery as well as not get the surgery, so like all matters, this is a personal choice that must be made.

General mind-pattern of cancer:

*Held resentment over a long period of time.*

Where the cancer develops is a clue to the type of resentment that the person has held over a long period of time. For example, liver, breast, ovarian, and prostate are common types of cancers.

## Liver Cancer

Mind-pattern:

*Processing current life experiences and having the energy to deal with them.*

Liver Cancer:

*I am unhappy and resentful of my life experiences.*

Generally, cancer does not initially develop in the liver. Usually cancer develops somewhere else and metastasizes to the liver as it moves through the lymph system. For this reason, liver cancer is rarely treated by medical doctors because when it reaches the liver, there are usually numerous underlying cancers throughout the body.

There is also an energetic reason why liver cancer is usually secondary. In most cases, resentment comes from another issue that is causing current life experiences. For example, if the initial tumor is in the colon.

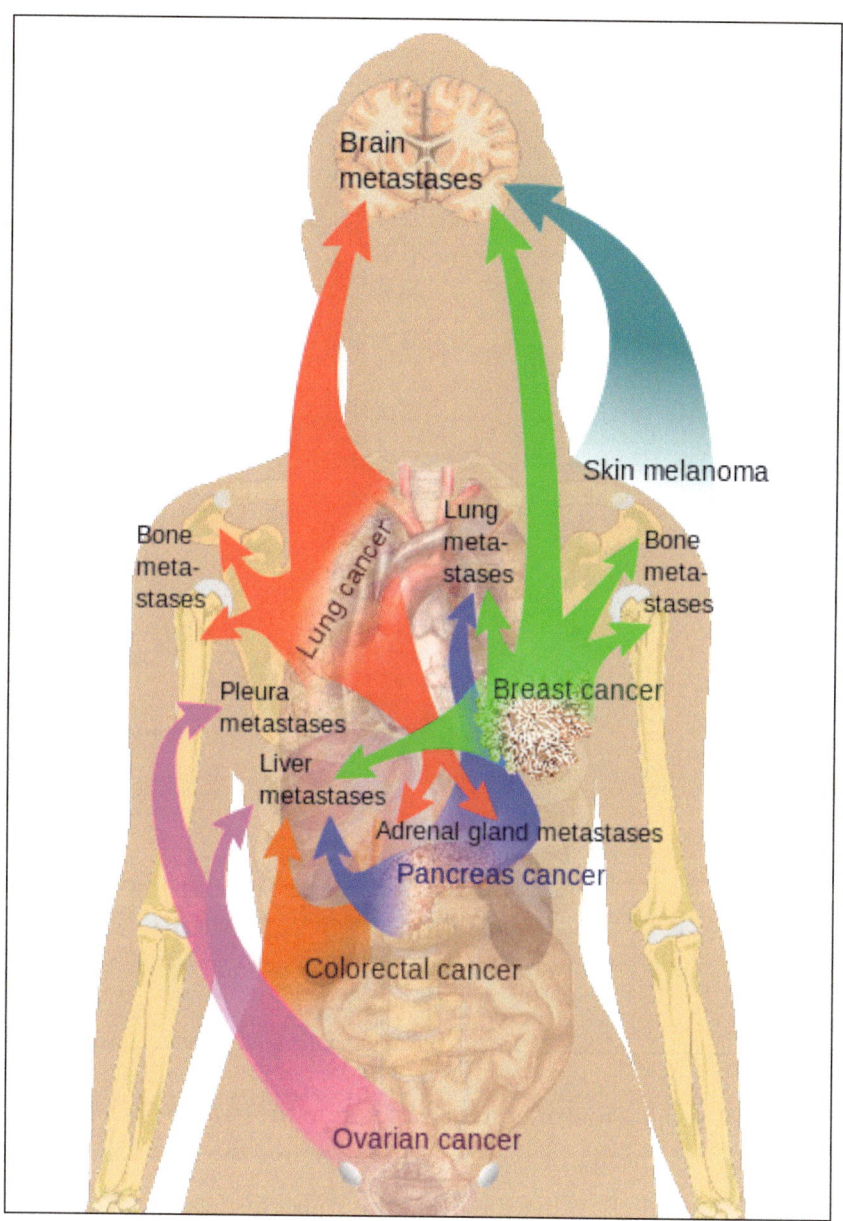

Colon Cancer:

*I am unable to release past experiences.*
*I am resentful of the past and I hold onto it.*

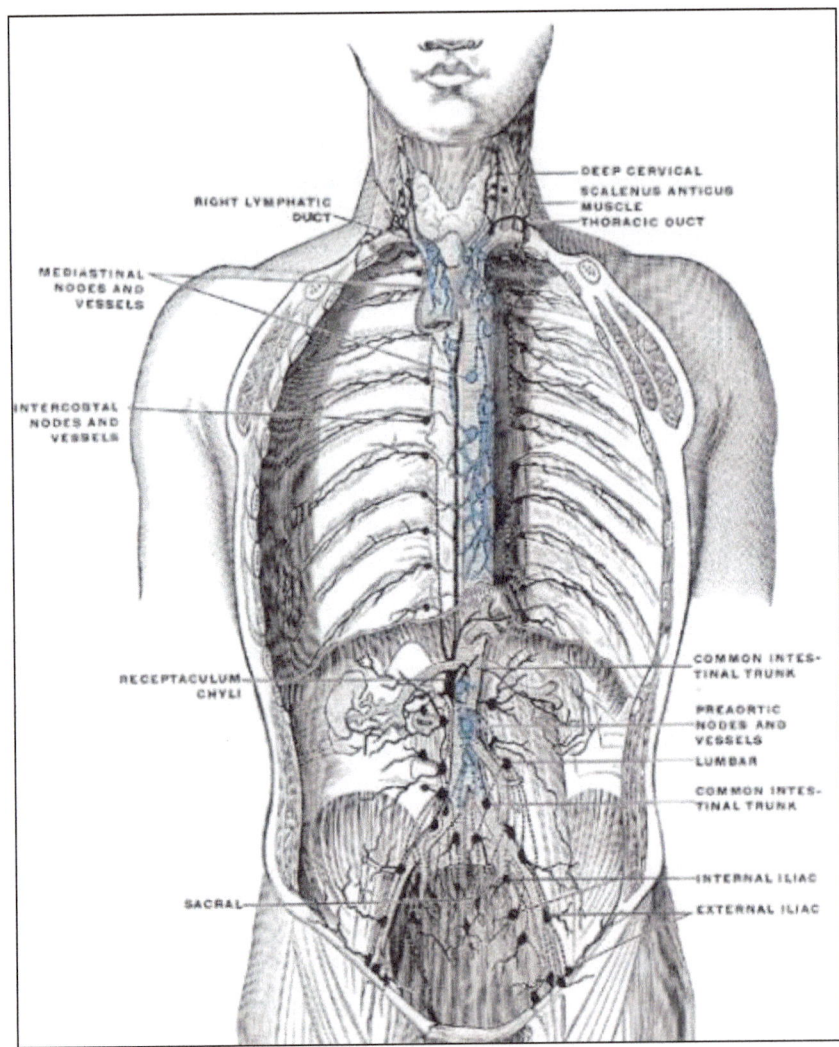

The person has to work on the issues from the past that are resented to improve the health of the colon and therefore the liver, too.

Flushing and cleansing the liver with milk thistle, dandelion root, apple cider vinegar, and lemon water; eating any bitter greens; and taking liver glandulars are all beneficial as a boost to mind-pattern release work.

Glandular treatments should only be taken for a period of time, then stopped for a while before starting again. Otherwise, they may cause wild cellular growth.

Drinking strong black coffee without any sugar or dairy can help cleanse the liver. Coffee enemas have a limited role in healing. Coffee colonics may be helpful. However, if the person is in a weakened condition you must know what you are doing or more harm can be done than good.

As with any cancer tumor, you can visualize a Violet hose vacuuming the liver, or sweep/flush the liver in Violet. The key is to work on the held resentment and eliminate it. Remember, in general the liver is only secondary and not the initial cause of the center of the tumor.

### Breast Cancer

Mind-pattern:

*I resent that my nurturing ability is rejected and/or suppressed.*

Breast cancer in a female happens when she no longer feels needed or her nurturing abilities are rejected/suppressed.

Breast cancer is increasing among males for the same reason. Physically, it can be due to an increase in estrogen in the body, but the mind-pattern is the same.

When you do not take the time to nurture yourself, resentment builds that you are not being nurtured. Be mindful to not let this happen to you.

### Ovarian Cancer

Mind-pattern for the ovaries:

*Creative and productive energies.*

Ovarian Cancer:

*I resent not being able to creatively and productively express in my life.*

Many women are dying from ovarian cancer unnecessarily, mainly because they do not take care of themselves or check on the symptoms until it is much too late. Ovarian cancer generally metastasizes very rapidly, virulently, and can spread over the body quickly.

For this reason, the medical profession removes the ovaries because you can live without them, but the result of this procedure is a plethora of hormonal issues.

Ovarian and breast cancers can both be corrected by balancing the estrogen levels of the body. There are estrogen and progesterone receptors in the body. If there is little or no progesterone, the progesterone receptors pick up the estrogen instead, causing wild cellular growth because estrogen creates growth in the body. The progesterone levels need to be boosted to match the estrogen levels so there is a balance without conflict.

However, once a person has an illness, it is important to increase the progesterone to exceed the estrogen levels until the illness goes away. Do this with wild yam root, homeopathic progesterone, and ovary glandulars.

## Prostate Cancer

Prostate cancer in men is the equivalent to ovarian cancer in women.

Mind-pattern:

*I resent that I am no longer creative or productive in my life.*

This is why prostate cancer is more prevalent in older men.

To eliminate Prostate Cancer, visualize the color Violet flushing the area. Also visualize Medium Green to oxygenate the area because cancer is an anaerobic cell and it dies in oxygen. If you oxygenate it, it will die. I also encourage a person to take liquid oxygen drops in their water or juice and a higher amount of COQ10 and ozone treatments. Taking hyssop herb, Pau d'Arco, Chapparell, and turmeric will kill the cancer virus. Use the Golden Altar release technique daily. Shark cartilage can be taken to reduce tumors; it will eventually reduce and eliminate cancerous or non-cancerous growths in the body. You can also use these as a preventative measure.

Take pumpkin seeds, saw palmetto, and eleuthero root/Siberian ginseng. There are all kinds of ginseng, but Siberian needed is for this issue. An acquaintance cured his prostate cancer with Ojibwa/Esiak extract. High doses of Vitamin C (10,000-12,000) daily will also shrink cancer tumors.

Radionic treatments are also beneficial. You can have an elixir developed for your particular issue.

# Regeneration vs. Removal and Cryropreservation

It is interesting and curious that most surgeries that involve the complete removal of an organ are women's organs. This is what the medical profession does—pluck them out.

Even if you have an organ physically removed, what does it say about that mind-pattern?

Mind-pattern:

*I am removing it from this lifetime;*
*I am not dealing with that mind-pattern.*

The only organ in the human body that can completely regenerate is the liver. The skin, nails, and hair also regenerate. Brain cells have been known to regenerate. In the thoracic region the thyroid has the potential to regenerate as well.

When someone has thyroid cancer, surgeons remove the thyroid gland. The reason is that the medical industry is concerned the thyroid will regenerate. So, radiation treatments and chemotherapy are administered to kill the cells to prevent this from happening.

Why? Because if your organ regenerates, you would not need to be on hormones and treatments the rest of your life. So, any organ that regenerates that you can live without, the medical and insurance complex wants to ensure does not grow back so you need to depend on them forever. If part of your organ regenerates, they will tell you it must be removed. Unfortunately this is because the medical profession has become a big business interested mostly in profit, not well-being.

Remember, the medical profession believes if you can live without an organ, it is expendable and should be removed. In medical school, surgeons are encouraged to expedite operations before the patient gets better.

On CNN a doctor admitted that doctors generally do not listen to their patients. The doctor said, "It is an economic problem and they cannot make money if they spend more time with patients. In medical school they teach that spending more than 10-15 minutes with a patient significantly decreases profits."

This program recommended that patients take notes and ask questions when visiting a doctor. Of course the doctor probably will not answer all of your questions. In a small village in China doctors earn approximately USD200 per month to keep people well. If someone gets ill, the doctor does not get paid.

In the near future, all organs will be artificially regenerated. There is a concept that when a person is born, cells are taken from the body so they can clone whatever is needed. This way you know there is always a perfect donor for you at any time in case you need an organ or limb. Scientists speculate if they can shut off the DNA that creates the head, what is left would no longer be considered a "real human being." Instead it would be a vessel for organ manufacturing. Would it have a soul? Yes, rudimentary Soul-Personality would not require a brain. It would be part of the Oversoul of that person because it is the same body.

This brings up the question of morality. Morally, should this be allowed to exist? There will be warehouses where these organ vessels will be stored. The government and elite and wealthy individuals would primarily be the only people able to do this.

You may have heard about cryonic centers where they freeze human bodies or heads for future use in the event you die so they will be able to regenerate or resuscitate you. The problem with this is no one has ever been successfully defrosted and revived to see if the cells are still viable.

Preserved DNA from frozen mammoths has been found under glacial ice and permafrost in Siberia. Cloning experiments are currently being conducted by Japanese scientists. The theory is when a living being or animal is quickly frozen, the cells and DNA go into a state of suspended animation with the potential to be cloned in the future.

What happens if your brain is neuropreserved or the body is cryopreserved? Then, centuries or millennia later, you are revived and brought back to life? What happens to your Soul-Personality? You created the DNA of the body through your mind-pattern.

What happens linearly from the moment of being frozen to the point of being awakened? During this interim could your Soul-Personality create other bodies in which to live?

There is not a definite answer; however there are the experiences of others. There are numerous people who were in comas for long periods of time that remember the interim period before being awakened. Many of these people distinctly recall an attachment to the body and were unable to progress onwards because of the attachment.

Had time for these individuals stopped? In actuality there is no time; progress was stifled due to the physical attachment. Assume the Soul-Personality progresses, continuing to learn and grow. Then, 5,000 years later when the body awakens, the Soul-Personality no longer matches the body. What happens if another Soul-Personality or an astral/demonic entity enters the body?

Another aspect to consider is that the world's population is approximately 7 billion people. Why would you wake up? Why would you be needed when there are billions of people already? My feeling is a majority of people would never be awakened because they would be superfluous.

What about all the ancient people that have been found frozen under glaciers?

Ötzi the Iceman was discovered in the Austrian Alps in 1991 on the border between Austria and Italy. The DNA of four other people were also found on the body of this one man. So, the DNA of five people were found on just that one body. Theoretically, all five of these people can now be cloned.

Is Ötzi the Iceman still attached to his body and cannot move on after being frozen for thousands of years?

No, because he died and then was frozen. He was not frozen at the point of death. He died of an injury and then froze. People that are cryogenically frozen are instantly frozen at death or right before they die. Once the body dies it starts to degenerate and decompose quite rapidly.

There is no significant difference in the body structure of human beings in the last 30-40,000 years.

This implies that there is not much progress in the mind-pattern because humans have not adapted or changed very much over the last 30-40,000 years. People still have five fingers and toes. Height and density have changed. Height is really a function of nutrition. Most of the diets of our forebears were high in protein with very little carbohydrates, fruits, or vegetables.

Scientists also observed sections of the brain that are different in ancient humans. The nonverbal centers are more powerful than ours. According to a renegade scientist, these people had more psychic abilities since they could not verbally communicate as well with others. They needed more mental capacity for communication due to the different languages/dialects and cultures.

Most had digestive issues. When researchers recreated their bodies through forensic science, which is 90% accurate, they found evidence in the visceral organs that people in that time period had three-foot-long tapeworms in their stomachs. They also found degenerative viruses and substantial dental problems. European cultures had an especially rough time. Bodies from Egyptian, Central, and South American cultures have been found with most of their teeth with minimal dental decay. Obviously whatever food and drink they consumed gave them the necessary Calcium and Vitamin D to maintain their bone structure and density.

DNA is important to body systems; you can tell so much about a person from one little cellular structure, and that can recreate all the others. The bodies of human beings are a hologram; each cell or pixel in a hologram contains the whole picture. This is why you can take one cell and recreate the whole body.

One day, you will be able to put live cells in an inkjet printer to duplicate them. Scientists already know how to open up DNA strands for regeneration or continuation, so any organ or limb can be regenerated completely. If someone loses an arm they can go to the cells of the injury and begin the regeneration program so it can grow again. Remember, the sympathetic system is still there. Think of phantom limbs.

In Kirlian photography, if you cut a leaf in half, the whole leaf still appears on the photograph, the pattern remains. You cannot separate the energy pattern from the mind-pattern of the body. So, no matter what you lose or damage, it can be regenerated because the pattern is still there, always. Even when you look energetically at a person who is missing an organ, the organ still shows energetically, even if the physical organ itself is removed.

# Part II

# Health Conditions & Treatments

## GENERAL STATEMENT

Not all specific health issues can be listed due to the massive volume of health concerns. Knowing the mind-pattern of the body part gives you a place to begin decoding your specific issues.

In addition, if the issue is on the left side of the body, the mind-pattern involves a female (which may include you if you are female), logic, and physical reality.

If the issue is on the right side of the body, the mind-pattern involves a male (which may include you if you are male), emotions, spirituality, and nonphysical reality.

Begin all Visualizations by first balancing your T-Bar; end all Visualizations by surrounding the body in Brown to seal and bring the healing into the present.

Vitamin and supplement dosages vary depending upon each person's unique configuration. Some people may need more; some people may need less. In all cases, stay away from soy, microwaved food, processed food, and refined sugars. For any hormone level, only saliva testing is accurate.

All far-infrared treatments must begin with minimal time in the sauna and at low heat. Every other day, increase the time by two minutes. Every other day, increase the temperature by two degrees until you reach a maximum of 30 minutes per session.

Please also refer to ***Healer's Handbook*** for specific health visualizations and meditations as well as ***Template of God-Mind; King Bee, Queen Bee; Healing Archetypes & Symbols; Hyperspace Plus***; and ***Hyperspace Helper***.

In all cases, affirmations may be applied to all illnesses and diseases to correct, balance, and reverse them. Use ***1099 Daily Affirmations for Self-Change*** as your beginning point as well as ***Decoding Your Life***.

Regardless of your course of treatment, always remember that all healing begins in the Mind. Everything else is a boost to your mind-pattern.

As a reminder, this book is not intended to diagnose, treat, or cure any illness or disease. The information contained herein is a result of decades of Hyperspace/Oversoul research and the testimonials of thousands of clients.

## Medical Disclaimer

The information provided in this publication is not an attempt to practice medicine or provide specific medical advice, nor is it a substitute for medical care.

We always recommend consulting with a healthcare professional before starting any diet, exercise, supplementation, or medication program.

You assume full responsibility for using any information provided and agree that we are not responsible or liable for any claim resulting from its use by you or any user.

## ACID REFLUX

### Mind-pattern

*I learned something but I am not keeping it; here it comes back.
I am not holding that information in me.*

### Treatment

- Medium Green in the esophagus, surrounded by Ice Blue
- Organic aloe vera juice (100 ml 3x/day)
- 1000 mg each of berberine and turmeric

## ACNE

### Mind-pattern

*I am not a good person.
I have a lot of bad things I am showing you.
I feel dirty in what I face in the world.*

### Treatment

- Visualize clear skin, then mentally surround in Brown
- Silver on skin surface where acne is located
- Turmeric cream and/or Solomon's Seal Deep Penetration Salve
- Organic castor oil at night
- Olive Gold Dental during the day
- Sea salt bath with contact to face
- Stay hydrated with distilled water, may add organic lemon/lime juice
- Aloe vera juice or take aloe vera capsules

## ADD (Attention Deficit Disorder)

### Mind-pattern

*I am overloaded with programming.*
*I am cycling through my alters.*

### Treatment

- Brown Merger/Self-Reintegration Archetype at the Pineal Gland and Reptilian Brainstem
- T-Bar balanced and/or Pineal Gland Archetype
- Silver Infinity Archetype above the Crown Chakra
- Basic deprogramming techniques
- Surround Self in Brown
- Sea salt baths
- Hyperbaric chamber
- Vision Therapy; www.wowvision.net to find a recommended provider in your area

## ADDICTION, ALCOHOL

### Mind-pattern

*I am trying to blot out or divert my attention from my reality so I do not have to deal with it.*

### Treatment

- Golden Altar, Child Within, Green Spiral Staircase to determine where the issues began
- Oversoul work
- Deprogramming
- Methylene Blue Plus
- Steam-distilled water
- Sea salt baths

## ADDICTION, DRUG

### Mind-pattern

*There is something about my reality that I want to blot out; there is something in my life or past that I do not want to deal with or remember.*

### Treatment

- Golden Altar, Child Within, Green Spiral Staircase to determine where the issues began
- Oversoul work
- Deprogramming
- Methylene Blue Plus
- Steam-distilled water
- Sea salt baths

## ADDICTION, SUGAR

(may be due to hormonal imbalance, parasites, and/or your system lacks sugar)

### Mind-pattern

*I am trying to fill mental/emotional holes with sweetness.*

### Treatment

- Golden Altar, Child Within, Oversoul Release work
- Stop all sugar, replace with limited amounts of organic raw honey
- Alpha Lipoic Acid (500 mg/day)
- 1 teaspoon of raw organic cinnamon to regulate blood sugar levels
- L-Carnitine, up to 1000 mg per day

## ADENOIDS (Pharyngeal Tonsils)

### Mind-pattern

*I filter and monitor what I have already expressed.*

### Treatment

- Royal Blue in area
- Violet vacuum to clear out the organ

## ADHD (Attention Deficit Hyperactivity Disorder)

### Mind-pattern

*I died suddenly in my last linear lifeline and did not complete my goals.*

*I came back immediately and I am frustrated.*

### Treatment

- Talk to the child like an adult
- Green Spiral Staircase Visualization before in mother's womb
- Self surrounded in Brown
- High protein diet
- No refined sugars, maintain a low carb diet
- Minimize dairy
- Hyperbaric oxygen chamber
- Vision Therapy; www.wowvision.net to find a recommended provider in your area

## ADRENAL GLANDS

### Mind-pattern

*My ability to cope with all life experiences.*

## ADRENAL GLANDS, FAILURE IN FEMALES
(due to production cessation of specific uterine hormones)

### Mind-pattern

*My creative support and development has stopped; I cannot cope with my life experiences.*

### Treatment

- Refer to UTERINE Treatment

## ADRENAL GLANDS, FAILURE
(involving Thyroid and Larynx, sometimes Kidneys)

### Mind-pattern

*I cannot speak about how I feel.*

### Treatment

- Pale Yellow in Solar Plexus Chakra Band
- Adrenal Support Formula
- Vitamin C, large doses daily

## AGORAPHOBIA

### Mind-pattern

*I am afraid of the outside world.*

### Treatment

- Green Spiral Staircase Visualization to identify where/when this issue began
- Oversoul release, Brown X negative mind-patterns, Brown Shelf
- Visualization Color Therapy
- Visualize a layer of Maroon around body, then a layer of Pale Red
- Depending upon the severity, you can then layer with Violet, then Silver, then Gold
- Valerian root and/or kava kava Root to calm

## ALLERGIES, DAIRY

### Mind-pattern

*I reject nurturing.*

## ALLERGIES, NATURE

### Mind-pattern

*This is my punishment for lifelines where I abuse Nature.*

## ALLERGIES, POLLEN

### Mind-pattern

*I am irritated with the world; what I see bothers me.*

## ALLERGIES, SEAFOOD

### Mind-pattern

*I reject the spiritual side of life.*

## ALLERGIES, WHEAT

### Mind-pattern

*I reject life.*

### Treatment/All Allergies

- Mentally flush affected area with Medium Green followed by flushing with Violet.
- Merge with alternative selves that have no allergies (as in **Hyperspace Helper** book).
- Identify your specific allergy, then release up to your Oversoul.
- Mentally place Ice Blue over/in any irritated area
- Keep Violet around your body to filter out any airborne allergens.
- Local organic honey
- Quercetin (enzyme that blocks histamine) all year
- Peppermint essential oil via nostrils as needed
- Organic castor oil on/around affected areas.

## ACQUIRED IMMUNE DEFICIENCY SYNDROME/HUMAN IMMUNODEFICIENCY (AIDS/HIV)

### Mind-pattern

*I have sexual guilt and sexual anger.*

### Treatment

- Identify and release guilt regarding past sexual activity
- Flush body in Violet
- Flush body in Medium Green
- Methylene Blue Plus or MMS
- Food grade hydrogen peroxide in bath
- Far-infrared sauna treatments (build up to 30 minutes every day)
- Thymus glandulars to boost T cells
- 2-3 Liters of steam-distilled water daily
- Vitamin C IV treatments of 40,000+ mg 2x weekly

## ALZHEIMER'S DISEASE

### Mind-pattern

*I see something I used in the past, but now I do not know what it is.*

*I disassociate from my life.*

*I am worried about death, afterlife judgment, and/or leaving someone behind.*

### Treatment

- Flush brain with Violet
- Hold Royal Blue in brain
- Vitamin C, large doses/day
- Vitamin K2, up to 200 mcg/day
- Shankhapushpi powder, ½ teaspoon up to 3x/day
- Methylene Blue Plus
- Gingko biloba (only effective before Alzheimer's Disease sets in heavily)
- Micro-current treatments on the head, such as Jade Machine
- Chelation therapy
- Hyperbaric chamber treatments
- Far-infrared treatments; build up slowly

## AMPUTATION

### Mind-pattern

*I do not have the support of (what organ or limb was removed).*

## ANOREXIA

### Mind-pattern

*I am trying to make my Self disappear; I feel "less than" and I am trying to Self-destruct. I am trying to slowly commit suicide.*

### Treatment

- Identify why the individual wants to disappear
- Green Spiral Staircase Visualization to identify points of trauma
- Oversoul and Golden Altar Release work
- Child Within Visualization
- Basic Deprogramming
- Surround person with Pale Pink then a layer of Brown to seal it in
- Keep Silver Infinity over Crown Chakra
- Visualize Pale Yellow in Solar Plexus area to help retain what they are digesting
- Eat proteins, good fats (nuts, organic butter, cheese)

## APPENDIX

### Mind-pattern

*I have a need to purge ancient genetic past.*

## APPENDIX, RUPTURED, INFECTED

### Mind-pattern

*The information I learned about my ancient genetic past is hurtful to me.*

*I cannot process the information.*

### Treatment/Infected

- Flush with Violet, then put Pale Yellow into the area
- Chaga mushroom tablets (500 mg 2x/day)
- If time, take massive doses of Vitamin C
- Seek immediate medical attention

## ARRTHYTHMIA

### (Disruption of myelin sheathing)

### Mind-pattern

*I am fearful of things in life, especially my emotions.*

### Treatment

- Visualize the arrhythmia at the Pineal Gland. Slow it down to normal rate. Set the normal rate in Medium Green. Surround in Brown. Push a "Set" button to hold it.
- Omega-3 fish oil (3000 mg/day) depending upon person's weight
- Organic virgin coconut oil (1 to 3 tablespoons per day)
- Nattokinase 200-500 mg/day (organic blood thinner) to replace blood thinners

## ARTERIES, ARTERITIS

### Mind-Pattern

*I am irritated in the pathways and methods that try to bring me happiness.*

## ARTERIES, PLAQUE

### Mind-pattern

*I insulate and protect my Self from life.*

### Treatment

- Flush the arteries and veins with Purple to pull the plaque out of the body.
- Odorless garlic scrubs the arteries and keeps them clean
- Visualize arteries in perfect condition. Surround in Brown.
- 1 scoop minimum per day of ProArgi9 to open arteries and normalize arterial wall. ProArgi9 produces Nitric Oxide, which prevents cholesterol plaque.
- Myrrh gum (300 mg/day)
- Organic blueberry and/or black cherry juice to normalize arterial wall
- CoQ10 (300 mg/day) to help regenerate cellular structure
- Vitamin K2 (100 mcg/day)

## ARTHRITIS

### Mind-pattern

*I feel hurt by my support structures in life.*

## ARTHRITIS, RHEUMATOID

### Mind-pattern

*I am hurt by my support structures in my life.*

*I feel my support structure in my life is out of control and not helping me.*

### Treatment

- Visualize Shiny Copper in your bones for a minimum of 45 seconds per day, 2-3 times per day. Use a Shiny Copper penny as a visual aid if needed.
- Visualize Ice Blue over Shiny Copper to remove pain and inflammation
- Use this affirmation:
   *I now feel totally supported in every area in my life.*
- 1500 mg calcium + 3000 IU of Vitamin D
- Far-infrared sauna
- Jade Machine treatments
- Organic collagen ointment over area affected

## ASTHMA

### Mind-pattern

*I am emotionally overwhelmed by a parent.*

## ASTHMA, REACTIVE

### Mind-pattern

*There is an emotional coldness, isolation or distance that takes my breath away. I had a sudden emotional trauma event. I cannot catch my breath when I am reminded of this event.*

## ASTHMA, SPORTS INDUCED

### Mind-pattern

*I feel emotionally stressed by someone pressuring me to achieve something I cannot.*

### Treatment

- Use the Green Spiral Staircase to identify when you felt warm and happy emotionally, then what made you feel cold and took your breath away? Usually this is a parent of the opposite sex.
- Release work on any person you find, such as Oversoul or Golden Altar
- Infuse Medium Green into both lungs
- Breathe in sea salt baths or sea salt ocean air.
- Rye grass extract (20 drops under tongue once a day) oralmat.com
- Liquid oxygen may help

## AUTISM

### Mind-pattern

*I have a Dolphin Mind in a Human Body.*

### Treatment

- Use Dolphin Archetype to connect person to Dolphins using a Royal Blue Frequency line
- Refer to **Healer's Handbook** for more detailed information
- Surround person with Brown when agitated
- Keep water around person, such as a fish tank
- Keep ocean sounds around person
- Sea salt baths
- Hyperbaric chambers
- Vision therapy www.wowvision.net to find a reputable one in your area

## BACK, LOWER, PAIN

### Mind-pattern

*I feel pressured by my creative abilities in life.*
*My creativity and/or children are hurting me.*

*I have concerns about material and financial things.*

### Treatment

- Visualize Shiny Copper in the area of discomfort. Hold for a minimum of 45 seconds. Surround the area in Ice Blue for pain.
- Determine underlying issues
- Myrrh gum capsules to reduce swelling
- Arnica
- Coconut oil (1 tbsp daily) and North Atlantic fish oil (2000-5000 mg/day) if discs are fading
- Organic peanut oil topically on area to feed cells for regeneration
- Lie on flat surface, bring knees to chest, pulling knees toward body with arms

## BALDNESS

### Mind-pattern

*I feel I am losing my person strength.*
*I feel stress, tense, and like I am being put down.*

### Treatment

- Visualize Violet on scalp
- Visualize Power Archetype in Violet on the scalp
- Merge Self with other Simultaneous Existences where you have hair
- Eat heavy proteins
- Folic Acid (400-800 mcg/day)
- Biotin (400 mg/day)
- Rub Jojoba oil on scalp daily and/or use Jojoba shampoo
- Cayenne paste on scalp and leave for 20-30 minutes then wash off
- Shampoo of egg yolks
- Light coating of organic castor oil on scalp, adding in cedar wood, lemongrass or lavender essential oils

## BARETT SYNDROME

### Mind-pattern

*I reject what I need to learn. I am angry at the outer world.*
*I do not feel in control of my environment.*

### Treatment

- Green Spiral Staircase Visualization to determine why the person is so angry. Use this affirmation daily:

*I now accept my daily experiences; I am able to handle all my daily experiences to help negate these mind-patterns.*

## BIPOLAR DISORDER

### Mind-pattern

*I flip flop between left and right hemisphere of my brain.*
*My logic and emotions are not balanced.*

### Treatment

- Balance T-Bar at Pineal Gland or use the Pineal Gland Archetype
- Visualization: Center at Pineal Gland. See a hallway with doorways on either side representing left and right brain. Enter first one side and then the other, each time taking a statue or symbol into the hallway. This helps to balance the mind-pattern and thoughts.
- Add a middle name or initial that is culturally appropriate if the person does not have a middle name.
- Flush brain in Royal Blue
- Put legs and feet in Brown for grounding
- Eat heavier proteins for grounding
- Physical exercises to stimulate the left brain
- Pineal gland or pituitary glandulars
- Breathe in sea salt baths or ocean air to help open the mind
- Frankincense oil to energize the pineal gland
- St. John's Wort to stimulate the brain and bring forward suppressed issues
- Use treatment for Myelin Sheath Deficiency
- Kava kava to relax, calm, and balance
- Valerian root to calm and relax

## BED-WETTING

### Mind-pattern

*I am angry at my parents (usually the father).*

### Treatment
- Release issues related to father

## BLADDER, URINARY TRACT

### Mind-pattern

*I am releasing anger.*

## BLADDER, URINARY TRACT BLOCKAGE

### Mind-pattern

*I refuse to release my anger.*

## BLADDER, URINARY TRACT INFECTION

(The darker the urine the angrier the person)

### Mind-pattern

*I am angry about being angry.*

### Treatment/All Bladder Issues
- Send up all anger issues to Oversoul
- Do release work on the people who made you angry
- Grow Up Angry Child Within
- Flush bladder first with Violet, then fill with Pale Orange
- Eat organic watermelon, hydrangea root, and uva ursi
- Cranberry capsules, organic cranberry juice, steam-distilled water

## BLOATING, HORMONAL

### Mind-pattern

*I am fearful about creative issues so I insulate against this.*

## BLOATING, INDIGESTION

### Mind-pattern

*I have fear about what I am learning so I insulate against it.*

### Treatment

- Maca Root (500 mg/day)
- Forskohlii root extract (250 mg/day)
- L-Theanine (100 mg/day)
- Boron (10 mg/day)
- Males only add:
  - Zinc (50 mg 2x/day)
  - Tribulus (750 mg/day)

## BLOOD

### Mind-pattern

*The flow of happiness and joy in life.*

## BLOOD, ANEMIA

### Mind-pattern

*I refuse to accept the power in my flow of life.*

### Treatment

- Visualize Medium Green in circulation system
- Visualize Pale Red Archetype in Heart Chakra Band
- Use Setting the Dial Visualization in **Healer's Handbook** to set the Dial to Normal Red Blood Cell Count
- Betaine HCL (600 mg/day)
- Organic Chlorella (500 mg/day)
- 1 cup coconut water
- Methylene Blue Plus
- Increase organic red meats, liver, shellfish, eggs, dark leafy greens

## BLOOD, CLOTS

### Mind-pattern

*Something is blocking my happiness*

### Treatment

- Visualize Violet arrows in bloodstream piercing clots followed by Violet vacuum sucking out the clots
- Vitamin K2 (200 mcg/day)
- Vitamin D (5000 IU/day minimum)
- Red yeast rice (1000 mg/day until clot is dissolved)
- Niacin (100 mg/day minimum, increase slowly every couple of days until you feel a Niacin Flush, then stop the niacin)
- Far-infrared sauna
- Micro-current treatments like Jade Machine

# BLOOD, CHOLESTEROL/PLAQUE

### Mind-pattern

*I need to protect myself in life.*

### Treatment

- Purple to flush the arteries to dissolve cholesterol/plaque
- Using the Color Code of Purple to flush the arteries also dissolves cholesterol/plaque.
- Vitamin B-3/Niacin. Begin with 100 mg of niacin for two weeks. If you do not have a flush, increase to 200 mg. As soon as you experience the flush, stop taking the niacin.
- Niacin loosens the cholesterol/plaque from your arterial walls, literally allowing it to slide out of the veins and the arteries. When you feel a niacin flush, this is the sensation you get when the cholesterol/plaque slides out of your circulatory system. This is why you must stop taking the niacin, or the vascular walls may collapse.
- Once this happens, replace the niacin with odorless garlic, which scrubs the arteries, helping to keep them clean and clear.
- Cayenne pepper helps to remove cholesterol/plaque
- Calcium and Vitamin D pull cholesterol/plaque out of the system and build your skeletal structure at the same time.
- Red wine, preferably Pinot Noir, because it has the highest capacity to reduce cholesterol/plaque

## BLOOD PRESSURE

### Mind-pattern

*I feel constantly pressured in my life.*

### Treatment

- Use the Set the Dial visualization putting "Low, Normal High" on the dial. Set the dial to "Normal" because everyone's normal is different
- Red yeast rice
- Garlic
- Red wine, preferably Pinot Noir because it has the highest capacity to reduce cholesterol/plaque
- Eat wild rice

## BRAIN, SHRINKAGE

### Mind-pattern

*I am losing my mind.*

### Treatment

- Royal Blue in Brain
- Increase fat consumption
- Hyperbaric chamber treatments
- Live cells

## BREASTS, FEMALE

### Mind-pattern

*My ability to Self-nurture and nurture others.*

## BUNIONS

### Mind-pattern

*I am not focusing properly on my future support structures.*

### Treatment

- Visualize the bone in its correct shape to reshape it. Mentally hold the correct shape in Shiny Copper. Surround it in Ice Blue to reduce pain.

## BROKEN BONE

### Mind-pattern

*I feel that there is damage to a support structure in my life.*

## CANCER

### Mind-pattern

*I have held resentment over a long period of time.*

### Treatment

- All cancer treatments have the same basics and are listed at the end of the "CANCER" section, with Additional Treatments listed for specific Cancers.

## CANCER, ADRENAL

### Mind-pattern

*I resent the stress and tensions in my life.*

### Additional Treatment

- Berberine

## CANCER, ANAL

(more intense level than Colorectal Cancer)

**Mind-pattern**

*I resent the past and refuse to let the past go.*

## CANCER, ANAL WARTS

**Mind-pattern**

*I am willing to let go of some things, but I am still holding on to other things that I resent.*

## CANCER, BASAL CELL CARCINOMA (BCC); SQUAMOUS CELL CARCINOMA (SCC)

**Mind-pattern**

*I resent the issues right in front of me that everyone has to see; I am embarrassed by what I show the world.*

## CANCER, BILE DUCT

**Mind-pattern**

*I resent the harsh/bitter overtones/undertones in my life.*

## CANCER, BLADDER

**Mind-pattern**

*I resent that I am angry and hurt. I resent that these feelings do not go away.*

## CANCER, BONE

**Mind-pattern**

*I resent my support structure in life.*

## CANCER, BONE, ARM

**Mind-pattern**

*I resent my current support structure in life.*

## CANCER, BONE, LEGS

**Mind-pattern**

*I resent my future support structure in life.*

## CANCER, BONE, RIBCAGE

**Mind-pattern**

*I resent how I protect my emotions.*

## CANCER, BRAIN

**Mind-pattern**

*I resentfully think negatively on a specific topic or issue; I resent my own thoughts.*

## CANCER, BRAIN, LEFT

**Mind-pattern**

*I resentfully think about physical reality, females, and/or logic.*

## CANCER, BRAIN, RIGHT

**Mind-pattern**

*I resentfully think about spirituality, males, and/or emotions.*

## CANCER, BREAST

**Mind-pattern**

*I resent that my nurturing ability is rejected and/or suppressed.*

## CANCER, BREAST, MALE

**Mind-pattern**

*I resent that I am not receiving nurturing from others.*

## CANCER, BREAST, NIPPLE

**Mind-pattern**

*I resent that I cannot nurture anyone.*

## CANCER, CERVICAL

**Mind-pattern**

*I resent the result of my creative abilities; what I try to create never comes out the way I want.*

## CANCER, COLON

**Mind-pattern**

*I resent my past experiences; I do not want to release my past experiences because I am angry about them and I cannot deal with them.*

## CANCER, COLORECTAL

**Mind-pattern**

*I resent and regret what I have not yet released and/or what I have released too much of; this is the result of not letting go; a part of me enjoys my suffering and pain.*

## CANCER, ESOPHAGEAL

**Mind-pattern**

*I resent the process by which I get my learning experiences.*

## CANCER, GALLBLADDER

**Mind-pattern**

*I resent my bitter/nasty experiences in life.*

## CANCER, INTESTINE, SMALL

**Mind-pattern**

*I resent the process of what I had to go through to learn.*

## CANCER, KIDNEY

**Mind-pattern**

*I resent my past experiences that I have not processed and am stuck in the past.*

## CANCER, LARYNGEAL

### Mind-pattern

*I resent not speaking up for my Self;*
*I resent holding in what I needed to say.*

## CANCER, LEUKEMIA

### Mind-pattern

*I resent that I am unhappy with my whole life.*

## CANCER, LIVER

### Mind-pattern

*I resent my repetitive current experiences and cannot process them.*
*I am unhappy and resentful of my life experiences.*

### Additional Treatment

- Flush and cleanse the liver with milk thistle, dandelion root, apple cider vinegar, and lemon water
- Bitter greens
- Liver glandulars
- Strong black coffee without any sugar or dairy. Sweeten with stevia if necessary.
- Gentle colonics with or without coffee

## CANCER, LUNG

### Mind-pattern

*I resent my emotional interactions with others and my environment; I resent my incorrect expressions of emotions by holding back what I need to emotionally share.*

### Additional Treatment

- Berberine, hyssop, and marshmallow herb
- Inhale sea salt from ocean air or sea salt baths

## CANCER, LYMPHOMA, AXILLA

### Mind-pattern

*I resent the negativity that I have hidden that has hurt others in the past.*

## CANCER, LYMPHOMA, GROIN

### Mind-pattern

*I resent my sexual actions.*

## CANCER, LYMPHOMA, NECK

### Mind-pattern

*I resent the collateral damage of my verbalizations. I resent that my past words hurt others.*

## CANCER, OROPHARYNGEAL

### Mind-pattern

*I resent my words and verbalizations as well as the effect of what I have said.*

## CANCER, OVARIAN

### Mind-pattern

*I resent not being able to creatively and productively express in my life.*

### Additional Treatment

- Increase the progesterone to exceed the estrogen levels by taking wild yam root, homeopathic progesterone, and ovarian glandulars until the condition improves.

## CANCER, PANCREATIC

### Mind-pattern

*I resent my inability to have happiness in life.*

## CANCER, PROSTATE

### (equivalent to Ovarian Cancer in Women)

### Mind-pattern

*I resent that I am no longer creative or productive in my life.*

### Additional Treatment

- Pumpkin seeds, saw palmetto, and eleuthero root/Siberian ginseng.

## CANCER, SALIVARY GLAND

### Mind-pattern

*I resent initial information that I need to understand.*

## CANCER, SARCOMA

### Mind-pattern

*I resent my personal strength in life; I feel weak or that I have overpowered others.*

## CANCER, SKIN/MELANOMA

### Mind-pattern

*I resent what I show the world about my Self.*

## CANCER, SKIN/MELANOMA, BACK

### Mind-pattern

*I resent my support structure and what I have shown the world in my past.*

### Additional Treatment/All Skin Cancers

- Topically apply tea tree oil followed by castor oil
- Elicina cream from Chile, which is snail residue http://elicina.us/
- Solomon's seal deep penetrating cream www.expansions.com
- Organic Vitamin C cream
- Calendula ointment

## CANCER, STOMACH

### Mind-pattern

*I resent what I have learned in life.*

### Additional Treatment

- Oil of oregano and olive leaf

## CANCER, TESTICULAR

### Mind-pattern

*I resent my creative abilities.
My creative abilities have not met my expectations.*

## CANCER, THYMOMA

**Mind-pattern**

*I resent being vulnerable in the world*

## CANCER, THYROID

**Mind-pattern**

*I resent the verbalizations and how I communicated that hurt others.*

## CANCER, TONGUE

**Mind-pattern**

*I resent what I held back from saying.*

## CANCER, UTERINE

**Mind-pattern**

*I resent my creative abilities as well as the products of my creations.*

## Treatment/All Cancers

- Do Golden Altar and Hyperspace/Oversoul Release work on resentment
- Mentally flush the area with Violet
- Visualize Violet vacuum hose to remove physical debris and cancer cells, and then put proper chakra color in that area of the body. Finally, surround the entire body in Brown to hold the healing work.
- Then, flush the area with Medium Green to oxygenate the areas because cancer is an anaerobic cell that cannot survive in oxygen.
- Mentally do Hyperspace surgery by visualizing a Royal Blue laser device that emits a Pale Red laser beam to dissolve tumors.
- Use the Overall Healing Archetype in that area of the body or in/over tumors.
- Use the Silver Oversoul Archetype in/over that area because Silver purifies.
- COQ10, hyssop herb, Pau d'Arco, Chapparell, turmeric, shark cartilage, berberine
- High doses of Vitamin C, IV treatments are best, but powdered Vitamin C is okay
- Ojibwa/Esiak/Essiac tea or extract
- Comfrey herb (3 teaspoons/day)
- Herbal Chelation
- Methylene Blue Plus
- Modifilan (start at two and work up to eight capsules/day until cancer is gone unless you have amalgam teeth fillings or metal implants in your body as Modifilan pulls metal out)
- Add liquid oxygen to steam-distilled water
- Ozone/hyperbaric treatments if possible
- Far-infrared sauna

## CARTILAGE, DAMAGED

### Mind-pattern

*My structural support system is weak.*

### Treatment

- Use this affirmation:
  *I now strengthen the connections to my body.*
- Visualize it in Shiny Copper because it is soft tissue, therefore similar to bone.
- Calcium with Vitamin D

## CELLULITE

### Mind-pattern

*I have some deep fears I will not release.*

## CELLULITE, ABDOMEN/STOMACH

### Mind-pattern

*I am anxious and worrying about what I am learning, digesting, and assimilating.*

## CELLULITE, BUTTOCKS

### Mind-pattern

*I carry the weight of my past with me.*

## CELLULITE, HIPS

*I always feel out of balance, especially with thoughts of my future.*

## CELLULITE, THIGHS

### Mind-pattern

*I have childhood trauma and abuse issues that I carry with me.*

### Treatment/All Cellulite

- Release work
- Visualize Violet vacuum hosing out the cellulite
- Steam-distilled water fast one day each week and three days every three months to help rid body of toxins

## CHICKEN POX/MEASLES

### Mind-pattern

*I feel irritated, weak, and vulnerable in an adult world.*

### Treatment

- Flush the body with Ice Blue and Violet
- Chaga mushrooms capsules 2x/day
- Immuplex and Congaplex
- Methylene Blue
- As much Vitamin C powder as possible until diarrhea occurs, then back the dosage down
- One drop of frankincense oil under tongue 1x/day
- Calendula cream and Solomon's seal salve
- Dead Sea salt baths 2x/day, 20 minutes each
- Steam-distilled water

## CHRONIC FATIGUE SYNDROME/ EPSTEIN BARR

### Mind-pattern

*I am tired of life; I am tired of what I feel.*

### Treatment

- Release mind-pattern of low Self-worth, Self-punishment, Self-sabotage
- Visualize Pale Red through the body, followed by Medium Green, followed by Violet
- Visualize Pale Red Archetype throughout the body
- B-Complex
- Alpha lipoic acid (1000 mg/day)
- Taurine (1000 mg/day)
- Coconut oil (2000-4000 mg/day)
- High protein organic diet
- Far-infrared sauna

## CHRONIC OBSTRUCTIVE PULMONARY DISEASE (COPD)

### Mind-pattern

*I have overwhelming emotional fear; fear takes my breath away.*

### Treatment

- Flush lungs with Medium Green
- Lung glandulars
- Marshmallow herb: 1000 mg/day (fortifies alveoli and lining of lungs)
- Deep breathe in sea salt air

## CIRCULATION, POOR

### Mind-pattern

*I do not receive any zest out of life;
I need something to perk me up.*

*I do not allow joy and happiness to circulate through my life.*

### Treatment

- Visualize Medium Green in Heart Chakra Band with Pale Red Archetype over the heart
- Visualize Purple flushing through veins and arteries
- Hawthorne berry herb, folic acid, organic Vitamin E, organic coconut oil, Cardiotrophin PMG, Vitamin K2
- Low impact aerobic exercises, 3-5 days/week, minimum 15 minutes each, work up to 30-45 minutes

## CLEFT PALATE

### Mind-pattern

*I am not able to communicate properly and I am not able to adjust to my life.*

### Treatment

- Surgery

## COLDS, FREQUENT

### Mind-pattern

*I am aimless about what I want to do/accomplish in life; I have a need to reset and receive attention.*

### Treatment

- Flush body with Medium Green and then Violet
- Vitamin C powder (5000-6000 mg/day if diarrhea, back dosage down)
- Immuplex and Congaplex
- Echinacea, Goldenseal
- Apply organic castor oil over sinuses
- Steam-distilled water
- Sea salt baths
- Far-infrared sauna

## COLITIS, ULCERATIVE

### Mind-pattern

*I do not want to accept, hold onto, or assimilate my experiences.*

### Treatment

- Use this affirmation to reverse the condition:
  *I now accept all that I learn about myself and others.*
- Visualize Pale Yellow in intestinal system for easier absorption while intestines heal
- Seal with Violet so everything eaten passes through the protected lining
- Tienchi tea or as pills or tablets

## COLON

### Mind-pattern

*My ability to release unnecessary past experiences.*

## COLON, CONSTIPATION

### Mind-pattern

*I unnecessarily hold onto the past and allow the past to hurt me; I spend too much time analyzing my past without any action. I am afraid of losing my past.*

### Treatment

- Push Violet through entire colon
- Use Violet vacuum to hose out the colon
- Place Pale Yellow in Solar Plexus Chakra Band
- Place Pale Orange in Sacral Chakra Band
- Fast with steam-distilled water, lemon and lime juice, sea salt
- Do a series of gentle colonics
- Aloe vera juice (100 ml 2x daily) to recondition digestive tract. Use daily for at least two weeks to long-term.
- Eat raw vegetables
- Olive leaf (330-900 mg/day) to reorganize environment of digestive system
- Oregano oil (300 mg/day) to kill bacteria or virus causing the backup
- Spicy food to stimulate metabolism
- Coconut oil (500-1000 mg/day)
- Vitamin C (3000-5000 mg/day, capsule or powder) as a temporary solution
- Chlorella (1 teaspoon/day)
- Castor oil (1 tbsp/day)
- Avoid foods with thick consistency like nuts, nut butters, and cheese

## COLON, LARGE INTESTINE

### Mind-pattern

*I am getting every opportunity to absorb and understand the main points of my experiences.*

## CRYING

### Mind-pattern

*I purge and cleanse what I see/experience in my life.*

## CYSTS

### Mind-pattern

*I am overwhelmed/adamant in a specific area of life (refer to where the cyst is located on/in the body).*

### Treatment

- Visualize Medium Red laser attacking the cyst, then vacuum up the debris with Violet hose
- Visualize pair of Violet scissors in right hand, then cut the cyst away
- Methylene Blue Plus
- Turmeric, berberine, black cumin seed oil
- Micro-current treatments such as Jade Machine
- Far-infrared sauna treatments

# DEMENTIA

## Mind-pattern

*I no longer feel a desire to interact with humanity;
I have fear of leaving the body/dying;
my mind has gone but I still am attached to the body.*

## Treatment

- Flush brain with Violet
- Then hold Royal Blue in brain
- Vitamin C, large doses/day
- Vitamin K2, up to 200 mcg/day
- Shankhapushpi powder, ½ teaspoon up to 3x/day
- Methylene Blue Plus
- Gingko Biloba (only effective before Alzheimer's Disease sets in heavily)
- Micro-current treatments on the head, such as Jade Machine
- Chelation therapy
- Hyperbaric chamber treatments
- Far-infrared treatments; build up slowly

## DEPRESSION

### Mind-pattern

*I am overwhelmed by my life;
I feel like I cannot accomplish my goals and the world is against me.*

### Treatment

- Release sad feelings into Oversoul
- Merge with alternate selves that are not sad/depressed
- Immerse Self in Pale Pink
- Golden Altar
- Do something that makes you happy every day
- Eat an organic diet
- Red wine with dinner
- St. John's Wort, valerian root, kava kava
- 

## DIABETES, TYPE I

### Mind-pattern

*I do not know how to generate happiness or make my Self happy;
I am unwilling to accept happiness.*

### Treatment

- Use the Dial Visualization from **Healer's Handbook** to set desired blood sugar number
- Determine underlying cause through extensive blood and urine tests
- Detox the body
- Build up the body
- High protein, low/slow carb diet
- Regular exercise

## DIABETES, TYPE II

### Mind-pattern

*I refuse to accept and keep any happiness that I create; I am unwilling to accept happiness, so I try to control and manipulate life to make my Self happy.*

### Treatment

- Use the Dial Visualization from **Healer's Handbook** to set desired blood sugar number
- Visualize Pale Yellow in Solar Plexus Chakra Band
- Eat high protein, low carb diet
- Organic cinnamon in the morning to regulate blood sugar
- Organic peppermint tea in the evening to increase insulin production
- Jerusalem artichokes every other day to help body absorb sugar
- Gymnema sylvestre to help body absorb blood sugar
- Insulin powder daily
- Live cell and stem cell therapy
- Pancreas glandulars
- L- Carnitine and Alpha Lipoic acid (500 mg/day)

## DIABETES, GESTATIONAL

### Mind-pattern

*I am not happy about being a mother.*

### Treatment

- Release the mind-pattern of why you are not happy about pregnancy
- Take insulin until pregnancy is over

## DISSOCIATIVE IDENTITY DISORDER (DID)

### Mind-pattern

*I have programming overload;
I am insecure in my own Self-identity.*

### Treatment

- Use Brown Merger Archetype to reintegrate personality
- Identify and release trauma
- Visualize Ice Blue, then Violet through body when traumatic memories resurface
- Eat heavy protein to ground in present moment
- Deprogramming

## DIGESTIVE ENZYMES, LACK OF

### Mind-pattern

*I no longer analyze or understand what I learn in life.*

### Treatment

- Flood digestive area with Pale Yellow
- Eat pineapple, papaya acidophilus, lemon, and lime
- Stomach exercises like crunches and leg-lifts to energize this area.

## DOWN SYNDROME
### (a lower-level species takes over the body)

### Mind-pattern

*I am a mismatch of human and alien genetics.*

### Treatment

- Visualize Royal Blue in brain
- Caregiver communicates with them using Dolphin Frequency Archetype, same as with Autism
- Caregiver visualizes Pineal Gland Archetype for Self and patient, and then connects both people with a Pale Yellow Frequency line to transmit and receive information.
- Royal Blue, Violet, Silver, and Gold
- Live cell treatments
- Hyperbaric chamber to enhance mental function

## DYSLEXIA
### (Crossover in corpus callosum is distorted. They perceive the nonphysical form of things; everything in physical reality is a mirror image of nonphysical reality)

### Mind-pattern

*I refuse to see the world logically.*

### Treatment

- Visualize a Royal Blue T-Bar Archetype in each eye
- Identify and release why they choose to rebel against everything
- Pick a letter or number. Mentally reverse it in the mind without looking at it. This teaches them to reverse what they are looking at.
- Wear Dark Red colored glasses
- Brain glandulars

## EARS/AUDITORY SYSTEM

**Mind-pattern**

*What I hear in my experiences.*

## EARACHE, CHILDREN

**Mind-pattern**

*I have an issue with one or both parents that I do not want to hear about any more.*

## EARS, CLOSED/DEAF

**Mind-pattern**

*I do not want to hear any more.*

## EAR, FLUID IN

**Mind-pattern**

*I feel emotionally overwhelmed by what I hear.*

## EARS, GROWING BIGGER

(with age)

**Mind-pattern**

*I want to hear more.*

## EAR, LEFT, PAIN

### Mind-pattern

*What I hear from a female figure or what I hear about my logical thoughts is hurtful to me.*

## EAR, RIGHT, PAIN

### Mind-pattern

*What I hear hurts me from a male figure or what I hear about my emotions or creativity is hurtful to me.*

## EAR, PIERCED

### Mind-pattern

*What I hear can pierce me or hurt me.*

### Treatment/All Ear Conditions
- Visualize Royal Blue in ears
- Identify what you do not want to hear and release them from mind-pattern
- Use 3% hydrogen peroxide in ear, followed by mullein oil in ear
- Use organic castor oil in ear at night

## EATING, DIRECTING ENERGY

### Mind-pattern

*I direct my body-intelligence to tell the food where to go.*

## EATING, DRINKING TOO MUCH LIQUID WHILE

### Mind-pattern

*I am diluting information, washing it out and getting rid of it because it is too much for me to absorb.*

## EATING, FALLING ASLEEP AFTER

### Mind-pattern

*I refuse to pay attention to what I am learning in life.*

## EATING, SPEED OF, FAST

### Mind-pattern

*I am trying to fill empty mental/emotional spaces without absorbing it.*

## EATING, SPEED OF, SECTION EATER

(eating one food at a time)

### Mind-pattern

*I am structured and focused; I am not a multitasking person; I finish one thing before I go on to the next.*

## EATING, SPEED OF, SLOW

### Mind-pattern

*I am trying to absorb, assimilate, and digest my mental and emotional food that I am learning in life.*

## ECZEMA/PSORIASIS

### Mind-pattern

*I have severe nervous agitation brought on by stress*

### Treatment

- Sea salt baths to bring the skin irritation to the surface.
- Castor oil to help the skin irritation heal.

## ENDOMETRIOSIS

### Mind-pattern

*I feel like my creative abilities go in the wrong direction; they are wild, serve no purpose, and are detrimental.*

### Treatment

- Use a Violet hose to vacuum out the excess material
- Visualize Pale Orange in the uterine area.
- Wild yam root, maca (after the estrogen comes down to normal levels)
- Blue cohosh in the early stages to purge the built up uterine lining
- 7-Keto DHEA (25 to 50 mg daily)
- Castor oil packs over the uterine area
- Do not eat soy, microwaved food, or preservatives/fillers

## ERECTILE DYSFUNCTION

### Mind-pattern

*I have fear of sex and creating; I have low Self-worth and feel that my power has been taken away from me.*

### Treatment

- Identify and release underlying issues
- Visualize Pale Red Male Erection Archetype in penis
- Outpicture erect penis in Pale Red
- Zinc (50 mg 2x daily)
- Tribulus (750 mg daily)
- Yohimbe (bark of a tree in Africa) 350 mg only before sexual activity; do not take for more than three days in a row to avoid toxic buildup in liver
- Horny goat weed (250 mg two days before sexual activity and that day)
- Siberian ginseng (1000 mg daily)
- Coca tea & yerba matte tea (vasodilators); 1 cup each per day
- ProArgi9 to clear out blood vessels
- Ashwaganda powder (½ tsp daily)
- Shilajit (300 mg daily)

## ESOPHAGUS

### Mind-pattern

*Allowing understanding of information to flow properly.*

## ESOPHAGUS, ACID REFLUX

### Mind-pattern

*I learned something but I am not keeping it;
I am not holding that information in me.*

## ESOPHAGUS, ACID REFLUX & SINUS ISSUES

### Mind-pattern

*I am not holding that information inside me. I see people and things that annoy and anger me, therefore I am getting mad at it.*

## ESOPHAGUS, BLOCKAGES

### Mind-pattern

*I reject what I am taking in; I do not want to understand it;
I want to get rid of it.*

## ESOPHAGUS, HIATIAL HERNIA

### Mind-pattern

*I do not want to understand this,
I am not even going to let it go this far.*

## ESOPHAGUS, INFLAMMATION/ ESOPHAGITIS

### Mind-pattern

*I have held resentment.*

## ESOPHAGUS, VOMITING

### Mind-pattern

*I am losing my recent happiness; I am blocking or getting rid of it.*

### Treatment/All Esophagus Issues

- Visualize Ice Blue in esophagus
- Organic aloe vera juice (100 ml to 300 ml daily)

## EYES

### Mind-pattern

*What I see and direct in my experience in physical reality.*

## EYES, CATARACTS

### Mind-pattern

*I no longer see things clearly in life.*

## EYES, FLOATERS

### Mind-pattern

*I tend to see things in life that should not be there.
I am easily distracted by what I see in life.*

## EYE, LEFT

### Mind-pattern

*My female issues, logic, and physical reality.*

## EYES, MACULAR DEGENERATION

**Mind-pattern**

*I do not want to see the whole picture in life situations.*

## EYE, RIGHT

**Mind-pattern**

*My male issues, emotions, and spirituality.*

## EYE, THIRD EYE/PINEAL GLAND

**Mind-pattern**

*What I see in nonphysical reality.*

## EYES, CROSSED

**Mind-pattern**

*I do not want to see anything that is in front of me; I am very troubled and traumatized.*

## EYES, FAR-SIGHTED

**Mind-pattern**

*I do not want to see what is around me right now. I want to go way out there.*

### Treatment/All Eye Issues

- Visualize Royal Blue in and around eyes daily for minimum of 33 seconds each time
- Bilberry herb, eyebright, lutein, and possibly eye glandulars

## FARET SYMDROME

### Mind-pattern

*I get agitated and hurt from what I start to learn in life.*

### Treatment

- Organic aloe vera juice daily
- Olive leaf, oregano oil and ginger tea

## FEET/LEGS

### Mind-pattern

*I am stepping into the future with my support structure.*

## FIBROID TUMORS

### Mind-pattern

*I create the wrong things in life for me:*
*I am afraid to make another version of myself.*

### Treatment

- Visualize Violet hose to vacuum out fibroids
- Royal Blue surgical knife to cut out tumor
- Pale Orange in the uterine area and then surround with Brown
- Vitamin D (2000-6000 IUs)
- Daily castor oil packs over uterine area
- Avoid soy and microwaved products
- Wild yam root and maca daily
- Shark cartilage

## FIBROMYALGIA

### (Caused by mycoplasmas)

### Mind-pattern

*I vibrate at a low frequency; my life pains me and everything hurts me.*

### Treatment
- Learn to vibrate at a higher frequency
- Violet, Silver, Gold, Medium Green
- Chaga mushroom capsules, 500 mg daily
- Olive leaf, 400 mg daily
- One drop of frankincense essential oil, 2x daily
- Far-infrared sauna

## FLUORIDE

### Mind-pattern

*I want to deaden/numb my brain.*

### Treatment
- Flush the body with Violet several times daily
- Organic tamarind in any form daily
- Sea salt baths often
- Modifilan tablets for 1-2 weeks
- Chelation therapy
- Far-infrared sauna

## GALLBLADDER

### Mind-pattern

*I feel bitterness in my life; I am bitter about my life.*

## GALLSTONES

### Mind-pattern

*I hold on to the bitterness in life.*

### Treatment

- Identify source of bitterness and release
- Visualize a Violet hose to vacuum out the stones
- Calcium and Vitamin D pull cholesterol/plaque out of the system as well as builds skeletal structure
- Flush gallbladder with Violet, and then visualize Pale Yellow in the gallbladder
- Vitamin D (4000 IU/day)
- Corn silk tea (3 cups/day for a few weeks) to strengthen gallbladder
- Bitter green leafy vegetables every day (spinach, kale, turnip greens, etc.)
- Castor oil on gallbladder area
- Gallbladder glandulars for two to four months

## GASTROESOPHAGEAL REFLEX DISEASE (GERD)

### Mind-pattern

*I reject what I learn in life.*

### Treatment

- Use same visualization as for gallbladder
- Aloe vera juice (100 ml 2x or more daily)
- Ginger capsules or tea
- Olive leaf (2 capsules/day)

## GENERALIZED ANXIETY DISORDER (GAD)

### Mind-pattern

*I have fear or trauma*

### Treatment

- Release the fear
- Maroon for courage
- Royal Blue to balance your brain
- Brown for grounding and balance
- Golden Altar and Child Within exercises to completion
- Valerian root (150 mg/day) to start, as it is the most mild
- If valerian root does not work, take kava kava (150 mg/day)
- If kava kava does not work, take St. John's Wort (200 mg/day)
- Omega-3 fish oil (1000-3000 mg/day) to build myelin sheathing
- Coconut oil (1000-4000 mg/day) to coat nerves and purge bloodstream and intestines
- B-Complex (1000 mg/day) to strengthen nerves
- Do low-impact exercise: walking, biking, swimming
- Take sea salt baths

## GENITALIA, MALE

### Mind-pattern

*My creative power and energy for physical and nonphysical.*

## GENITALIA, FEMALE

### Mind-pattern

*I am receiving energy for creative power for physical and nonphysical.*

## GOUT, LEFT SIDE

### Mind-pattern

*Female issues are irritating me in my support structure, which affects my future.*

## GOUT, RIGHT SIDE

### Mind-pattern

*Male issues are irritating me in my support structure, which affects my future.*

### Treatment/Both Sides

- Engulf area in Ice Blue and surround it in Brown
- Identify and correct the mind-pattern
- Golden Altar and Oversoul release work
- Move your center of consciousness from Pineal Gland to the gout location; observe what comes into your mind to understand the underlying mind-pattern
- Medium Green as a flush through the affected area daily to oxygenate
- B-Complex (1 capsule/day)
- Castor oil packs over digestive system
- Coconut oil (2000 to 4000 mg/day)

## GYNOPLASTIA

### Mind-pattern

*I am not nurtured by feminine energy; I will not let anyone in.*

### Treatment

- DHEA (25 mg/day)
- Sarsaparilla and nettles
- Weight training specifically for the chest.

## HASHIMOTO SYNDROME

### Mind-pattern

*I am attacking and trying to kill my own Self-expression; I am ashamed, embarrassed and fearful of saying what is inside of me.*

### Treatment

- Blue-green algae, kelp
- Thyroid glandulars
- Flush thyroid with Ice Blue
- Golden Altar and Oversoul Release work
- Learn to speak up tactfully and honestly

## HAIR LOSS

### Mind-pattern

*I no longer feel my personal strength or power.*

### Treatment

- Use topicals like jojoba oil, organic castor oil, yarrow and rosemary essential oils, cayenne pepper
- Massage scalp frequently

## HEART

### Mind-pattern

*My flowing joy and happiness in life.*

## HEART, AORTA, COLLAPSED

### Mind-pattern

*I have a broken heart; something deeply emotional hurts me.*

## HEART ATTACK

### Mind-pattern

*I am emotionally overwhelmed so I create a blockage in my heart to stop the flow of my emotions. I am stressed out by something that I do not want to deal with. I do not want to look at my Self. I want to blame others for causing my emotional distress and upheaval.*

### Treatment

- Golden Altar and Oversoul release work
- Oxygenate heart with Medium Green
- Visualize Violet around heart to protect it
- Visualize Medium Green and Violet all surrounded by Brown to seal in the healing and bring it into the present
- COQ10 (100 mg or more/day)
- Folic acid daily
- Vitamin E daily
- Hawthorne berry daily

## HEELS

### Mind-pattern

*I am vulnerable in the present, which affects the future.*

## HEMORRHOIDS

### Mind-pattern

*I do not want to release something that is painful from the past; the past hurts me.*

### Treatment

- Visualize a Royal Blue scalpel to remove them and then surround that area in Brown
- Flush them in Ice Blue to reduce swelling and help alleviate pain
- Put the inside of a banana peel on the area
- Castor oil on the area at night
- Organic blueberry juice (½ to 1 cup/day)
- Use Solomon's seal on the area
- Flush

## HIATIAL HERNIA

### Mind-pattern

*I do not want to understand something; I am not going to let anything I do not want to understand go very far.*

### Treatment

- Use same treatment as for Esophagus

## HERPES (virus)

### Mind-pattern

*I am hurt and angry about sexual unions; I am a bad person because of my sexual ideas and I need to be punished for my sexual thoughts and behavior.*

### Treatment

- Release the mind-pattern of shame around sexuality
- Golden Altar and Oversoul release work
- Hyssop
- Larreastat (made from cactus, may get worse as virus is pulled out of body but then will get better)
- For outbreaks use tea tree oil topically followed by castor oil
- Sea salt baths
- Far-infrared sauna
- Steam-distilled water
- Garlic

## HIPS

### Mind-pattern

*I am worried that I cannot move forward with balance into my future.*

# HORMONAL IMBALANCE

## Mind-pattern

*I do not feel creative in life.*

## Treatment

- Take a saliva test to determine estrogen levels
- Balance estrogen and progesterone ratio
- Maca root to balance estrogen with progesterone (400 mg/day)
- 7-Keto DHEA (25 to 50 mg daily) to start the process of creating needed hormones.

## Women

- Most women have high estrogen.
- Heavier women may have too much estrogen and no progesterone; may be under stress; many have been sexually abused.
- Thinner women may have no estrogen or progesterone
- The best source of progesterone for women is wild yam root.
- Black cohosh for extremely low estrogen levels
- Do not take ovarian glandulars
- Place warm castor oil packs over uterine area

## Men

- Heavy men may have higher estrogen.
- Thinner men may have low testosterone.
- With low testosterone levels, the precursors start converting to estrogen rather than testosterone in andropause.
- Zinc (50 mg/day)
- Tribulus (600 mg/day)

## Both Men and Women

- Avoid soy products because they increase estrogen
- Microwave creates estrogen compounds in foods
- Processed foods (preservatives, coloring, flavor enhancers) are estrogen based

## HUNTINGTON'S DISEASE

### Mind-pattern

*I no longer want to think or be in control of my life.*

### Treatment

- Visualize Royal Blue in the brain daily for 45 seconds or more
- Eat organic proteins daily
- Hyperbaric chamber treatments for 30 minutes 2x/week.
- Brain glandulars
- Stem cell treatments

## HYDROTHERAPY TREATMENT

- Helps move the body when it is in pain.
- Use cool to cold water to help increase mind function.
- Use warm to hot water to help increase body function.
- Good for spinal conditions to help take pressure off of the body.

## HYPERTENSION

### Mind-pattern

*I feel pressured in life; happiness is being squeezed out of me.*

### Treatment

- Visualize Ice Blue in the Heart Chakra Band, hold for 2-3 minutes, and then immediately replace with Medium Green
- Visualize a Blood Pressure Dial in Royal Blue with a button set to "Normal." Surround this with Brown
- ProArgi9 (1-3 scoops/day in coconut water/distilled water) to create nitric oxide in bloodstream to normalize circulatory system and reduce cholesterol
- 4-6 ounces daily organic blueberry juice
- Red wine, 1-2 glasses/day for resveratrol, preferably Pinot Noir
- 4-6 ounces daily organic black cherry juice
- Red yeast rice (300 mg/day) for 10-14 days at a time, then wait a month and repeat if necessary
- Taurine (500 mg/day), an enzyme that strengthens vascular system and reduces blood pressure
- L-Lysine (500 mg/day)
- 4-6 ounces of organic beet juice daily

## HYPOTHALAMUS

### Mind-pattern

*I cannot think of ways to regulate my life.*

### Treatment

- Use same treatment as for Huntington's Syndrome
- Add hypothalamus glandulars

## HYPERTHYROID

### Mind-pattern

*I have anger, hatred, and anxiety that I need to verbalize, but sometimes I hold it in. Sometimes I speak too much in a rude way.*

### Treatment

- Center consciousness at the thyroid to determine anger, hatred, and anxiety issues.
- Balance T-Bar
- Flush thyroid with Medium Green to neutralize Red energy
- Flush and hold thyroid in Ice Blue once Red energy is neutralized.
- Surround thyroid in Brown to hold the Ice Blue in place.
- Valerian root (200 mg/day)
- Castor oil on throat
- Do not eat seafood or sea salt
- Eat heavier proteins and fats until issue goes away.

## HYPERVENTILATING

### Mind-pattern

*I am always in fear and afraid of many situations.*

*I feel smothered, often by my overprotective mother.*

### Treatment

- Golden Altar release work, Child Within, Oversoul Communications, and possibly deprogramming exercises.

## HYPOTHYROIDISM

### Mind-pattern

*I am confused about what I should say, how to say it; I am confused about how to communicate.
I have bad relationships and jealousy issues.*

### Treatment

- Flush thyroid for a few seconds in Pale Red
- Then, put an Ice Blue Power Archetype over the thyroid
- Ice Blue T-Bar Archetype over the thyroid to balance it
- ¼ to ½ teaspoon sea salt 2x/day
- North Atlantic kelp (300 mcg iodine/day)
- Thyroid glandulars for two months
- Men—Tribulus (750 mg/day), zinc, use castor oil over scrotum
- Women—Take saliva test to determine estrogen levels
- Boron (3 mg/day), Maca, and reduce stress.

## INFLAMMATORY BOWEL DISEASE (IBD), includes CROHN'S DISEASE & ULCERATIVE COLITIS

### Mind-pattern

*What I am learning in life is too painful.*

# IRRITABLE BOWEL SYNDROME (IBS)

## Mind-pattern

*I either cannot hold onto something that I need to learn or I hold onto it too much.*

## Treatment

- Digestive enzymes as well as lemon, lime, and pineapple juices
- Visualize Ice Blue in the entire small and large intestines if painful and/or bleeding.
- Flush Pale Yellow through entire small and large intestines
- Oregano oil (300 mg/day)
- Olive leaf capsules (2 capsules/day)
- Aloe vera juice (100 ml 2x/day)
- Tien Shen tea (add raw organic honey if necessary to mitigate taste)
- Eat high protein low carb diet, including organic liver
- Organic ginger tea
- Use castor oil over afflicted area, wool flannel on top of castor oil, and then a hot water bottle on top of that for 20-30 minutes at least one time per day)

## ISCHEMIC HEART DISEASE (IHD)

### Mind-pattern

*I have long-term overwhelming emotions regarding a relationship that I need to stop.*

### Treatment

- Golden Altar and Child Within visualizations
- Flush Chakra Band with Violet for cleansing
- Visualize Medium Green into the heart muscle to oxygenate
- Then flush heart muscle with Pale Pink
- Hawthorne berry (300 mg/day to help repair heart muscle)
- CoQ10 (400 mg/day to rebuild muscle tissue)
- ProArgi9
- Vitamin E (400 mg/day)
- Folic acid (400-800 mcg/day)
- Resveratrol (1000 mg/day)
- Red wine, two glasses/day preferably Pinot Noir
- Vitamin D (5000 IU/day for men; 3000 IU for women to pull plaque and cholesterol into the bones)
- Red yeast rice (300 mg/day to pull out cholesterol/plaque, 30 days only or could damage liver)

## IMPLANT, ORGANIC

### Mind-pattern

*I have a need for outside help in my life and do not do things for myself.*

### Treatment

- Visualize Violet laser to eliminate the implant
- Possible physical implant

## INFERTILITY

### Mind-pattern

*I am afraid to be creative in life; I am afraid of Self- re-creation.*

### Treatment

- Visualize Pale Orange Fertility Archetype in uterus at time of ovulation
- Visualize Sperm and Egg Archetypes at pineal gland by both partners during sexual intercourse
- Females visualize Pale Orange in uterine area to strengthen it, eat a diet rich in good fats, eggs, and red meat
- Males visual Pale Red in Sacral Chakra Band to strengthen it, eat a diet rich in protein as well as avocados to promote sperm health, take zinc (50 mg 2x/day), Tribulus, and use castor oil on scrotum
- Refer to Fertility chapter in **Hyperspace Helper** book

## INFLUENZA

### Mind-pattern

*I need a reset from the world so I can focus on my Self.*

### Treatment

- Alternate flushing the body with Medium Green and Violet
- Add Ice Blue to stop fever/swelling
- MMS or Methylene Blue Plus
- 2 liters of distilled water daily
- Chaga mushroom (500 mg/day)
- Vitamin C powder (4000-10,000 mg/day)
- Immuplex and Congaplex (3 capsules each, every 3 hours)
- Sea salt baths daily

## INTESTINE, SMALL

### Mind-pattern

*Digesting the smaller details of an experience. To take new and learned ideas, keep what is necessary and eliminate the rest.*

*This is my last chance to get the final bit of understanding from what I have taken in.*

## INVERSION THERAPY

Not good for the brain;
blood could pool in the head and lead to health issues.

## JAW/MANDIBLE

### Mind-pattern

*How I communicate my strength of character.*

## JOGGING/RUNNING

### Mind-pattern

*I am running away from life.*

## JOINTS

### Mind-pattern

*I am flexible with strength for my life experiences.*

## KIDNEYS

### Mind-pattern

*How I process my past experiences.*

## KIDNEY, RENAL FAILURE

### Mind-pattern

*I refuse to release and process the past, especially my anger issues.*

## KIDNEY, RENAL FAILURE, LEFT

### Mind-pattern

*I refuse to release and process the past, especially my anger issues dealing with females, including Self if female.*

## KIDNEY, RENAL FAILURE, RIGHT

### Mind-pattern

*I refuse to release and process the past, especially my anger issues dealing with males, including Self if male.*

### Treatment

- Flush Kidneys with Violet, then Pale Orange, and then surround all of this in Brown.
- Organic pink grapefruit juice every three months; the enzyme loosens any residue in kidney tubule; drink steam-distilled water to flush out
- Hydrangea root (300 mg/day for one month)
- Uva ursi (250-300 mg/day for one month)
- Organic watermelon and cranberries

## KIDNEY STONES

### Mind-pattern

*I am unable to process my past experiences.*

### Treatment

- Calcium and Vitamin D pull cholesterol/plaque out of the system and build your skeletal structure at the same time.
- Taking sufficient Vitamin D is protection against kidney stones

## KNEECAP DETERIORATION, BACK

### Mind-pattern

*Issues of flexibility about the future.*

## KNEECAP DETERIORATION, LEFT

### Mind-pattern

*I am not flexible in the future with a female/logic, including Self.*

## KNEECAP DETERIORATION, RIGHT

### Mind-pattern

*I am not flexible in the future with a male/creativity, including Self.*

### Treatment

- Glucosamine and Chondroitin
- Vitamin D and calcium
- Castor oil on kneecaps daily
- Flush legs in Brown
- Weight training exercise to increase bone density and strengthen bones

## KNEE, WATER ON

### Mind-pattern

*Inflexibility and feeling pressured with the thought of being flexible. The thought of being flexible is too much for me to handle.*

### Treatment

- Release work on the issues that make you inflexible with the future and you feel a need to insulate from them
- Use organic castor oil packs on knee
- Topically apply Solomon's seal salve, deep penetrating formula

## LACTIC ACID

### Treatment

- Flush kidneys and bladder by drinking stream-distilled water.

## LARYNX

### Mind-pattern

*How I express and communicate my thoughts.*

## LARYNX, EYES CROSS WHEN SPEAKING

### Mind-pattern

*I do not want to see anything in front of me, so I mirror the translation.*

## LARYNX, VOICE, NASAL

### Mind-pattern

*I have congested emotional irritations under my nose that I want to convey, but I am doing my best to block it out.*

## LARYNX, VOICE, SQUEAKY

### Mind-pattern

*Do not take seriously what I am expressing.*

*Make light of my expressions (of any issue).*

*I am still a child stuck in my childhood.*

### Treatment

- Visualize Ice Blue in the throat for 45 seconds or more daily
- Organic castor oil topically over the area
- Gargle with Celtic sea salt
- 1 or 2 drops of organic frankincense essential oil daily

## LEGS & FEET

### Mind-pattern

*I use my support structure to step into the future.*

## LEG, LEFT

### Mind-pattern

*Female figure, including Self, logic and physical reality.*

## LEPROSY (manufactured virus)

### Mind-pattern

*I feel like I am a rotten person and want to fall apart.*

### Treatment

- Release past traumas
- Organic silica
- Collagen powder in steam-distilled water
- Microcurrent treatments (2-3x/week)
- Sea salt baths
- Far-infrared sauna

## LEUKEMIA

### Mind-pattern

*I resent not having happiness in the flow of life.*

### Treatment

- Chelation therapy (2-3x/week)
- IV Vitamin C
- Spleen glandulars
- Methylene Blue drops daily
- Ozone treatments
- Radionics sessions weekly
- Far-infrared sauna

## LEUKOPLAKIA

### Mind-pattern

*I hold back what I need to say.*

## LEUKOPLAKIA, LEFT SIDE

### Mind-pattern

*I hold back what I need to say to a female.*

## LEUKOPLAKIA, RIGHT SIDE

### Mind-pattern

*I hold back what I need to say to a male.*

### Treatment/All Leukoplakia

- Release the issue
- Violet hose to vacuum out the area
- Ice Blue for pain and swelling
- Visualize Shiny Copper in teeth
- Swish virgin organic coconut oil in mouth 20-30 minutes without swallowing; spit in waste receptacle, as it will clog sink
- Rinse mouth with organic tea tree oil (2x/day)
- Vitamin D (3000 IU/day)
- Organic calcium citrate (2000 mg/day)

## LIVER

### Mind-pattern

*Detoxing and processing current life experiences and having the energy to deal with them.*

## LIVER, CIRRHOSIS

*I am trying to blot out my current experiences
because I do not want to deal with them.*

### Treatment

- Eat organic foods with natural iron such as spinach, liver, kelp, and eggs
- Liver glandulars
- Far-infrared sauna
- Live cell therapy

## LIVER, DISEASE

### Mind-pattern

*I cannot process my life past or current life experiences.
I cannot filter or process them;
I have no energy left to deal with them anymore.*

## LIVER, RIGHT LOWER LOBE

### Mind-pattern

*How I process my non-emotional life experiences.*

## LIVER, HEPATITIS

### Mind-pattern

*I cannot learn from my current experiences because I cannot handle/process it.*

### Treatment

- Violet vacuum to vacuum out the liver
- Liver in Ice Blue if it is inflamed
- Royal Blue scalpel to excise tumors if present
- Immerse lower liver (below rib line) in Pale Yellow and upper liver in Medium Green
- Visualize the entire liver in Liquid Silver, and then flush with Violet
- Next, flush the upper lobes in Medium Green and the lower lobes in Pale Yellow
- Drink black coffee
- Milk thistle herb (300 mg/day for 10 days only)
- Dandelion root (400 mg/day)
- Organic apple cider vinegar (2 tablespoons, 2x daily)
- Lemon juice in steam-distilled water
- Immuplex
- Liver glandulars for three months
- MMS for viral infections or Methylene Blue Plus

## LUNGS

### Mind-pattern

*I energize my Self and expel negative spiritual ideas.*

## LUNGS, FLUID ON, PNEUMONIA

### Mind-pattern

*I am so emotionally overwhelmed that I cannot take in or release any more ideas of Self-expression; I am overwhelmed by what I have done so far in life.*

### Treatment

- Golden Altar release work
- Violet vacuum hose to remove fluids
- Warm organic castor oil compresses
- Ginger tea
- Marshmallow herb and hyssop daily
- Citrus essential oils as a topical; ingest 1-2 drops daily
- Inhale Olio Del Re as needed; use a few drops over bronchial tubes and chest
- Far-infrared sauna treatments

## LUPUS

### Mind-pattern

*I hate my Self; I have had devastating and humiliating experiences.*

### Treatment

- Balance T-Bar Archetype and surround person in Brown
- Logos Christos Archetype in each Chakra Band, in the color of each respective Chakra Color Band
- Flush the body in Violet, then White for a few seconds only, several times each day
- Thymus glandulars (2 capsules 3x/day) for 3-6 months
- Radionics treatments
- Rife machine
- Far-infrared sauna

## LYMPH GLANDS

### Mind-pattern

*I need to remove/clean the negative thoughts out of my body.*

## LYMPHOMA

### Mind-pattern

*The negative thoughts I am holding onto are festering inside of me.*

### Treatment

- Do release work for held resentment
- Visualize Violet knife cutting away growth
- Flush body alternating with Medium Green followed by Violet
- Comfrey tea
- Chapparel tea
- Esiak tea
- Shark cartilage and Pau d'Arco
- Vitamin C IV treatments (3x/week)
- Frankincense injections directly into growth area
- Hyperbaric chamber treatments (3x/week)
- Ozone treatments
- Radionics treatments
- Sea salt baths
- Far-infrared sauna

## MAD COW DISEASE

### Mind-pattern

*My mind is turning to jelly;, I cannot think properly.*

### Treatment

- Same as for Huntington's Disease

## MIGRAINE HEADACHE

### Mind-pattern

*I Self-denigrate and hate my Self.*

### Treatment

- Resolve and release why person hates Self; usually has had severe childhood emotional, mental, or physical trauma
- Visualize Ice Blue in the head during an attack, followed by Royal Blue in the Royal Blue Chakra Band
- Myrrh gum (2 capsules 2x/day if Migraines are frequent)
- Arnica (2 pills sublingually/day)
- White birch bark as needed
- Feverfew as needed
- Topically use Olio Del Re Oil during an attack
- Masturbation stops migraine at onset as it pulls the blood with muscular contractions to the other end of the body
- Micro-current treatments such as Jade Machine

## MOLES
### (Wild cellular growth caused by viruses)

**Mind-pattern** (Location on body determines specific mind-pattern)

*I show the world that I have negative growth that I need to understand*

### Treatment
- Topically apply organic castor oil, Solomon's seal salve, organic aloe vera gel
- Chaga mushroom capsules daily

## MONONUCLEOSIS/Related to EPSTEIN BARR

### Mind-pattern

*I am tired of life.*

### Treatment
- Chaga mushroom, Immuplex, Congaplex, Astragalus, Resveratrol, and kelp with 300 mcg of iodine, all daily.
- Vitamin C IV treatments 3x/week
- Far-infrared Sauna

## MORNING SICKNESS

**(Indicates abundance of hormones for a strong pregnancy)**

### Mind-pattern

*Whatever I create in life makes me sick; I am disappointed in what I have created in life. I am sick of recreating my Self.*

### Treatment

- Flush uterine area with Violet to protect and filter
- Visualize Pale Orange Pregnancy Archetype in uterine area
- Chew on raw ginger root
- Sip on ginger tea
- Olive leaf (1 capsule/day)
- Oregano oil (1 capsule/day)
- Sauerkraut juice (1 teaspoon/day)
- Organic apple cider vinegar (½ teaspoon/day)

## MUSCLES, CRAMPS

### Mind-pattern

*I am pained when I exert my physical powers.*

### Treatment

- Increase steam-distilled water intake
- Organic calcium in citrate form.
- Magnesium (400 mg 1-2x/day)

## MUSCULAR ATROPHY & DYSTROPHY

### Mind-pattern

*The way I move through life hurts me.*

### Treatment

- Daily release work and Oversoul Communication
- Increase consumption of organic proteins
- HCL Betaine with meals to aid digestion
- Collagen powder in steam-distilled water daily
- Topically rub organic castor oil and Solomon's seal deep penetrating salve into affected areas
- Consider stem cell and live cell treatments
- Light weight-bearing exercises every other day

## MUSCLES, LITTLE DEVELOPMENT

### Mind-pattern

*I am weak in my life and I have no way of moving through it.*

## MUSCLES, LOTS OF DEVELOPMENT

### Mind-pattern

*I have power and strength to move through life.*

## MULTIPLE SCLEROSIS (MS)

### Mind-pattern

*I no longer wish to physically interact with life;
I would rather only observe.*

### Treatment

- Balance Brain using Pineal Gland Archetype
- Green Spiral Staircase Visualization
- Visualize "MS" in Brown block letters at the pineal gland to determine origin of MS in this or other lifelines
- Do DNA Opening Visualization
- Visualize entire nervous system in Shiny Copper
- Visualize Shiny Copper and Pale Yellow in and through the body.
- Omega-3 (coconut oil, fish oil, olive oil, peanut oil) in large amounts
- Vitamin B12
- CoQ10 (600 mg/day)
- Eat red meats (especially buffalo)
- Live cell and stem cell therapy
- Hyperbaric chamber treatments

## MYELIN SHEATH DEFICIENCY/ DEGENERATION

### Mind-pattern

*I feel short-circuited in life.*

### Treatment

- Increase consumption of organic meats
- High doses of organic fish oil and organic coconut oil
- Taurine, B-Complex, Resveratrol, organic silica, and collagen daily
- Organic lemon essential oil (1-2 drops daily)

## NAILS

**Mind-pattern**

*I am protecting my Self.*

## NAILS, BITING

**Mind-pattern**

*I am a very vulnerable person who allows others to hurt and abuse me.*

## NAILS, FINGERNAILS

**Mind-pattern**

*I am protecting my life, right now.*

## NAILS, LONG CLAW-LIKE

**Mind-pattern**

*Stay away from me; I am protecting my Self from you.*

## NAILS, TOE, TOO LONG

**Mind-pattern**

*I am protecting my Self from the future; I do not want to go there.*

## NARCOLEPSY

### Mind-pattern

*I want to sleep away my life.*

### Treatment

- Release the mind-patterns that make you want to avoid life
- Deprogramming may be necessary
- Drink two cups of organic black coffee in the morning
- Eat organic dark chocolate daily
- Keep home temperature at a cooler setting
- Take cold showers daily
- B-Complex daily
- Aerobic exercises 3x/daily

## NECK PAIN

### Mind-pattern

*I am stubborn and not willing to see alternate solutions.*

### Treatment

- Determine burdens from childhood that need to be released if Trapezius muscle is pulling
- Shiny Copper in spine to strengthen bones
- Ice Blue to lessen pain and swelling
- Chiropractic adjustments

## NERVES

### Mind-pattern

*I overreact to life circumstances all the time.*

### Treatment

- Shiny Copper in spine and skeletal structure
- Royal Blue in brain
- Pale Yellow from the neck down in the spinal cord and nervous system to regenerate nerve tissue and maintain optimal nerve function

## NERVES, INFLAMED

### Mind-pattern

*I overreact to life circumstances all the time.*

### Treatment

- Ice Blue on pain to stop swelling
- Fresh pineapple
- Myrrh gum capsules
- Use cold compress for 15-20 minutes; remove, repeat until irritation stops
- Then, apply warm compress to get electrical flow moving

## NERVES, REGENERATION

### Mind-pattern

*I need to feel my emotions properly.*

### Treatment

- Pale Yellow surrounded by Shiny Copper tube from the neck down
- Visualize Royal Blue in brain

## NOSE

### Mind-pattern

*What is right in front of my face; what is obvious to me.*
*I, me, it is all about me, everything is about me.*
*The world is made for me.*

## NOSE, BREAKING

### Mind-pattern

*It has been a long time since I took the obvious into consideration.*

## NOSE, SLIGHT INJURY

### Mind-pattern

*I am not paying attention to the most obvious things in my life;*
*I need to pay attention to them.*

## OBESITY

### Mind-pattern

*I am insulating and putting up walls between me and the outside world.*

### Treatment

- Visualize Violet vacuum hose to suck out fat
- Use affirmations to slim down and remove insulating mind-patterns
- Release work of Golden Altar and Child Within daily
- Stay on a strict high protein, low carb diet
- Drink steam-distilled water to help flush toxins from body; add in organic lemon/lime/grapefruit juice with stevia to help balance blood sugar if needed
- Exercise with weights every other day
- Low impact aerobic exercises daily
- Drink organic black coffee in the morning
- Fast 24-48 hours weekly, drinking only steam-distilled water, organic herbal teas and/or organic black coffee

## ORGAN, REMOVAL

### Mind-pattern

*I am removing this organ's mind-pattern from my body; I am not dealing with this mind-pattern in this lifeline.*

### Treatment

- Determine mind-pattern of removed organ
- Determine why the mind-pattern was so challenging that you needed its physical organ removed
- Work on the mind-pattern as the energy pattern of the organ remains

## ORGANS, REVERSED PLACEMENT

### Mind-pattern

*I am here to learn the opposite of what most others expect; I am creatively different than others.*

### Treatment

- Draw/paint your ideas of the world.
- Determine how your view is opposite of others.

## OSTEOPOROSIS

### Mind-pattern

*My support structure in life is weak.*

### Treatment

- Shiny Copper in entire skeleton for 45 seconds (3x/day)
- Release work and affirmations for support structures in life
- Increase organic meat consumption
- Organic calcium in citrate form with Vitamin K2 daily
- Weight-training exercises 3-4x/week

## OVARIES

### Mind-pattern

*Creative/productive energy or power for physical and nonphysical experience.*

## OVERHYDRATING

### Mind-pattern

*I am overwhelmed in life; I am drowning from the inside out.*

### Treatment

- Drink the amount of steam-distilled water for your body size/type
- Supplement with digestive enzymes/probiotics
- Increase your mineral consumption using high quality sea salt

## PERITONEAL DIALYSIS (PD)

### Mind-pattern

*I cannot understand or accept past experience.*

### Treatment

- Same treatment as for Kidney Issues

## PICA DISORDER

(This illness is usually in dually diagnosed individuals with a mental incapacity that makes it challenging to change the mind-patterns using alternative methods)

### Mind-pattern

*I am never satisfied in life and I understand information inappropriately.*

### Treatment

- Must look at Simultaneous Existence life influences as well as animal mind influences.
- Must remain in a strictly controlled environment with 24/7 monitoring.

## PANCREAS

**Mind-pattern**

Understanding and accepting the happiness or sweetness in life.

## PANCREAS, NORMAL INSULIN PRODUCTION

### Cannot absorb blood sugar

**Mind-pattern**

I do not accept happiness; I can get and have happiness but I do not accept it. I have low self-worth; low self-esteem; I self-punish and self-sabotage; I feel guilty.

## PANCREAS, INSULIN OVERPRODUCTION

**Mind-pattern**

I cannot hold onto happiness in life; happiness is slipping away from me.

## PANCREAS, INSULIN UNDERPRODUCTION

**Mind-pattern**

I can see the happiness in life, but I cannot feel it; I know that it is there but I cannot appreciate it.

### Treatment

- Stevia to help regulate insulin production
- Peppermint tea to aid blood sugar absorption
- Pancreas glandulars

## PARALYZATION

### Mind-pattern

*I feel I have no future, no support structure, nothing. I need to be guided and steered all the time; I cannot move forward in life on my own.*

### Treatment

- Pale Red flushing through the body 3x/day
- Merging of White Winged Lion/White Winged Dragon Archetypes 3x/day
- Collagen and silica capsules daily
- High doses of B-Complex and Taurine
- Hyperbaric chamber treatments (30 minutes, 3x/week)
- Live cell and/or stem cell injections
- Far-infrared sauna treatments daily

## PARATHYROID GLANDS

### Mind-pattern

*Supporting life structures and expressing support. No one listens to or pays attention to me.*

### Treatment

- Ice Blue in the throat for 33 seconds (minimum 2x/day)
- High doses of Vitamin D
- Parathyroid glandulars
- Kelp with iodine

## PARKINSON'S DISEASE

### Mind-pattern

*I can no longer direct my life path and thoughts.*

### Treatment

- Same as for Huntington's Disease

## PERIPHERAL VASCULAR DISEASE/PVD

### Mind-pattern

*I stay outside of the flow and joys of life.*

### Treatment

- Pale Red, Purple, and Medium Green in the body
- Nattokinase, organic coconut oil capsules, Omega-3 fish oil capsules daily
- Topically apply organic coconut on the affected areas of the skin

## PETS, ISSUES WITH

### Mind-pattern

*My pet's health/behavior issues are reflective of my own mind-patterns.*

### Treatment

- Pay attention!

## PELVIS

### Mind-pattern

*Balancing into the future.*

## PELVIS, CHRONIC PAIN

### Mind-pattern

*My future looks out of balance and I do not know what to do about it.*

### Treatment

- Identify and deal with worries about the future to feel secure in support structure in life
- Shiny Copper in pelvic bones and coccyx
- Pale Red in lower pelvis and Pale Orange in upper pelvis
- Wild yam root
- Organic calcium citrate (1000-15,000 mg/day)
- Vitamin D
- Omega-3
- Maca
- B-Complex with B12 to strengthen nerves
- Walk and use light leg weights

## PEPTIC ULCER DISEASE (PUD)

### Mind-pattern

*Specific recent emotional issues cause me to lose happiness in life.*

### Treatment

- Ice Blue over the ulcer to stop pain/bleeding, and then Brown over the ulcer as a patch. To conclude, place Pale Yellow over entire area
- Aloe vera juice (100 ml 2x or more/day)
- Ginger capsules or tea
- Olive leaf (2 capsules/day)
- Tien Shen tea
- Coconut water (8 oz/day)

## PERSPIRATION GLANDS

### Mind-pattern

*What I present to the world. I keep my Self emotionally cool;
I keep my anger in check.*

## PERSPIRATION GLANDS, EXCESSIVE SWEAT

### Mind-pattern

*I am angry, stressed and frustrated;
I cannot mentally cool off so my body does it for me.*

### Treatment

- Ice Blue in and around the body at all times
- Release work and Child Within on fear issues in life
- Dial Visualization as listed in **Healer's Handbook** to reset body temperature
- Stay in cool temperature environments

## PH, ACID

(Body must be more acidic to prohibit growth of viruses/bacteria)

### Mind-pattern

*I am always reacting aggressively in all situations.*

### Treatment

- Dial Visualization as listed in **Healer's Handbook** to reset pH
- Two liters of steam-distilled water daily
- Methylene Blue drops morning and evening
- NADH (10 mg to 20 mg/day)
- Frequent sea salt baths
- Organic dairy products

## PH, ALKALINE

### Mind-pattern

*I tend to be mild and bland all the time.*

### Treatment

- Eat fermented foods and more spices in your foods daily
- Red wine at dinner

## PINEAL

### Mind-pattern

*How I balance and create experiences.*

### Treatment/Decalcification

- Rub frankincense essential oil on hands, feet and/or forehead
- Comfrey herb as a tea

## PLASTIC SURGERY

### Mind-pattern

*I artificially express my mind-pattern: I want a quick fix and I am not willing to do mental work to correct my Self; I live in a virtual world.*

### Treatment

- Change the mind-pattern so plastic surgery is not needed

## POISON IVY

### Mind-pattern

*I have inner angers and irritations that I want to show the world; there is something about the natural environment that angers and irritates me.*

### Treatment

- Tea tree oil
- Castor oil
- Sea salt baths

## PNEUMONIA

### Mind-pattern

*I have overwhelming emotional congestion; my emotions are clogged and I cannot move them.*

## PNEUMONIA, WALKING

### Mind-pattern

*I am so used to my overwhelming clogged emotions that I do not even realize how bad I feel.*

### Treatment

- Identify and release the specific emotions
- Violet hose to vacuum out fluids
- Flush lungs with Violet to cleanse followed by Medium Green to oxygenate
- Ice Blue wherever fever is present
- Echinacea (200-500 mg/day)
- Vitamin C (5000-6000 mg/day)
- Hyssop herb (500 mg/day to clear out lungs)
- Marshmallow herb (1000 mg/day to fortify alveoli and lining of lungs)
- Organic castor oil packs over chest for 20 to 30 minutes/day
- Deep breathe in sea salt baths
- Far-infrared sauna

## POLIO

### Mind-pattern

*I no longer wish to control my movements and directions in life.*

### Treatment

- Same as for Nerve Issues
- Stem cell treatments and hyperbaric chamber 3x/week

## POLYCYSTIC OVARY SYNDROME (PCOS)

### Mind-pattern

*My stress and need to insulate my creative abilities lead me to enhance my male characteristics so I can fight off external circumstances. In the past, my creative abilities have been criticized and unappreciated.*

### Treatment

- Identify and remove source of foundational negative mind-pattern
- Do something creative to completion
- Visualize Pale Orange in the affected area and then visualize the Overall Healing Archetype and the Logos Christos Archetype in the area
- Visualize ovaries absorbing the cysts
- Estrogen-dominant people may also have adrenal, thyroid, and bone density issues; correct with wild yam root, Maca
- Vitamin D to help dissolve cysts
- Organic castor oil over abdomen

## PRADER WILLI SYNDROME

**(A form of retardation combined with mental illnesses originating from Simultaneous Existences as an animal or insect; the person must be monitored 24/7 in a strictly controlled environment)**

### Mind-Pattern

*I have no self-control. I self-destruct by ingesting more than I need or can use. I do not understand anything in life, so I go to extremes in trying to absorb all I can with no conclusion.*

### Treatment

- DNA work can be done by others for the person, including releasing influences of Simultaneous Existences

## PREMATURE EJACULATION

### Mind-pattern

*I have inherited memory, or from another lifeline, where I had to flee quickly and often; I have fear of being caught; I have fear of sexual activity and intimacy.*

### Treatment

- Green Spiral Staircase Visualization to identify and release fear
- Ice Blue in genital area when you sense a need to ejaculate
- Tribulus (750 mg/day to enhance sexual capabilities)
- Kegel exercises to tighten and release the muscles near the genitals that relate to urination and orgasm to strengthen for greater control

## PREMENSTRUAL SYNDROME (PMS)

### Mind-pattern

*I am angry and distraught at how I have created my life.*

### Treatment

- Pale Orange in affected area surrounded by Ice Blue
- Balance Pale Orange T-Bar Archetype in uterine area
- Take saliva test to determine estrogen and progesterone levels
- When estrogen-dominant, take wild yam root (1500 mg/day) to increase progesterone
- Maca root (250-400 mg/day) to balance estrogen with progesterone
- Castor oil over lower abdomen at night
- Black cohosh (300 mg/day) if there is no cycle. If the cycle does not begin take blue cohosh (will cause cramping and seem like hemorrhage but lining is being expelled). This is only to be taken if uterine lining needs to be expelled because menstrual cycle is blocked
- Eat foods without added hormones
- Avoid all microwaved and soy foods

## PROGERIA

### Mind-pattern

*I must get through this lifeline quickly because I do not have much time; I am an ancient Soul; I have something important to experience/say and then I must leave.*

### Treatment

- DNA work to reverse the aging process
- Resveratrol
- Stem cells and live cells

## PROSTATE

**(correlates to the uterus)**

### Mind-pattern

*To create support and development.*

## PROSTATE, BENIGN TUMOR

### Mind-pattern

*I reject/suppress my male creative energy.*

### Treatment

- Violet hose to vacuum out excess tissue
- Royal Blue scalpel to remove excess tissue
- Flush area in Pale Orange
- Affirmations
- Selenium (200 mcg/day)
- Pumpkin seed oil (600 mg/day)
- Saw palmetto (300 mg/day)
- Siberian ginseng (1000 mg/day)
- Zinc (50 mg 2x/day)
- Prostate glandulars
- Lycopene (20 mg/day)

## PSORIASIS

(Deterioration of myelin sheathing that alters cellular replication in skin; a form of shape-shifting; people with this have a higher percentage of Reptilian DNA)

### Mind-pattern

*I feel so agitated by the world that I exude anger from my body; subconscious memories from other lifelines trigger my anger, Sfear, and disgust of the world.*

### Treatment

- Golden Altar, Child Within, Oversoul Release work to remove anger, fear, and disgust
- Reptilian Brainstem Archetype at the Reptilian brainstem to balance it
- Flush affected area with Chakra Band color where affected area is located
- Omega-3 oils (3000-6000 mg/day)
- B-complex (2000 mg/day)
- Topically use aloe vera gel and Olive Gold
- Topically use Solomon's seal salve-deep penetrating over affected areas

## RASH

### Mind-pattern

*I have emotional irritation that I want people to see.*

### Treatment

- Identify and release emotion
- Flush rash in Ice Blue
- Topically use organic aloe vera gel on affected area
- Topically use organic coconut oil to prevent bacterial infections
- Castor oil on rash at night
- Olive Gold topically
- Calendula cream topically
- Pure zinc oxide topically

## REJUVENATION/AGING

### Mind-pattern

*I do not want to stay long on Earth.*

### Treatment

- Infuse pineal gland with Royal Blue
- Reset biological clock using visualization in **Healer's Handbook**
- Spin Chakra Bands to flush out unhealthy colors
- Siberian ginseng (1000 mg/day)
- Modifilan/Siberian brown seaweed (4 capsules/day, build up to 8/day, take 8/day for one month, stop for two months and repeat as needed)
- Frequency numbers for rejuvenation (requires Frequency Activator Report)—numbers must be thought, said, or looked at 21x/day to install a new mind-pattern/frequency.
- Herbal Chelation: Add to 4 liter jug of steam-distilled water 1 tablespoon each blueberry extract, black cherry extract, elderberry extract, and 1 cup aloe vera juice. Drink throughout the day without adding any other food or liquid except more steam-distilled water. Add 1 Tablespoon of Vitamin C powder to cleanse colon.
- Note: Just as the liver can regenerate, there are instructions present in all areas of the body to do the same. Use your mind-pattern to activate the genes that will regrow other body parts as well.

## REPTILIAN BRAINSTEAM ACTIVATION

### Mind-pattern

*I have a high percentage of activated Reptilian genetics.*

### Treatment

- Royal Blue at the brain to connect to Hyperspace energies
- Reptilian Brainstem Archetype along the spinal column
- Balance T-Bar Archetype at the pineal gland
- Deprogramming work; in addition bring Reptilian Brainstem Archetype and T-Bar Archetype together so they meet at midbrain
- Visualize Pale Pink throughout energy field to install Unconditional Love and Acceptance of Self
- Visualize Pale Yellow throughout the energy field for Understanding; Ice Blue for Communication; Brown for Grounding, all as needed
- If drug addict, must detox

## ROSACEA/RHINOPHYMA

### Mind-pattern

*I have a particular anger issues for which I blame others.*

### Treatment

- Green Spiral Staircase to identify anger issue or move consciousness to affected area of skin to determine anger issue
- Ice Blue over irritated area
- Omega-3, coconut oil, turmeric
- Silica (500-2000 mg/day)
- Apply Vitamin C cream on RHINOPHYMA
- Apply castor oil at night
- Apply Solomon's seal salve-deep penetrating during day
- Eat organic proteins
- Avoid dairy products, which can cause skin congestion

## SACRAL ULCER

### Mind-pattern

*I feel financially and materialistically vulnerable.*

### Treatment

- Identify and release issues
- Flush with Violet, then Pale Orange; seal by visualizing Brown around the area.
- Visualize area healed with Brown around it
- If open ulcer, apply white sugar or organic raw honey
- Organic coconut oil capsules and aloe vera gel or capsules to kill germs (antifungal and antibacterial)
- Use cold laser

## SALIVARY/PAROTID GLANDS

### Mind-pattern
*I need to deal with the pieces instead of the whole.*

## SALIVARY/PAROTID GLANDS, BLOCKAGES

### Mind-pattern
*I am not going to make my life easier.*
*I refuse to accept an easier way of doing this; I want it the hard way.*

### Treatment
- Oil pull using organic coconut oil mixed with 1-2 drops organic frankincense essential oil 15-30 minutes 2x/day
- Note: Be sure to spit the oil into a waste receptacle because if you spit the oil into your sink it will eventually clog the drain

# SCHIZOPHRENIA

## Mind-pattern

*I am afraid of my logical mind and I am afraid of my creativity/emotions.*

## Treatment

- If no middle name, add one that is culturally appropriate such as the mother's maiden name
- Use given first name, never middle name as the first name
- Balance T-Bar at pineal gland or use the Pineal Gland Archetype
- Visualization: Center at Pineal Gland. See a hallway with doorways on either side representing left and right brain. Enter first one side and then the other, each time taking a statue or symbol into the hallway. This helps to balance the mind-pattern and thoughts.
- Royal Blue to stimulate proper brain activity and function
- Brown to ground and balance the brain
- Eat heavier proteins for grounding
- Pineal gland or pituitary glandulars
- Breathe in sea salt bath or ocean air to help open the mind
- Frankincense oil to energize the pineal gland
- St. John's Wort to stimulate the brain and bring forward suppressed issues
- Treatment for Myelin Sheath Deficiency
- Kava kava to relax, calm, and balance
- Valerian root to calm and relax
- Physical exercises to stimulate the left brain

## SEASONAL AFFECTIVE DISORDER (SAD)

### Mind-pattern

*Feeling abandoned by God-Mind and detached from spiritual energies.*

### Treatment

- Spend 15 minutes outside in sun/day
- Do not wear sunglasses
- Take Vitamin D

## SEIZURES

### Mind-pattern

*I have an overwhelmingly intense mind-pattern.*

### Treatment

- Balance T-Bar at pineal gland
- Visualize and hold Dolphin Frequency Archetype at pineal gland
- Emphasize Royal Blue in Royal Blue Chakra Band
- Wear 3 microns copper foil on head and in shoes
- Keep Shiny Copper of some kind on your body at all times, such as in your pockets
- Eat fish, lamb, buffalo, raw nuts
- Vitamin A, Omega-3, Vitamin D, Vitamin E (400 IU/day)
- Brain glandulars

## SEXUAL DYSFUNCTION, FEMALE

### Mind-pattern

*I have fear of sex and men.*

### Treatment

- Identify and release the issues/look for abuse by men
- Hold Pale Red in Root Chakra Band
- Lubricate vaginal walls and cervix with mixture of virgin coconut oil, organic castor oil, lemon juice, and olive oil 1x/day

## SEXUAL DYSFUNCTION, MALE

### Mind-pattern

*Fear of union with others;*
*feeling inadequate creatively and fear of reproducing.*

### Treatment

- Deprogramming may be needed
- Zinc (100 mg) and sarsaparilla (1000 mg) to increase testosterone
- Vascular issues may be involved, which need to be addressed

## SEXUALLY TRANSMITTED DISEASE (STD)/ CHLAMYDIA, SYPHILIS, GENITAL WARTS, GONORRHEA

### Mind-pattern

*I am angry, frustrated, and hurt in sexual activity and intimacy.*

### Treatment

- Identify and release feelings
- Flush area with intense burst of White followed by Violet, then put in Pale Red
- Violet hose to vacuum out viruses
- Royal Blue scalpel to remove warts/growths
- MMS or Methylene Blue
- Strong sea salt baths with baking soda, pharmacy-grade hydrogen peroxide, 1 cup of each; females need to make sure the bath water goes into the vagina
- Apply organic castor oil over genitals
- Olive leaf (500 mg/day)
- Elderberry (500 mg/day to kill pathogens)
- Echinacea (1000 mg/day to kill pathogens)
- Immuplex several times per day
- Chaga mushroom capsules (500 mg/day)
- Far-infrared sauna daily

## SEX CHANGE OPERATION

### Mind-pattern/Programming

*My mind-pattern creates the correct body, so I am following a programming alter*

### Treatment

- Deprogramming
- In-depth search of childhood and other lifetime issues that need to be released

### Mind-pattern/Gestational Demonization

*Demonization happened during gestation and I have an astral attachment causing a need to change sexes.*

### Treatment

- Deprogramming

### Mind-pattern/Taking Body With Permission

*The original Soul Personality from my Oversoul decided not to enter the body, so I have taken it with permission.*

### Treatment

- Sex change operation may be necessary

### Mind-pattern/High-Level Soul-Personality

*I am a high-level Soul Personality, aware of my multi-dimensional Selves; I need a switch-over of genders to fulfill my mission and function on Earth.*

### Treatment

- Acknowledge bisexuality
- All persons considering sex change operations must consider programming and emotional traumas, coupled with Simultaneous Lifetime Influences, to effectively determine what treatments are most correct and beneficial.

## SHINGLES

### Mind-pattern

*I am extremely angry and irritated so I put up a rough external front.*

### Treatment

- Identify and release issue
- Ice Blue in the area
- Pale Yellow and Violet flushing in, through, and around the body
- Apply Olive Gold, organic virgin coconut oil, organic castor oil at night; may initially make it worse as it pulls out the virus
- Apply organic apple cider vinegar and aloe vera gel to soothe area
- Methylene Blue
- Organic cocoa powder (1 tablespoon/day) to kill pathogens
- Raw organic honey (1 tablespoon/day) to kill pathogens
- Apply raw organic honey to area to promote healing

## SINUSITIS, CHRONIC

### Mind-pattern

*Someone under my nose is irritating and annoying me; I see my Self in that person and I do not want to admit it.*

### Treatment

- Do release work on those who annoy you.
- Topically use organic castor oil over the sinus areas of the face and a little inside the nostril
- Use a neti pot with warm sea salt water to flush out excess mucus
- Increase citrus to cut phlegm and mucus
- Avoid all dairy foods

## SKELETON SYSTEM

### Mind-pattern

*My general support structure in life.*

## BONES, BROKEN/FRACTURED

### Mind-pattern

*My support structure is broken/fractured.*

### Treatment

- See Bone Treatment in Bone section

## BONE, MARROW

(may also have spleen issue)

### Mind-pattern

*I have a problem with the depth of my support structure.*

### Treatment

- Identify and release issue from the past
- Visualize the spinal column as a tube made of Shiny Copper; fill inside tube with Pale Yellow, the color of nerves
- Eat organic red meats
- Bone marrow soup
- Red wine, preferably Pinot Noir

## BONES, OSTEOPOROSIS

### Mind-pattern

*My support structure in life is weak.*

### Treatment

- Increase organic meat consumption
- Organic bone marrow
- Spleen glandulars
- Stem cells

## SKIN

### Mind-pattern

*What I present to the world;
my first impression to the world; my physical border.*

## SLEEPWALKING

### Mind-pattern

*I am afraid that I will die when I am asleep.*

### Treatment

- Contact the Oversoul of the person to ask if the person could be allowed to leave his/her body, or if he/she needs to stay.
- Look at the objects/people who are forgotten to determine why the person wants to disassociate from life.
- Put the Silver Infinity Archetype over the Crown Chakra and connect it to the Pineal Gland via Silver Frequency Line
- Then, put Brown around legs and feet to ground to the Earth
- Chelation or cleanse to remove heavy metal in the system

## SMOKING

### Mind-pattern

*I am trying to calm and balance my Self.*

### Treatment

- Visualize Brown throughout the entire energy field to ground and balance

## SNORING

### Mind-pattern

*I am very stubborn, will not change my mind-pattern, and subliminally I need attention. I am afraid of conscious attention.*

### Treatment

- Determine where you are inappropriately stubborn in life and release that
- Kava kava, St. John's Wort or valerian root about one hour before bed
- Sleep on your side or elevate upper body

## SPINE, DISK CARTILAGE DEGENERATION or HERNIATED DISK

### Mind-pattern

*Feeling your main support structure in life is weak and hurtful.*

### Treatment

- Chiropractic adjustments
- Omega-3, horsetail herb, olive oil, and calcium in citrate form with Vitamin D all to rebuild cartilage
- Vitamin K2
- Have a massage using combination of peanut oil, castor oil, and olive oil, all of which will help build and regenerate cellular tissue
- Shiny Copper in and around the spine for 45 seconds, 3x/day.

## SPINE, SCOLIOSIS

### Mind-pattern

*I feel weighted down; I feel completely overwhelmed in my support structure in life; I cannot support anything.*

### Treatment

- Same as above.

## SPINE, SHRINKING DUE TO DISC DEGENERATION

### Mind-pattern

*I am not important any more: I am less than I used to be; from my perspective I am not as high-powered as I used to be; I feel put down.*

### Treatment

- Do stretching exercises
- Take calcium with Vitamin D
- Take Omega-3, horsetail herb, olive oil
- Massage area with combination of peanut oil, castor oil and olive oil to regenerate cellular tissue
- Receive occasional chiropractic adjustments to separates bones

## SPINE, SUBLUXATIONS, CERVICAL

### Mind-pattern

*I am stubborn*

## SPINE, SUBLUXATIONS, LUMBAR

### Mind-pattern

*I feel unsupported in life.*

## SPINE, SUBLUXATIONS, SACRAL/COCCYX

### Mind-pattern

*I am concerned with finances and materiality.*

## SPINE, SUBLUXATIONS, THORACIC

### Mind-pattern

*I am shouldering burdens from childhood that I have not released.*

## SPLEEN

### Mind-pattern

*Keeping happiness and joy in life Self-protected.*

## STOMACH

### Mind-pattern

*Holding onto information until it is ready to be understood.*

## STOMACH, MALABSORPTION DUE TO BLEEDING/ULCERS

### Mind-pattern

*I cannot retain information; the information is painful and hurtful to me; I do not want to hold onto anything.*

## STOMACH, RUPTURED

### Mind-pattern

*I do not want to store information for understanding later; I do not even want to be here.*

## STOMACH, STAPLED/GASTRIC BYPASS SURGERY

### Mind-pattern

*I cannot handle any more information; just a little bit of information at a time.*

### Treatment

- Visualize Pale Yellow in and around the stomach; then visualize a layer of Brown around that
- Take organic silica (1000 mg daily)
- Take organic aloe vera juice (200 ml 3x/day)

## SUDDEN INFANT DEATH SYNDROME (SIDS)

### Mind-pattern

*I am not in the situation I expected or needed; I need to leave; my parents are making me unhappy.*

### Treatment/Parents

- Need to release the negative mind-patterns of abandonment, self-punishment, self-sabotage and judgment.
- Perform Golden Altar, Child Within, Oversoul Communication

## SWEAT GLANDS

### Mind-pattern

*What I present to the world; I keep my Self emotionally cool and my anger in check.*

## SWEAT GLANDS, BLOCKED

### Mind-pattern

*I refuse to release my fears and angers.*

### Treatment

- Release work
- Topically apply Neem oil on skin
- Far-infrared sauna

## TEETH

### Mind-pattern

*How I adjust to life.*

## TEETH, BACK

### Mind-pattern

*How I relate to the past.*

## TEETH, BOTTOM

### Mind-pattern

*How I adjust to past and present situations.*

## TEETH, CAVITIES/FILLINGS

### Mind-pattern

*I am a victim and need artificial assistance to adjust to life.*

## TEETH, CLEANING

**Mind-pattern**

*There is a layer of adjustment I need to remove to continue.*

## TEETH, CROOKED

**Mind-pattern**

*I am incorrectly adjusting to my current life situation.*

## TEETH, CROWNS/IMPLANTS/VENEERS

**Mind-pattern**

*I am artificially covering up or replacing an issue.*

## TEETH, DECAY

**Mind-pattern**

*I have difficulty adjusting to life issues.*

## TEETH, EXTRACTION

**Mind-pattern**

*I am not going to deal with the issue; I am just getting rid of it.*

## TEETH, FRONT

**Mind-pattern**

*How I relate to the present.*

## TEETH, GUMS

**Mind-pattern**

*How I hold my life path/adjustments together.*

## TEETH, LEFT SIDE

**Mind-pattern**

*How I adjust to female issues.*

## TEETH, NERVES

**Mind-pattern**

*My life adjustments make me jumpy, jittery, and short-circuited.*

## TEETH, NUMB

(during dental work)

**Mind-pattern**

*I do not want to talk about the adjustment process.*

## TEETH, OVERBITE

**Mind-pattern**

*I am trying to adjust to my future instead of what is in front of me now.*

## TEETH, RIGHT SIDE

**Mind-pattern**

*How I adjust to male issues.*

## TEETH, ROOT CANAL

**Mind-pattern**

*I do not have the nerve to make this adjustment.*

## TEETH, SENSITIVE

**Mind-pattern**

*I am too sensitive; I cannot adjust to any situation.*

## TEETH, TOP

**Mind-pattern**

*How I adjust to future situations.*

# TEETH, UNDERBITE

## Mind-pattern

*I only assimilate and adjust to my past;
I do not adjust to my present or my future.*

## Treatment/All Teeth Issues

- Visualize your teeth in Shiny Copper to strengthen them
- Surround teeth/gums in Ice Blue to mitigate any pain
- Take B-Complex for nerve health
- Take CoQ10 (400-600 mg/day) to improve gum health
- Take calcium citrate and Vitamin D to strengthen bones/teeth
- Use coconut, olive, or peanut oil Plus Olive Gold Dental to swish in mouth for 3-10 minutes; spit in waste receptacle, as it will clog sink
- Brushing teeth is a form of reflexology
- Only use organic mouthwash if necessary
- Take berberine and/or myrrh gum to reduce pain/swelling, including before and after dental work/surgery of any kind
- Before dental work/surgery, eat ⅓ fresh pineapple one and two days before surgery; eat the last ⅓ of the pineapple after surgery; pineapple can be frozen and put in blender to be consumed as a slushy; cold also helps reduce swelling

## TEMPOROMANDIBULAR JOINT DYSFUNCTION (TMJ)

### Mind-pattern

*I must hold back what I need to say or it will hurt me in some way.*

### Treatment

- Identify and release issue (if it involves a relationship the left side represents female; right side represents male)
- Use Ice Blue to help with pain
- Take homeopathic Arnica (2-3 drops under tongue/day) to help with pain
- Take myrrh gum (2 capsules up to 3x/day for pain)
- Take coconut oil or fish oil if bone is rubbing on bone
- Take Vitamin D if due to calcification

## TINNITUS

### Mind-pattern

*I am disturbed by what I am hearing; I do not want to hear it anymore; I am trying to change what I hear.*

## TINNITUS, LEFT EAR

### Mind-pattern

*My hearing disturbances concern female issues.*

## TINNITUS, RIGHT EAR

### Mind-pattern

*My hearing disturbances concern male issues.*

### Treatment

- Resolve what you do not want to hear anymore
- Flush outer and inner ear with Royal Blue
- Put T-Bar Archetype in inner ear to balance energy
- Visualize Royal Blue in ear
- Visualize Pale Yellow to help receive information for those with hearing loss
- Take Omega-3 (2000-5000 mg/day) to build myelin sheathing of nerves
- While lying on each side, place two drops 2-3% hydrogen peroxide in one ear at a time 1-2x/day to remove wax buildup and organisms
- Use a drop of organic castor oil at night in affected ear
- Use mulein oil with garlic in affected ear

## THALAMUS

### Mind-pattern

*What I expect from others or myself, my habits and inherited mind-patterns and genetically-encoded memory.*

## THROAT ILLNESS

### Mind-pattern

*I have anger and frustration because I am holding back what I need to say.*

### Treatment

- Visualize Ice Blue in the throat several times per day
- Gargle with sea salt 3x/day
- Oil pull with organic coconut oil daily
- Note: Be sure to spit the oil into a waste receptacle because if you spit the oil into your sink it will eventually clog the drain

## THROAT, STREP

### Mind-pattern

*What I already experienced is festering and unspoken, making me angry and hurt.*

### Treatment

- Same as above

### Additional Treatment

- Take Immuplex and Congaplex
- Take Chaga mushroom capsules
- Dead Sea salt baths
- Far-infrared sauna

## THROMBOSIS, ARMS

### Mind-pattern
*I have experienced a traumatic event of an immediate current nature.*

## THROMBOSIS, LEGS

### Mind-pattern
*I have a complete fear of unhappiness in my future life and support structure.*

## THROMBOSIS, LUNG

### Mind-pattern
*I have a complete stoppage of emotional happiness in life*

### Treatment
- Flush area of blockage with Purple, and then follow with Medium Green to oxygenate affected cells
- Visualize a Violet piston pushing through vein to push through and open the blood flow.
- Visualize the clot dissolving via a Violet beam dissolving the clot to nothingness; then flush the entire area with Violet.
- Take fish oil (3000-6000 mg/day for three weeks, then drop down to 1000-3000 mg/day)
- Increase steam-distilled water consumption to decrease blood viscosity
- Take Nattokinase, a natural organic blood thinner, until there is a release of the block of happiness
- Use organic castor oil over the area
- Take ProArgi9
- Far-infrared sauna

## THYMUS GLAND

**Mind-pattern**

*Fighting for what is good or protected for me.*

## THYROID GLAND

**Mind-pattern**

*Supporting expressions of learned information.*

## THYROID GLAND, HYPERTHYROIDISM

**Mind-pattern**

*I talk too much and belittle myself.*

## THYROID GLAND, HYPOTHYROIDISM

**Mind-pattern**

*I do not speak up for myself; instead I insulate.*

### Treatment

- Same as for throat issues
- Additional Treatment
- Do the Dial Visualization as listed in **Healer's Handbook**
- Take thyroid glandulars
- Take organic kelp (300 mcg of iodine 2x/day)
- Topically apply organic castor oil over the throat 3x/day

## TONGUE

**Mind-pattern**

*How I taste life expressions of myself.*

## TONGUE, BURNED

**Mind-pattern**

*I am angry I said that.*

## TONGUE, PIERCED

**Mind-pattern**

*I am clamping down on the things I need to verbalize.*

## TONGUE, TASTE, BITTER

**Mind-pattern**

*I do not like bitter food; I have a very bitter life.*

*I like bitter food; I get pleasure from rough, bitter life experiences.*

## TONGUE, TASTE, BLAND

**Mind-pattern**

*I am afraid of unfamiliar experiences.*

## TONGUE, TASTE, DRY

### Mind-pattern

*I like dry foods because I like my information "cut and dried."*

## TONGUE, TASTE, SALTY

### Mind-pattern

*I crave salty foods because I am trying to clean up my life experiences.*

## TONGUE, TASTE, SPICY

### Mind-pattern

*I like spice in my life; I enjoy fast, hot, and exciting experiences.*

## TONGUE, TASTE, SWEET

### Mind-pattern

*I crave sweets because I am looking for pleasure and sweetness in life. I do not like foods that are too sweet or rich because I restrict my own happiness in life; I do not think I deserve sweetness or riches.*

## TONGUE, TASTE, TEXTURE

### Mind-pattern

*I eat smooth, creamy foods because I desire a smooth life. I eat textured food because I like the variety of texture in life. I like to eat meat from the bone because I like to gnaw on my experiences.*

## TOURETTE SYNDROME

### Mind-pattern

*I do not think properly. I am always inappropriate.*

### Treatment

- Release work on traumas that created the condition
- Visualize Royal Blue in the brain
- Visualize Ice Blue in the throat
- Balance your T-Bar Archetype frequently before speaking.
- Use the Green Spiral Staircase Visualization to determine when the issue began and the cause.
- Deprogramming work may be necessary.

## ULCERS

### Mind-pattern

*I feel hurt by what I have understood in life.*

### Treatment

- Flush ulcers with Violet, then Pale Yellow frequently
- Take organic aloe vera juice (300 ml 3x/day)
- Drink Tienchi raw powder tea several times per day
- Take oregano oil capsules 3x/day
- Take stomach/intestine glandulars if stomach ulcers
- Take Methylene Blue drops morning and evening.

## ULCER COLITIS

### Mind-pattern

*I cannot retain information because it is hurtful and painful to me; I do not want to hold onto it.*

### Treatment

- Same Treatment as above.

### Additional Treatment

- Take silica capsules
- Drink collagen powder in steam-distilled water each morning

## UTERUS

### Mind-pattern

*Creative support and development.*

## UTERUS, HYSTERECTOMY

### Mind-pattern

*I am noncreative with low self-worth. I have issues of creative support and development, so I am useless and rejected by others.*

### Treatment

- Surgery
- Rub organic castor oil over the area.

## VARICOSE VEINS

### Mind-pattern

*I have stagnated happiness in life involving my support structure.*

### Treatment

- Visualize Purple flushing through the affected veins
- Use Ice Blue to reduce swelling and pain
- Flush with Brown, which is the natural energetic color of the legs
- Take ProArgi9
- Take myrrh gum (300 mg/day)
- Apply organic castor oil over area at night
- Apply Solomon's seal salve-deep penetrating over affected area

## VISCERA

### Mind-pattern

*I have all I need to function properly.*

### Visual Recognition Mind-pattern

*I recognize something but I cannot determine what to do with/about what I see.*

### Treatment

- This depends on which parts of the viscera are disturbed. Viscera are simply the internal organs of the body and connecting tissues.

## VITILIGO

### Mind-pattern

*I am unsure of my self-identity. I do not present myself in a consolidated manner.*

### Treatment

- Visualize skin as one continuous color, then put entire body in Brown
- DNA work as outlined in **Hyperspace Plus**
- Topically apply neem oil/cream on the skin in combination with pure Vitamin C cream
- Topically apply Methylene Blue to affected areas
- Expose affected areas to UVA and UVB light

## WEIGHT, EXCESS

### Mind-pattern

*I am insulating against the world.*

## WEIGHT, EXCESS, BACKSIDE

### Mind-pattern

*I am carrying around the weight of my past that I cannot release.*

## WEIGHT, EXCESS, HIPS

### Mind-pattern

*I feel like I am out of balance, especially when I think about the future.*

## WEIGHT, EXCESS, STOMACH

### Mind-pattern

*I cannot assimilate and digest my life.*

# WEIGHT, EXCESS, THIGHS

## Mind-pattern

*I have childhood abuse issues that I carry with me.*

## Treatment/All Excess Weight

- Do Golden Altar, Child Within, Oversoul Release work
- Merge with alternate Selves who do not have weight issues
- Visualize Violet hose to vacuum out excess fat
- Visualize Pale Red flame to burn off excess fat
- Visualize Pale Red in excess fat to boost metabolism only if heart and blood pressures are normal
- Take Alpha Lipoic Acid and L-Carnitine combination capsule (500-1000 mg/2x per day)
- Eat proteins and low carbohydrates
- Drink 1-3 liters of steam-distilled water
- Drink ¼-½ teaspoon of sea salt in warm water to curb sugar cravings and kill parasites
- Eat jalapenos (2/day to boost metabolism)
- Avoid soy, microwaved, and processed foods
- Take L-Glutamine (500-1000 mg/2x/day)
- Men take zinc and tribulus to increase testosterone
- Women take wild yam root to increase progesterone as well as Maca root to balance estrogen and progesterone
- Both Men/Women with excess estrogen, take boron to slowly decrease estrogen levels (1 mg/day)
- Take a series of colonics
- Do low-impact aerobic exercises combined with weight-training to strengthen bone

## WEIGHT, UNDERWEIGHT

### Mind-Pattern

*I want to be "less than"; I have low Self-worth issues.*

### Treatment

- Do Golden Altar release work
- Grow Up The Child Within
- Eat more carbohydrates than proteins
- Eat whole organic dairy
- Avoid excess sugar and processed wheat
- Do weight-training exercises 3x/week

# General Supplements with General Information

**Aloe Vera Gel**: Topically apply to heal skin

**Aloe Vera Juice**: For digestive system, reconditions intestinal wall; eliminates pathogens; take 100 ml 2x/day

**Alpha Lipoic Acid**: Aids absorption of blood sugar properly: curbs appetite

**Apple Cider Vinegar**: Cleanses liver; alkalizes body

**Arnica**: Anti-inflammatory

**Beet Juice**: Reduces blood pressure

**Biotin**: Aids protein assimilation; aids hair/nail growth; take 500 mcg/day

**Black Cohosh**: Builds up level of estrogen for women who are devoid of hormonal activity with these types of characteristics: thin, frail, wrinkled, look older than age, facial hair, irritable; take 200 mg/day. Follow up with maca root for life (250-400 mg/day)

**Blueberry Juice**: Reduces blood pressure

**Blue Cohosh**: Purges uterus of built-up material; for women with fibroids, endometriosis, perimenopausal; take 250 mg/day for 3-5 days; may experience excessive bleeding and cramping; replaces need for D&C and hysterectomy

**Cilantro**: Pulls out heavy metal

**Cinnamon**: Helps regulate blood sugar; take 1 teaspoon in morning

**Coconut Oil**: Blood thinner, heals wounds, antiviral/antifungal; take 1 tablespoon/day and/or apply topically as needed

**Coconut Water**: Strengthens blood plasma because it is one molecule away from blood plasma; with the addition of Chlorella it is one molecule away from red blood cells; helps circulation issues

**Coffee, Black**: Cleanses liver; protects against cirrhosis

**Congaplex by Standard Process**: Relieves head and sinus congestion

**Chelation Oral or IV Therapy**: Deep detox; go slowly especially in anyone with weakened immune system

**CoQ10**: Regenerates muscle including heart and gum tissue; take 200-400 mg/day

**Cranberry Juice/Capsules**: Corrects bladder issues

**Dandelion Root**: Cleanses/strengthens liver

**Echinacea**: Kills pathogens in bloodstream; use for colds, sore throat, flu; do not take for more than two weeks at a row otherwise it builds up toxins in liver; take 500 mg 2x/day

**Far-Infrared Sauna**: Resets body's immune system and eliminates pathogens; build up time slowly over 6-8 weeks

**Folic Acid**: Strengthens heart; take 400-800 mcg/day

**Organic Ginger Tea/Capsules**: Quells nausea, reduces edema, aids digestion, kills pathogens in digestive tract; use for upset stomach and morning sickness; take 300 mg/day

**Gingko Biloba**: Removes aluminum from cellular structure of brain to improve memory and rewires neuron pathways; take 500-1000 mg/day

**Glandulars by Standard Process**: Feeds/strengthens internal organs; use specific glandular for specific organ

**Goldenseal Herb**: Kills pathogens toxins; take 2-4 capsules/day for 3-4 days only; repeat again in 30 days if needed

**Hawthorne Berry**: Repairs heart muscle; take 300 mg/day

**HCL Betaine**: Breaks down proteins; flushes toxins out; natural colonic

**Homogenization of Milk/Juice**: Produces sharp texture that damages arteries

**Honey, Raw/Organic**: Heals external ulcers/wounds; taken internally boosts energy and resets the body; local honey regularly taken internally helps eliminate/reduce allergies

**Hyssop Herb**: Recalibrates/clears cells of lungs to open breathing passages; take 300-500 mg/day

**Immuplex by Standard Process**: Use as antibiotic/antivirus

**Inulin Plant-based Powder**: Helps regulate blood sugar

**Iodine**: Blocks radiation uptake; take 1 teaspoon sea salt and North Atlantic kelp with 300 mcg of iodine

**Jerusalem Artichoke**: Helps body absorb blood sugar when eaten every other day

**L-Arginine**: Forms nitric oxide to open arteries and blood vessels, removes cholesterol/plaque

**L-Carnitine**: Weight loss, balances metabolism, improves digestion, aids blood sugar absorption; take 500 mg 2x/day; best when taken with Alpha Lipoic Acid

**L-Citrilline**: Use with L-Arginine to create nitric oxide in blood system

**L-Glutamine**: Increases metabolism, speeds up metabolic conversion of fat to muscle, diuretic; take 500 mg 2x/day or 2x/week for weight maintenance

**Lipoic Acid**: Absorbs blood sugar

**Maca Root:** Balances estrogen and progesterone; take 250-400 mg/day

**Marshmallow Herb:** Fortifies lung alveoli, helps COPD, lung fibrosis; take 1000 mg/day

**Milk Thistle:** Detoxes liver; take daily for 7-10 days every 3-6 months

**Modifilan/Russian Brown Seaweed:** Purges liver, pulls heavy metals from the entire body; take 4 capsules/day, do not take for more than 30 days; do not take if you have metal fillings or other metal body parts

**Myrrh Gum:** Anti-inflammatory

**Nattokinase:** Blood thinner; take 200-500 mg/day; do not take if taking prescription blood thinners

**Olive Leaf Capsules:** Use for intestinal or stomach viruses/bacteria/flu, including food poisoning, ulcers, IBS; take two capsules up to 3x/day

**Olive Gold or Olive Gold Dental Oxygenated Olive Oil:** Topically apply for all body ailments, skin care, deodorant, combine with Organic Coconut Oil for oil pulling in mouth

**Omega-3 Fish Oil:** Natural blood thinner; lubricates joints, aids healthy nerve tissue, promotes maintenance of heart tissue, clears arteries, lubricates the joints; take 2-3000 mg/day

**Oregano Oil:** For intestinal tract and same indications as Olive Leaf Capsule; take 300 mg/day

**Pasteurization Milk/Juice:** Kills nutritional value

**Peppermint Tea:** Helps increase insulin production, cleanses; take one cup in evening

**Pineapple, Fresh:** Reduces pain/swelling/inflammation and aids digestion; before surgery eat 1/3 of a pineapple for 3 days in a row to reduce pain/swelling/inflammation post-op

**ProArgi9**: Opens arteries, helps heart/vascular/blood pressure/triglyceride issues, creates Nitric Oxide to clear out arterial system and repair heart damage; take 1 scoop daily for maintenance or more depending upon severity of issue

**Quercetin**: Blocks allergic reactions from asthma/hay fever/pollen; take 300 mg/day throughout the year regardless of seasonal allergy conditions

**Resveratrol**: Rejuvenates body; revitalizes cells; found in red wine; drink red wine/Pinot Noir or take 1000-1500 mg/day

**Rye Grass Extract**: For asthma; take 20 drops/day under tongue

**Sauerkraut Juice**: For seasickness and nausea; 1 teaspoon/day

**Saw Palmetto**: For prostate health

**Siberian Ginseng**: Revitalizes males

**Silica/Horsetail Herb**: Builds and strengthens visceral body tissue; use for injury/illness; take 500 mg/day

**Stevia Herb Powder**: Balances blood sugar; natural sweetener

**Sylvestre Gymnema**: Aids in blood sugar absorption; take 2x/day but do not combine with other blood sugar-lowering supplements or medications

**Tamarind**: Removes fluoride from body and pineal gland

**Tien Shen Tea**: Stops intestinal bleeding; helps IBD, internal ulcers

**Tribulus**: Increases testosterone level and low sex drive; improves energy in males

**Turmeric**: Reduces body inflammation

**Watermelon, Fresh**: Promotes bladder health

**White Birch Bark**: Anti-inflammatory; take for headaches/migraines

**Wild Yam Root**: Increases progesterone; take 1500 mg/day

## Vitamins

**Vitamin B12:** For nerves, low energy, neuropathy, nerve damage, epileptics, MS; take 5000 mcg/day

**Vitamin C:** For adrenals, immune system; take 1-5 grams/day depending upon body weight and if illness is present; if diarrhea develops, reduce intake until diarrhea stops

**Vitamin C Cream:** Improves skin

**Vitamin D:** Helps bones absorb calcium; dissolves breast cysts, kidney stones, gallstones, eye floaters; take 1000-5000 mg/day depending upon body weight

**Vitamin E:** Improves circulation, arteries and skin: take 400 mg/day

## Essential Oils

Information from:
https://www.doterra.com/US/en   https://www.youngliving.com/en_US

**Frankincense:** Used for muscular aches and pains, scar tissue

**Helichrysum:** Used as an all-around healer, pain relief, bruises, cuts, including open wounds, tendons, scar tissue, burns

**Birch:** Helpful for bone repair, muscular aches and pains, stiffness and tightness, to increase range of motion (you can put this remedy on your bicep), cooling nature. Birch is replacing Wintergreen as a muscular pain relief and in many products it is largely replaced by synthetic methyl salicylate as that is cheaper. Birch contains 98% methyl salicylate. Not to be used if taking warfarin or other salicylate based medications

**Cypress:** Increases circulation

**Lemongrass:** Used for muscular aches and pains, tired and sore muscles, sprains, bruises; to strengthen connective tissue

**Marjoram**: Helpful for muscular and joint aches and pains; increases circulation

**Peppermint**: Used for muscular stiffness, aches and pains, tightness, pain, cooling

**Tea Tree**: Relieves tired, achy muscles and joints

**Rosemary**: Used as muscle relaxant, for aches and pains; also good for respiratory issues, headaches, and memory

## Recipes

### For Ripped Muscles

**Ingredients**

10 drops rosemary

10 drops eucalyptus

5 drops cypress

5 drops thyme

2 tbsp carrier oil (argan, coconut, sesame, sweet almond, jojoba, grapeseed, macadamia)

### Muscle Fatigue Massage Formula

**Ingredients**

10 drops rosemary

10 drops eucalyptus

5 drops cypress

5 drops thyme

2 tbsp carrier oil (argan, coconut, sesame, sweet almond, jojoba, grapeseed, macadamia)

## Muscle Relief Massage Oil

### Ingredients

15 drops juniper

15 drops marjoram

10 drops rosemary

5 drops black pepper

## Over-Exerted Muscles Massage Formula

### Ingredients

5 drops eucalyptus

5 drops ginger

5 drops peppermint

1 tbsp carrier oil (argan, coconut, sesame, sweet almond, jojoba, grapeseed, macadamia)

## Muscle Cramp Massage Oil

### Ingredients

15 drops geranium or lavender

15 drops rosemary

10 drops marjoram

5 drops black pepper or bay laurel

### Alternate blend

5 drops marjoram

5 drops rosemary

5 drops lavender

3 drops black pepper or ginger

5 tsp carrier oil (argan, coconut, sesame, sweet almond, jojoba, grapeseed, macadamia)

### Directions

In a 5 ml glass dropper bottle, combine your oils.

Shake to blend.

Massage a little of this blend into the affected muscles (walking and stretching the muscles will also help).

## SORE MUSCLE MARJORAM LEMON BATH

### Ingredients

3 drops marjoram

2 drops lemon

### Directions

Simply add the essential oils to your bath and enjoy. Be sure to massage your sore muscles while bathing.

## SORE MUSCLE SOAK

### Ingredients

1 cup Epsom salts

3 drops lavender

3 drops juniper

2 drops peppermint

2 drops black pepper

## Rheumatism Blend For Bath Or Massage

Sometimes our sore muscles can arise from inflammatory disorders of the joints and connective tissues (between tendon and bone, or between muscle and muscle).

If you are dealing with more that what you think could be an inflammatory bout of sore muscles, try this blend.

### Ingredients

24 drops cypress

16 drops rosemary or marjoram

12 drops juniper

12 drops roman chamomile

**Important note** —some essential oils are not suitable for pregnant women or people with certain medical conditions. Check with your doctor before using them.

## Oils For Hair Loss

Lavender, peppermint, bhringraj, sesame

Rosemary, argan, almond, castor

Cedarwood, coconut, jojoba, cayenne

Clary, sage

Lemongrass

## Essential Oils

**Chamomile:** is well known for its effective anti-inflammatory properties. Helps to relieve muscle pain and spasms, low back pain, headaches and pain caused by PMS.

**Sweet marjoram**: has sedative properties. Helps to relieve muscle pain and spasms, stiffness, rheumatism, osteoarthritis and migraine.

**Lavender**: this is probably the most famous essential oil for pain relief and relaxation. It has anti-inflammatory, anti-microbial and sedative properties and it helps to relieve muscle tension and spasms, joint pain and headache.

**Eucalyptus**: has analgesic and anti-inflammatory properties. It is one of the top five essential oils for allergy relief. Good for muscle pain and nerve pain. Use in small quantities.

**Peppermint**: good for muscle and joint pain, headache, and nerve pain. Also read my article about the top 10 uses for peppermint essential oil.

**Rosemary**: has analgesic and antispasmodic properties. Good for relieving back pain, muscle and joint pain, and headaches.

**Thyme**: antispasmodic, good for joint and muscle pain as well as backache.

**Clary sage**: has calming and soothing properties as well as anti-spasmodic and anti-inflammatory properties. Helps to ease muscle tension, spasms, and PMS pain. Use in small quantities.

**Sandalwood**: relieves muscle spasms. One of sandalwood's most important uses is to sedate the nervous system, so it helps to reduce nerve pain. Read more about this oil in my article about the best uses for sandalwood essential oil.

**Juniper**: has antispasmodic properties. Relieves nerve pain, joint and muscle aches, and spasms. Also read my article on how to make juniper berry ointment for joint, muscle and arthritis pain relief.

**Ginger**: can ease back pain and improves mobility. Can be used to treat arthritic and rheumatic pain, muscle pain, and sprains.

**Frankincense**: has anti-inflammatory properties and also acts as a mild sedative. It is also used to alleviate stress and relieve pain.

**Yarrow**: a powerful restorative and analgesic pain reliever with powerful anti-inflammatory properties. Good for muscle and joint aches and pains.

**Wintergreen**: this is not a well known essential oil, but it is very effective to treat painful conditions including headache, nerve pain, arthritis, and menstrual cramps. This essential oil is created by steam distilling the leaves, and it contains a very high percentage of methyl salicylate. This oil has pain-relieving properties similar to aspirin (salicylate is the principal component of aspirin).

**Vetiver**: not very known in the West, vetiver has been used since ancient times in Ayurvedic medicine. Vetiver essential oil is extracted from the roots of a grass known as *Vetiveria zizanoides*, which belongs to the same botanical family as lemongrass and citronella. It brings relief to general aches and pains, especially for rheumatism, arthritis, and muscular pain and headache.

**Helichrysum**: this essential oil is quite expensive and valued for its pain relief properties. It has anti-inflammatory, antispasmodic, and analgesic properties. It helps to relieve arthritis pain and supports the nervous system. Pain relief reported by most users happens nearly instantly : certainly within minutes of application. Read more about this oil in my article about the health benefits and best uses of helichrysum essential oil.

# The Top 8 Herbs for Andropause

BY DR. EDWARD GROUP DC, NP, DACBN, DCBCN, DABFM

Last Updated on May 19, 2014

Andropause, or male menopause, is a condition associated with a drop in sexual activity, testosterone levels, and a diminished frequency of normal erections. It is an age related problem and many men are in full swing by middle age. Thankfully, there are natural solutions for combatting the demoralizing effects of andropause. Herbs that have been used for centuries have demonstrated their potent abilities and received validation from modern science. Here are the top 8 herbs for promoting vitality during andropause.

## 1. TRIBULUS TERRESTRIS

A natural aphrodisiac, Tribulus terrestris has been used in various countries for centuries to stimulate libido and promote normal testosterone levels. The plant's active compound, protodioscin, is a precursor to testosterone. As a blood vessel dilator, protodioscin may allow more blood to reach the penis, resulting in a normal, full erection. In animal models, impotent male rats given Tribulus terrestris showed an increased erection frequency.

## 2. Suma

The suma root comes from the suma ground vine, typically found in the rain forests of South America. It is widely used as an herbal tonic for hormone activity and some evidence suggests it is effective for improving libido and sexual response. Ecdysterone, a bioactive compound in suma, may help promote normal hormone levels in men, particularly the sex hormone testosterone, which stimulates male sexual performance. Men suffering from andropause or general sexual dysfunction are among the most popular consumers of suma root.

## 3. Ashwagandha

Also known as "Indian ginseng," Ashwagandha has been used for over 3000 years to remedy various sexual issues. There is some research to suggest that Ashwagandha, especially when combined with Tribulus terrestris, may promote fertility in men. Researchers believe that Ashwagandha helps alleviate stress, which is essential for promoting sperm quality. The herb may also be helpful for encouraging normal energy levels, a common issue that plagues many infertile, impotent, and sexually inactive men.

## 4. Maca

Native to Peru, maca (also known as Peruvian ginseng) has been a favorite aphrodisiac and sexual endurance enhancer for thousands of years. Research has consistently shown maca to produce a significant erectile response. Positive effects on ejaculation rates have also been reported in animal models; and human studies confirm that maca may boost sperm quality.

## 5. Avena sativa

Avena sativa is a potent tool and its benefits for testosterone production, energy enhancement, endurance, and prostate health have been studied in the lab. Compounds in Avena sativa may stimulate luteinizing hormone, the hormone responsible for activating the production of testosterone. Examinations into the use of Avena sativa have found that it offers help for promoting a healthy sexual response, libido, and orgasm frequency.

## 6. Tongkat ali

Another herb with powerful aphrodisiac properties, Tongkat ali has been shown to stimulate libido, semen quality, and muscle growth. These effects are attributed to Tongkat ali's positive effects on testosterone levels. Middle-aged males experiencing menopause may see changes in their sexual health while supplementing with this Malaysian herb!

## 7. Catuaba

Similar to Tribulus terrestris, Catuaba bark promotes a strong and longer-lasting erection by increasing blood flow to the penis. Catuaba may also increase the brain's sensitivity to dopamine, a neurotransmitter that enhances the pleasurable effects experienced during sex.

## 8. Muira puama

Studies have shown that Muira puama, an herb native to Brazil, may promote blood flow to support the chances of having a normal erection. Men who are experiencing andropause often seek out Muira puama for this reason, and its ability to increase sexual desire and satisfaction.

## A Final Thought

Whether it is reducing stress or promoting blood flow or testosterone levels, there are plenty of natural aphrodisiacs for supporting sexual health. Getting enough exercise and sleep are also integral for battling the early onset of andropause symptoms.

# Part III

# Addicted to Addictions

Most people think addictions are just alcohol or drugs, but addictions cover many more categories.

An official definition of addiction according to the American Society of Addiction Medicine https://www.asam.org/resources/definition-of-addiction

> addiction is a primary chronic disease.
>
> Addiction is considered a disease of brain reward, motivation, memory and related circuitry. Dysfunction in these circuits leads to characteristic biological, psychological, social, and spiritual manifestations. Basically an addiction means that your brain is wired incorrectly and you have strange characteristics that lead to these addictions.
>
> This is reflected in an individual pathologically pursuing reward or relief by substance abuse or other behaviors.

Pathological in this case means you have a mental issue because of a brain malfunction. It is defined in this way so that a general diagnosis can be made. Next, the official definition says:

> addiction is characterized by the inability to consistently abstain impairment and behavioral control, craving diminished recognition of significant problems and one's

behaviors and interpersonal relationships and a dysfunctional emotional response.

Like other chronic diseases addiction often involves cycles of relapse and remission, so in a way addiction is kind of like cancer. Without treatment or engagement in recovery activities addiction is progressive and can result in disability or premature death. Genetic factors account for half of the likelihood that an individual will develop addiction.

This means that environmental factors interact with a person's biology, thus affecting the extent to which genetic vectors exert their influence. Additionally, this means that you have a genetic predisposition to be addicted to something and that your environment opens up that genetic factor.

Biological deficits, in other words factors in your body that make you want a certain thing. Neural adaptation which means as you get addicted your body and your brain rewire itself so that the addictive substance becomes part of your necessity. Cognitive distortions that appear as perceptions, so you think one thing but it really is not that.

Everyone has exposure to trauma and stressors. Addicted persons distort the meaning and purpose of their coping abilities as well as their thinking and behavior.

This official definition refers to the distortion of the connection of Self, often referred to as "God" by many, the "Higher Power" by the 12 steps groups or "higher consciousness" by others.

There is often the presence of co-occurring psychiatric disorders in persons who engage in substance use or other addictive behaviors, meaning that they have more than one mental issue.

Here are the general characteristics of addictions:

> An addicted person is unable to consistently abstain from their addiction, they have an impairment in behavioral control, they have a craving or increased hunger for drugs or rewarding experiences. Diminished recognition of significant problems with ones behaviors and interpersonal relationships, and they have a dysfunctional emotional response.

So basically they do not have the ability to make decisions or handle their life or other people and do not know how to interact with others.

It says also:

> in an addicted person there is an increased disorder in the hippocampus which involves the memory of previous euphoric or dysphoric experiences and that connects with the amadala with having motivation concentration on selecting behaviors.

They are just saying how addiction affects different parts of the brain and the different functions. There is also a persistent risk of reoccurrence or relapse. We know this is true; we will get to why.

And it continues on to say:

> impairment in executive functioning which they say represents perception, learning, impulse control, compulsivity and judgment. also manifests a lower readiness to change their dysfunction

In other words, these people are not ready or do not want to change their behavior despite the concerns of the significant others in their lives. So even when people warn them or try to help them it does not make a difference.

> And there is an apparent lack of appreciation of the magnitude of cumulative problems and complications.

They do not realize the damage they are doing to themselves and others and its cumulative effects. These are all the characteristics of addiction and of addictive personalities.

On the emotional level it says:

**there is increased anxiety, dysphoria**

which means the opposite of euphoria; they are very unhappy

**and there is emotional pain. There is also increased sensitivity to stressors**

This means life events that you might accept casually, an addict may react to intensely and with a great deal of trouble.

**And difficulty identifying feelings and distinguishing between feelings and bodily sensations.**

In other words, what their body feels and what they emotionally feel are the same. They do not make a distinction between hurting an arm or being harmed emotionally; to them it is all the same and they react in the same way, according to this official definition.

Official definitions correlate addictions to a brain malfunction rather than a thought/mind-pattern.

Now that you understand the official explanation of addictions, can you see yourself in any way? Do you have some sort of addiction?

Remember addiction does not mean, "I am addicted to a thing." Addictions can be spiritual, emotional, mental, and/or physical.

People with addictions have ambivalence, which means they can be angry one moment and happy the next minute, or they may not feel anything. They have a great deal of guilt, which is a primary factor in addictions.

People who are addicted to abuse actually feel guilty about betraying their abuser. That is why women do not leave their abusive husbands and vice versa. Abused people feel emptiness and isolation as well as a separation from their sense of Self. These people really do not know who they are; they have no self-identity so they feel isolated.

Many have sexual confusion; they may have impulses that are contradictory and conflicted because they do not have enough sense of identity as well as an impaired ability to trust.

They may have identity and role reversal, feeling that they are manipulated into their abuse and addiction. Most of them have suppressed rage because many addicted people are survivors of incest, rape, or physical abuse. Victims often must deny or suppress their anger.

A common factor that is extremely important is that they may not reveal the trauma they experienced that led them to the addiction. This may result in deep and powerful rage, which they are unable to talk about or even acknowledge.

When children are punished, some are punished a second time for reacting to the first punishment. They are never allowed to express themselves in the home. For example, a child who is slapped or hit, then cries, is told not to cry or he/she will be slapped or hit again for crying. If the child continues to cry, he/she is slapped or hit again, which continues the abuse.

This creates a cycle in which the person is stuck. Sometimes people do not even know they have anger because they were never allowed to express it. Suppressing anger becomes normal because it is all they have ever felt.

What you do not talk about gets suppressed. Like a spring, the more you push the spring down, the more force it gathers; when the spring finally does release, it explodes. Hyperspace/Oversoul work is so important because you must discover what underlies your issues.

If you were never allowed to express your angers, feelings, or thoughts or you just feel beaten down, you may have inner rage that you have not touched yet, buried so deep you do not really know it is there. These feelings and emotions can be crucial underlying factors.

Compare this to the analogy of a person who sits in an ice cold bath for so long that the body becomes so numb that he/she does not realize the extreme cold. When you have anger for so many years, the feeling is so normal that you do not realize it is there.

These underlying feelings and emotions can lead to depression as well as irrational guilt or shame; this then can lead to feelings of hopelessness, helplessness and suicidal thoughts.

People can become addicted to the depression, which then becomes cognitive dysfunction meaning not being able to think properly. They can lose the ability to concentrate, so focus lessens and they can become easily disturbed.

These people may have flashbacks, unbidden images, nightmares, intrusive thoughts, and symptoms of Post Traumatic Stress Syndrome (PTSD), all of which may or may not be programming. PTSD seems to be a common cover diagnosis that is used just like COPD.

When the medical community does not know the underlying cause of something, it often resorts to these types of diagnoses. Official information about addiction often focuses on abuse as the cause of addiction, saying that abuse can be exceedingly painful therefore a victim may deny, rationalize, minimize, or distort the meaning of the experience.

For this reason, addicted people turn to something else that provides immediate relief or comfort. When they receive that comfort they continually do that behavior even though they know it is incorrect and killing them. They do not want to feel the pain of the memory and experience.

Self-identity is also an issue for people with addictions. This often starts in childhood because in some way their identity is formed by people around them as they try to please others instead of themselves. For this reason they do not know who they are, thus prompting inner rage.

Their identity is now defined by what others made them so even when they explore their own deep energetic levels, they do not understand their addictions because their thoughts and feelings have been pushed down so deep for so long. Who they are now is all they know, meaning they create a looping cycle of Self-exploration that is extremely challenging to stop.

Addicted people often have significant low Self-esteem, lack Self-confidence, and may be exceedingly Self-critical and Self-blaming. If others have criticized and blamed them, the abused person continues the process to Self even in the absence of the abuser. This creates a cycle of guilt and shame that further entrenches them in the loop of addiction as they seek to find comfort somewhere from something or someone.

This looping creates addictions to such things as alcohol, drugs, and sex. Rather than understand or feel compassion for the addicted people, society judges and criticizes them even more for these behaviors. The societal judges give the impression that "we are perfect and you are not," so this further distorts the addicted feelings about what is right or wrong.

## BOUNDARIES

Boundaries are extremely important. As you read through this list, ask your Self if you have any signs of unhealthy boundaries.

1. Telling all. Loose lips sink ships.

2. Sharing intimate details with recent acquaintances or strangers.

3. Being overwhelmed by or preoccupied by another person.

4. Being sexual for others and not yourself.

5. Being nonsexual or asexual for others and not yourself.

6. Going against personal values or rights to please others.

7. Not noticing or disregarding when someone else displays inappropriate boundaries.

8. Not noticing or disregarding when someone invades your boundaries; if someone is touching you, puts their arms around you, gets right up in your face, and/or shares inappropriate verbiage.

9. Accepting food, gifts, touch, or sex that you do not want.

10. Being touched by another person without giving permission.

11. Giving as much as you can for the sake of giving.

12. Taking as much as you can for the sake of taking.

13. Allowing someone to take as much as they can from you.

14. Letting others direct your life or the lives of your children or other loved ones.

15. Letting others define you. This typically goes for everyone, especially when you were growing up if you had religious people telling you what to be.

16. Letting others describe your reality. When someone says, "Well, this is what you really are thinking."

17. Believing others can anticipate your needs.

18. Believing you must anticipate the needs of others, especially if you have children or are taking care of other people.

19. Practicing Self-abuse, Self-harm, or Self-mortification including cutting or some other way to hurt your Self.

20. Allowing sexual or physical abuse; you allow this to happen because you do not have boundaries.

21. Being deprived of food and/or sleep, either by others or via Self-deprivation.

22. Being unable to separate your needs from those of others.

How many of these types of boundary issues do you have?

Remember that you have a variety of Protection Techniques that you can use to create a secure energetic boundary. These can be found in **Hyperspace Helper, Hyperspace Plus, Healing Archetypes & Symbols**, and **Decoding Your Life**.

Most of the population has energy fields that are all over the place; people have no idea where they start or where they stop so they think that everything is theirs. You must learn and respect your own boundaries first; then you learn to respect the boundaries of others.

Many people are sensitive to even a slight touch because they have been inappropriately touched or physically abused. You have to stop and think about these possibilities when considering boundaries. What may be acceptable with you may not be tolerated by someone else.

Always remember to ask your Oversoul before you open your mouth or move your body. In this way, you are more likely to be respectful of the boundaries of others in the same way that you want others to be respectful of your boundaries.

For example, you may kindly put your arm around someone or touch his/her arm, thinking that you are making a friendly gesture. But what is positive to you may be negative to the other person, making them cringe and wish that you would stop touching them.

You may not know the reason, but you do need to follow whatever is most correct and beneficial in each and every situation. It only takes a nanosecond to ask your Oversoul so that you remain respectful of other people and what each uniquely requires.

Conversely, you can have Isolation Programming where you actually close everybody out to the point of paranoia. Or you may vacillate between strong boundaries and no boundaries. This is important to look at so you can understand why you react as you do.

People with boundary issues may walk around in fear, yet they do not want you to see what they are trying to hide. Abused people were/are the focal point of their abuser, so if you look at them they may feel threatened. As the focal point of their abuser, they may feel as if they are on stage waiting for something to happen.

If someone uninvitingly touches you, it is important to tell them to stop. You do not have to explain your Self to anyone. You can say, "Please don't," and then move away.

When someone starts touching you inappropriately, you may freeze and not know what to do; when you freeze you either hold your breath or your breathing becomes shallow.

Without enough oxygen, your brain cannot properly function so you cannot clearly respond. Remember that your brain is your most oxygen intensive organ. You must breathe deeply to give your brain oxygen for clear thinking to happen.

The breathing work taught in **Decoding Your Life** automatically pulls you into your center, grounding you in your Oversoul and God-Mind, thus giving you a ready reference point from which to appropriately respond.

Anytime you let someone else direct your response, they have control of you and your boundaries are overstepped. **Decoding Your Life** is an important book of Universal Law to give you practical direction to help smooth out your everyday life. This book teaches you how to handle what is in front of you now so that when bigger issues arise, your foundation is firmly in place. Please also watch the "Self-Healing Webinars" series based on this book, free to members of www.expansions.com

Hyperspace/Oversoul work helps you establish energetic boundaries that mean on some level your energetic boundaries are seen by others. Without physically saying anything, your boundaries are automatically respected.

Where in your life have your boundaries been breached?

Maybe to the point you felt like you could not have any boundaries, or you had inappropriate boundaries?

Perhaps you found comfort in the breach of your boundaries because this is what you knew/know?

A breach of boundaries is where you are invaded by something inappropriate that hurts you. Then that hurt leads to the addiction of comfort. This is why you need to think about your childhood and even recent events.

Where have your boundaries been affected that led you to think, "If I had this or that, this or that will make me feel better"?

You are always going to be affected until you fix your boundaries. Life will get "worse" because the magnification of your issue becomes bigger and bigger until you find a way to correct it. When you decide to correct your issue you must take a look at your weaknesses and strengths.

Determine your weaknesses so you can build them up. Use your strengths to help you, and then create a balance of body, mind, and soul. You, like most people, are likely unknowingly addicted to many, many things. This is why it is important to work on consciously developing an awareness of your addictions so you can correct them and balance the mind-pattern.

Even the words that you choose are clues to what is going on inside and why. The words you choose are frequencies that when combined with your physical actions create archetypes. Every way you express says something about you.

This is another reason to become an objective observer of Self as taught in **Decoding Your Life**. The idea is simple but you must be willing to see Self as is vs. how you think Self is. Once you understand what you are doing, saying, and why, then you realize that you have choices. It all starts with basic foundational inner level work.

As an adult, you may think that you are always supposed to know what to do. If you do not know what to do, then there is something wrong with you. As a child, you may have had expectations placed upon you by adults that you could not fulfill.

This is another mind-pattern that is then carried forward into adulthood. You feel like you must be in control of all situations, continuing to try to fulfill childhood expectations. There are always situations in life where you feel you have no control, so you find aspects that you can control. When you are in control in some way, somehow you feel you are okay.

## Addictions, Obsessions & Cravings

Addictions start deeply at the mind-pattern level, most often related to abuse of some kind. Addiction becomes a need; there is no alternative; there is no logic; there is only an amazingly strong impulse and compulsion that propels you.

Addiction is "I cannot live without something; I must have it," almost to the point of negating the rest of your life. Some people feel like they want to kill others to get whatever it is they think they need; some people become suicidal without it.

Addictions are all about other things having control or power over you. A gambler is going into a casino because the casino has power and control over him/her. A drug addict will take a drug if you place in on the table in front of him/her. If you cannot leave a piece of chocolate or sugar alone when it is in front of you, then that chocolate or sugar has power and control over you.

The outer world has power and control over you when you think that your happiness is dependent on something outside of your Self. You give your power to be happy, calm, satisfied, and so forth to something or someone else.

Most addictions involve the animal mind having more control of you than your Spiritual Mind. Then, you give your power to your animal mind. Removing addiction concerns your Spiritual Mind taking control and taking your power back. Anytime you depend on somebody or anything outside of "Self" you have an addiction.

When a person has an addiction to anything external from Self, if the individual can no longer access the object of their addiction, they may become violent or go into suicide mode.

An obsession can be controlled. You might have an obsession for coffee but if you do not have it, you can live without it. If you were addicted you would *have* to have it. If you crave coffee you just have a taste for it; tomorrow you may not desire it at all.

Obsessions can become addictions so it is important that you recognize these next categories to identify if you have a craving, obsession, or addiction. When you identify a craving you can monitor your Self so the craving does not turn into an obsession. In the same way, an obsession can turn into an addiction. Additionally, because programming is built upon what already exists within you, programming can kick in, which complicates removing whatever negative mind-pattern underlies it all.

Just as in programming, many of these addictions have overlaps as well as more than one addiction. A drug addict may also be a money addict because he/she needs money to get drugs. Or he/she might need sex to get drugs, alcohol, or whatever it is.

In a way an addiction can be a step to healing as long as you do not stay in the addiction. An addiction is really a loop from which you do not voluntarily extricate your Self.

When you are addicted to these old mind-patterns you might move from Point A to Point B. You might be better off at Point B, and think that you are "done" but you are not; you must keep your Self moving forward until you reach an inner balance.

Based on the following addictions, think about what addictions you have that you have not labeled as such. Is there any thing, place, or person that you cannot live without? If so, then that person, place, or thing has power and control over you, meaning you have an addiction that needs to be corrected.

When you observe others with addictions, it is important to remember that everyone is a reflection of you: past, present and/or future.

Be mindful not to judge or criticize because this person could be you or could have been you, or maybe was you depending upon where you are in your life. Have compassion for others as well as for Self at all times. No matter how high you are, you can fall back. You must always remain vigilant and grateful for your own internal progress. "There but for the Grace of God, go I."

## Physical Addictions

### Food

This could be either a specific food or food in general. If you have an addiction to a specific food, think about what that food represents to you. Put the image of the food at your pineal gland to see what images appear.

### Alcohol

What kind of alcohol? Is it specific or does it matter? Sometimes alcohol can be connected to childhood, either positive or negative, with a desire to recreate the memories.

### Smoking

Cigarettes, cigars, pipes, or hookahs? Some people smoke to reward themselves for something. Smoking grounds and balances but you can do the same thing by flooding the energetic field with the color Brown without any negative side effects.

## Drugs

If you are addicted to a drug, you may think that you are not. Some people believe they need an aspirin every day. Others may have a need for antacids, antihistamines, nasal spray, and/or laxatives. You may consider these harmless but they are drugs, too.

Marijuana is a separate category because it is legal in some places. Keep in mind that it destroys your chromosomes, brain cells, and the liver. Artificial/synthetic marijuana can be lethal as well as induce mental crises and brain damage from which people never fully recover.

Anyone with a drug addiction perceives they receive a benefit even though it may be a negative benefit. You must always ask what is this doing for you and what do you think you are getting from it?

## Prescriptions

Some people are addicted to collecting prescriptions; they just want to have them, even if the scripts are never filled. They have a need to go to a doctor and get something.

## Healthcare Professionals

Some people who are chronically ill are addicted to their doctors. They constantly must be in contact with their physician; perhaps they want constant medical testing whether they truly need it or not.

You can be addicted to your massage therapist or chiropractor; if you do not go every week or month then you have a problem. If you think, "If I miss an appointment I am going downhill," then you have an issue.

Some people are addicted to their kinesiologist; they cannot make a choice until they take their supplements or medications for testing. They are addicted to their supplements/medication, the methodology, and the kinesiologist.

Most people repeatedly describe the same problems to the same person to receive basically the same answers, when you really can answer your own questions. Use your healthcare professionals as needed but eventually your goal is to go within instead of without.

When you are whole and complete within, you do not need a person, place, or thing to feel fulfilled. You can use other people, places, and things to boost your mind-pattern or to help open new frequencies but eventually your goal is always about turning within.

Because you have an animal body you are dealing with what you need to get the body into balance. This is different than an addiction because you know that the ultimate answers always lie within.

## Diet

Diet means not only *what* you eat but also *how* you eat. This is different than a food addiction. Some people are so strict on their diets that they make themselves sick instead of healthy. Or they can only eat specific foods, or specific food combinations, or food can only be eaten in specific order. Some people get disturbed if one food touches another food.

## Sleep

People can be addicted to sleeping, usually because they do not want to participate in the world. Sleeping too much is a way to escape your life. This can also be a sign of severe depression.

## Exercise

Exercise can be a huge addiction. Some people exercise many hours every day. If they do not exercise they feel like something is wrong and they cannot function. Some people literally exercise themselves to death, shrinking away to nothing all the while thinking that they look great.

## VITAMINS & SUPPLEMENTS

If you cannot go a day or two without taking your vitamins and supplements then you have an addiction. If you fear running out of them or if you actually do run out of them and become panicky or paranoid that something bad will happen to you without them, you have an addiction.

## SEX

Sex addictions get many people into trouble. Please read ***True Reality of Sexuality*** to understand how the orgasmic release is really a replication of the creative process of the God-Mind. There is a reason sex has such a powerful hold not only on the mind but also on the body. When the animal mind is control, it must have sex to keep the species alive.

## TALKING

If you or someone you know cannot stop talking, there is a reason. Usually this type of person is full of fear; talking helps avoid facing Self or personal feelings; he/she may need to be the center of attention; perhaps there is a fear of silence, or all of these. There can also be a lack of filter from thought process to speaking that enhances the addiction.

## MONEY & FINANCES

People addicted to money often wind up without any or even without their health. They must learn that there are some things that money cannot buy; that health cannot be bought. Sometimes these kinds of people are dishonest; they take advantage of others but cannot admit that their actions are harmful.

## Material Objects

Hoarders are individuals who collect things incessantly. They must collect and hoard. What they are addicted to hoarding says something about their personalities. For example, someone who is addicted to tools has a mind-pattern of needing to fix Self. They get the physical tools to represent the inner tools that they do not have. Because they do not know how to fix the inner, they hoard the outer representation of their inner needs.

## Coupons

Some people only buy products with coupons or on sale, stocking the closets to the ceiling. Trying to get something for nothing indicates a mind-pattern of lack and low self-worth. You have no value for Self so nothing has value, therefore items must be purchased for nothing. These individuals feel undeserving and "less than" so they must purchase items for "less than" their worth.

Usually you will not find wealthy people shopping at discount stores or using coupons. If you are at a restaurant and have to ask the prices then you should not be there. This mind-pattern says that you always expect and know that you have as much as you want all the time.

## Debt

Feeling lack in your life makes you overcompensate by wanting and buying everything. To clear this mind-pattern you have to ask your Self to what or whom do you feel indebted?

## Saving & Preservation

This comes from a mind-pattern of lack and fear of losing what you have as well as distrust in Source to provide. In this case, people buy things and never/rarely use them. For example, a wealthy family from Germany and Austria lost everything in WWII so they came to America.

They bought a lovely three-story home but only lived in the basement; the rest of the house was like a museum. They covered everything in plastic; you could look in a room but you were not allowed to go in or touch anything. The family stayed in a small space during the day; at night they allowed themselves to go in the bedrooms.

Remember that objects do not have any life when they are preserved. Things do not grow; if that family would have utilized the house they might have opened up their mind-pattern to allow more in.

When wealthy people do not share or spend their money they can find themselves too sick to enjoy it or perhaps their life ends when they are too young to have enjoyed the fruits of their labor. Restrictive mind-patterns can be from low Self-worth/value.

Accumulation of anything without using it, even knowledge, is breaking Universal Law. Accumulation restricts or stops flow. God-Mind is about movement. Allowing movement/flow allows whatever you have to increase.

## Weather

People who are addicted to weather and weather information often operate out of fear. Perhaps as a child they lived in an area where there were tornadoes or hurricanes that caused power failure, destruction, and even death. Knowing what is going on with the weather may make the addict feel like he/she is more in control of his/her life. This can also be a result of programming; for example, tornadoes represent vortices. People who are addicted to chasing tornadoes may be reacting to internal programming.

## Clothing

Clothing represents what you present to the world, so if you have an issue with self-identity and you really do not know who you are, you want many different looks to show others who and what you are in that moment. If your addiction to clothing comes from programming, keep in mind that different alters wear different styles or colors of clothing.

## Travel

Travel addictions usually come from a mind-pattern of escapism or feelings of not belonging anywhere. Some people cannot stay home; they may travel around their neighborhood, state, country, or the world. They always have to be going somewhere.

Some people use travel as a reward. They often get home from one trip to plan another with the thought that they have something to which they can look forward. This is still living in the future/escapism vs. enjoying the Eternal Now. Travel becomes their motivation for living.

## Smell

You can be addicted to a variety of smells to the extent where the smell has control over you. The smell may be a trigger for a physical or emotional action/reaction.

Some people can intuitively "smell" if someone is a positive or negative person on the Oversoul level. You should be able to comfortably go anywhere regardless of positive or negative physical or intuitive smell.

## Color

If you can only wear one color, specific colors, or specific color combinations, you need to look at the mind-pattern behind the color/s that you choose. Ultimately the color, and/or the pattern on the clothing if there is one, is reflective of your mind-pattern.

Colors can pull your mind-pattern backwards, hold you where you are, or pull you forward. Once you know why you choose the color/s you do then you can make conscious choices.

## Pets

An addiction to pets is an addiction to animal mind. Maybe when you were a child you were not allowed to have pets, so you felt left out. Now as an adult you cannot stop collecting pets. Or, you may be addicted to only one pet.

This is because you are looking to the animal to love you instead of your Spiritual Mind as well as your Oversoul and God-Mind.

Pets love you unconditionally no matter what. Sometimes people have such a need to be loved that when they adopt a pet they burst out crying. The love they feel from the animal overwhelms them; the love they feel toward the animal overwhelms them. Feeling unconditional love for Self is the next step.

If you have a pet that is addicted to anything, you need to look at what this is because pets are always a reflection of the person to whom they belong.

## Plants

Plants represent whatever is growing within you. If you are addicted to plants you have to think about what mind-pattern they represent inside of you. Do you take time to bring your ideas to fruition? Do you have ideas growing inside that often die? Do you have so many ideas that you cannot take care of them all? Or do you have one or two ideas that are your sole focus in life?

Plants have to be watered, repotted, trimmed, fertilized, and planted in the correct soil in the correct environment with the correct temperatures and amount of light. Just like you!

## Friends & Family

People who are lonely with no self-identity are often addicted to connecting with other identities to feel like they are somebody. This means the more "friends" the better; these kinds of people may even be "for sale" meaning you can buy their loyalty with money, things, or even emotional rewards.

Animals travel in packs so if you are in your animal mind you need many animals around you, continuing to affirm your animal status rather than your status as a Spiritual Being.

Some people are especially addicted to their children or to other relatives. They must stay connected; they cannot let go even when it is correct to do so. Anytime you feel driven to stay connected to someone you must look at the mind-pattern that creates this within.

## BATHROOM & CLEANING

If you are addicted to using a bathroom every time you see one, you have a mind-pattern of needing to release old experiences.

If you must wash your hands or take showers constantly, you may have an addiction to washing and you may also have germophobia.

If you feel dirty for whatever reason it is highly likely that you had a trauma that left you feeling like you were unclean, even if the trauma was many years ago. You constantly try to clean the physical body because inside you feel dirty.

Sexually abused people often feel dirty. Sexual abuse does not necessarily mean that you had sex. Sexual abuse includes inappropriate touching as well as inappropriate verbiage.

People who feel dirty and/or violated do not want their space violated so they may be especially fastidious, always trying to clean up their environment.

## FIRE & PYROMANIA

Psychologically pyromania is a mental illness, but it is also an addiction to fire. Pyromaniacs need to see, feel, and know about fire. The mind-pattern that creates this is one of anger and the need to transmute something.

This means that there is something within that has to be changed related to anger. Since the individuals cannot or do not know how to change within, they must change what is around them with fire.

## TEMPERATURE

Some people must be in a specific temperature to be comfortable. They may need the thermostat set to an exact temperature that can never be changed. Or, they may always need to feel hot or always need to feel cold.

There can be many reasons for this. One reason may be an unwillingness to change. To determine the exact cause, place the temperature you require at your pineal gland and do the Green Spiral Staircase visualization from **Hyperspace Helper**. Do your best to remember when this addiction started where you could only find relief and security in this specific temperature.

## ICE

Some people must always have an ice cube in their mouth or their drink. Ice represents frozen emotions. People who always keep ice in their mouths are blocking what they have to say. If they do not have ice in their mouths they might say something they regret. Blood sugar issues can be present in people who need to constantly chew on ice, so anyone who does this should consult a healthcare professional.

## WATER

Constantly drinking or sipping water comes from a mind-pattern of trying to flush things out of your body and thus out of your mind. You most likely do not know exactly what it is, but it could be an emotion or a memory that goes back to using a bottle as a baby or something to do with mouth satisfaction.

People who always need to be around a body of water like an ocean, lake, pond, or river may be addicted to their emotions. However, water is also an amplifier so this can help you sort through emotions that you are releasing or against you to make your emotions even more painful.

## Technology

Technology includes computers, televisions, video games, cell phones, and mobile devices. Everywhere you go, people are texting, listening, speaking, or staring at a screen. This can be a lack of Self-identity so they must be connected to something at all times. Without a conscious internal connection they connect externally.

Technology addiction is a diversion that distracts your thinking so you do not have to face your Self.

Electronic devices can change your brainwaves; it is important for everyone to regularly take a break from technology for at least a short period of time.

## Gambling & Risk

Gambling and risk-taking provide excitement as well as an adrenaline rush, to which you can physically become addicted.

People who are addicted to gambling and risk-taking generally have a past or present filled with high drama and abuse. Additionally there is a sense of accomplishment or gratification that they survived the experience.

The mind-pattern behind this is Self-destruction and even suicide.

## Light & Dark

Some people can only be in the light or in the dark. Regardless of the time of day or weather outside, the inside light is always the same.

Someone who always needs the lights on is afraid of the dark, most likely because of trauma that happened in the dark.

On the contrary, people who have to be in the dark want to hide from something that is inside of Self.

## Profanity

Using foul language involves deep inner anger. Pay attention to the exact words the person uses, as these are clues to why he/she has to express this way in the outer world. Trauma somewhere along the way is being verbally expressed. He/she is telling you something about his/her past/present that you need to know. There is a need to get this inner trauma out, so saying these specific words becomes an addiction.

## Abuse

Self-abuse, being abused, and abusing others are all addictions. If you are abused since childhood, this is all you know and abuse becomes normal in your world.

Without the abuse these people feel like something is not right. They feel the need to be punished because they have always been punished. The abused person unconsciously creates the circumstance so they can continue to be abused/punished. With a mind-pattern of low Self-worth, abuse is what they feel they deserve.

## Depravation & Starvation

People who deprive or starve themselves have a mind-pattern of Self-punishment and low Self-worth. They may have money but will not buy food or anything else for themselves. They may buy for others, but not for themselves.

Anorexia may be a result of this addiction because the unconscious goal is to hurt Self. If someone else is not abusing or punishing you, you abuse and punish yourself. This turns into an addictive behavior because you feel relief after the punishment.

## Lying

Compulsive lying comes from many mind-patterns including low Self-worth and Self-preservation. Perhaps as a child you were accused of something you did not do, or perhaps you feared the punishment. Maybe lying was the only way you could get what you wanted. Success for any of these reasons means you do it again and again until it is a way of life—you are addicted to lying.

Some people lie so much that they lose the truth. Their lies become their truth until even they believe their own lies. The truth is now buried so deep within that they can no longer reach it.

## Fighting & Arguing

These people do not even care if they are right or wrong, they just want to fight. This means that there is an inner mental and/or emotional conflict within themselves that they are constantly battling. Their outer battling is a reflection of the inner battle that they cannot resolve. Perhaps they have been confronted all of their lives so they had to fight and argue for survival on some level. This can also indicate a childhood of some kind of abuse. These kinds of people may also be addicted to drama and manipulation.

## Emotional Addictions

### Low Self-Worth

When you feel you have no value, you attract abuse so you can continue to feel bad about your Self. This becomes a cycle to which you become addicted because this is what you know. Low Self-worth is the biggest emotional addiction, underlying almost all other addictions.

People who are chronically ill will say that they do not want to be chronically ill. Yet, this gets them attention. If you say, "You are chronically ill because you want attention," most likely that person will disagree.

In the same way, if you ask a person with low Self-worth "Do you really want to be this way?" the person will answer "No!" but continue with the same behaviors until he/she is able to really look at Self from deep within.

## FEAR

Fear underlies most addictions. People are afraid so they look for comfort in some person, place, or thing. Paranoia is a form of fear, including panic attacks that have physical symptoms. The physical symptoms are a projection of what is happening within the mind.

## ANGER & RAGE

Society is designed to make you angry and push you into rage. Media everywhere shows you something to feed your inner angers to the point where you violently do something about it. People talk about peace because this is what they are looking for; inside they have deep anger and rage or the media could not pull this out of them. In general, society is addicted to anger and rage.

## HURT

People who are hurt in childhood may especially feel like everyone is against them. They expect people to disappoint and hurt them, so this is what their mind-pattern pulls them. They think that they are supposed to feel hurt, so either they hurt themselves or they attract people who hurt them. This supports the addictive behavior of hurt.

## SELF-PUNISHMENT

Self-punishment includes such emotions as anger, hurt, fear, abuse, and low Self-worth is self-punishment. There are many forms of self-punishment. You can punish yourself by living in a place that does not match your frequency so you miserably struggle all the time. This is Self-punishment. You can move somewhere else; the only person stopping you is you.

Even when you live in a geographic location that matches your frequency, you may be unhappy. Here, you still have issues but the energies surrounding you are supportive of resolving these issues. Again, the only person stopping you from resolving your issues is you.

## Self-Sabotage

Self-sabotage happens when everything is going well and then on some level you do something that stops the positive direction from continuing. This stems from low Self-worth, the need to Self-punish, and even fear of success and/or change.

For example, people always say they want to come to Expansions' seminars and events, but something interferes and they cannot attend. They fear that if they attend life will change and they do not want to let go of old mind-patterns to which they are addicted.

## Guilt

People who are addicted to guilt often want you to be addicted to guilt, too. The person feels bad about him/her Self so he/she wants you to feel bad as well. The person may try to make you feel guilty that you made him/her feel bad even though the person did it to him/her Self. People who are addicted to guilt are often experts at perpetuating this loop not only for themselves but for others, too.

## Depression

Some people must be depressed to feel normal. This gets them attention and can be used as an excuse from participating in daily activities. This addiction can pull you in deeper and deeper until you can barely function. Some people rely on medications to help them cope, but sooner or later it is important to face the reason for the addiction to depression.

## ABANDONMENT & ISOLATION

Many people who are addicted to abandonment and isolation say that they are fine even when they are not. As stated in ***True Reality of Sexuality***, you are not meant to be "A-Lone" because on some level people are "All-One."

If this is your addiction, you have to look at where you abandon and isolate Self; where this imprinting came from and why; why you accept this as your fate; where you feel lost inside. As with all addictions, no one can do the inner work for you, but you are supported by your Oversoul and God-Mind at all times. Even when you feel abandoned and isolated you can never be separated from Source.

## VULNERABILITY

Being addicted to vulnerability fulfills other addictions of anger, hurt, sabotage, Self-punishment, abuse, abandonment, and isolation. You feel that no matter what you do or whom you help, you are the scapegoat for everyone and everything. This means on top of everything else, you need to look at your energetic and physical borders and boundaries so that you stop allowing others to take advantage of you.

## VICTIMIZATION

If you live on this planet, you are addicted to victimization. Overcoming victimization addiction means overcoming all of your other emotional and physical addictions as well.

Some people want to blame their victimization on others, even demonic forces. However, you cannot be a victim of anyone or anything unless there is something in your mind-pattern that allows it.

You always must look at the part your own mind-pattern plays in whatever situation you find your Self. Blaming others is the easy route; looking within takes fortitude and courage.

## Worry

Addiction to worry has the underlying addiction to fear; worry/fear that something is going to happen to someone or something that you love and care about, including Self. For this reason, addiction to worry is usually tied into love.

When you worry about someone you love, you are really trying to control their thoughts or actions. Everyone must have his/her experience. You have to give them to God for safe-keeping knowing that each person must do what is most correct and beneficial for him/her regardless of what you think should or should not happen to them.

Worry does not equal love.

## Confusion & Doubt

Some people are addicted to living in a state of confusion and/or doubt. The benefit to this addiction is that they do not have to make a decision. This often comes out of abusive relationships where Self-identity is lost. Therefore you cannot easily make a decision because any decision you make may lead to punishment of some kind.

## Shame & Embarrassment

Shame and/or embarrassment bring attention, so some people are addicted to these. Plus, it makes them feel bad at the same time, like a punishment that others watch.

Facial tattoos, for example, bring attention. People may not really like to have tattoos on their faces but this shame/embarrassment is worth it to gain the attention they seek. In this way, their shame/embarrassment actually makes them happy

Perhaps they were shamed as a child by someone they loved so they may even associate shame/embarrassment with love.

People who make fun of themselves in Self-deprecating ways were also often ridiculed in childhood, so they make fun of themselves first before someone else can do it.

## CRITICISM & JUDGMENT

If you must constantly criticize and/or judge, you are addicted to this behavior. No matter what anyone says or does, if you must always add a negative comment then you have an issue.

## FALSE SENSE OF SECURITY

False sense of security is an avoidance of truth. Rather than accept the reality of your situation so you can do something about it, you continue to tell Self and others that all is well, when it is not.

## HAPPINESS & HEDONISM

Some people laugh at everything, convincing themselves that they are happy when they are not. They have so many layers of issues buried so deeply that they cannot face that they simply tell themselves they are happy, no matter what.

Conversely, some people are addicted to finding happiness, usually from something outer rather than inner. They think, "I will be happy when…"

Hedonism is another addiction where you constantly look for pleasure as a means to happiness.

## JEALOUSY

Jealousy is never logical, as with all emotions. You want what others have, no matter what it is. You are jealous because you do not have it, think you cannot have it, or worry that you will never have it. You may even tell others that you do not want what others have because you think you can never have it, no matter how much you want it.

## BLAMING

Blaming is related to guilt and judgment. Constantly blaming Self or others and never taking responsibility becomes an addiction. Nothing is your fault. This can be the result of a child taking responsibility and being severely punished or hurt. You learn to blame others to avoid perceived punishment.

## HOPE

Hope means that you are waiting for something to happen in the future rather than "now." You become addicted to the feeling of hope rather than allowing what is meant to be to happen in the present. Even when what you want is trying to reach you, this mind-pattern keeps a distance between you and what is trying to get to you. Every time you get to the future, hope moves forward again, always dangling in front of you but never quite within reach.

## LOVE

Love is not the same as sex. Love is a neutral energy; how you apply it determines its function. For example, you can love someone unconditionally or you can love them to death. In the same way, you can take a pen to write beautiful poetry or stab someone with it; it is the same neutral pen. In the same way, love is the same neutral energy.

Some people say they love everyone and everything, using love as a mask so that they do not have to deal with their true inner feelings.

God is more than love. God is everything, including all negative emotion like rage and anger. If God was only love, then that is all that would exist. God created everything; nothing exists without It.

## Avoidance

There are people who avoid everything. If there is a conflict, they avoid it. It goes back to doubt and confusion; if you never make a decision then you never fail and you are never wrong.

## Forgetfulness

Forgetfulness is connected to avoidance as well as doubt and confusion. Regardless of mental condition or physical capabilities, this person forgets birthdays, anniversaries, dates, events, appointments, and so forth. This type of person does not want responsibility nor do they want to deal with reality. But most importantly, they want to forget Self, so they have a Self-identity issue.

Even with people who have dementia and senility, others may say it is because of their age, but it is really from their life experiences that they do not want to remember.

## Chronically Late

Mind-pattern behind this addiction:

*You cannot accomplish your goals; it is too late for you.*

You are late because time does not matter and you do not care anymore. Being chronically late also draws attention from others.

## Grief

Grief is a deep sadness. You may be grieve over many aspects of your childhood, perceived lost opportunities, finances, career, relationships, what you cannot have or control, and so forth. Some people are in a perpetual state of grief.

## Sadness

Sadness can be a reason for not accomplishing a goal. Sadness can become your identity when Self-identity is lacking. You wear a cloak of sadness for so long that eventually it is sadness that gives you your identity.

## Helplessness

Addiction to helplessness is often compounded with an addiction to hopelessness. The person feels that no matter what he/she does, nothing can be changed or made better. They feel helpless in life. This can further lead the person to believing that nothing is worth living for. The person must determine where the feelings of being helpless began so that these feelings can be released and the individual can finally move out of this addiction and into positive Self-growth.

## Spiritual Addictions

All of the addictions previously discussed are left-brain, ego based. Ego is the necessary interface with physical reality.

Spiritual addictions are right-brain and may be the least recognizable. Is it possible that God-Mind is addicted to Creation and this is the origination of the addiction of humans?

## Religion

People who are addicted to religion take no responsibility for their lives. They pray to a religious figure to fix whatever the issue. If no resolution is forthcoming the answer is always that it is "God's will."

## Angels & Demons

These people use these addictions to avoid responsibility. They will say that Angels protect and help them when all goes well; that Demons interfered or made them do something when things do not go well.

## Rapture

Rapture is an addiction; again, no responsibility. You just sit and wait to be raptured.

## Talking in Tongues

There are religions where people sing and dance themselves into a frenzy, which actually activates their psychic energy. Remember that psychic energy is the energy that the body uses to function; please review this in ***Decoding Your Life***.

These people lose themselves in the animal mind, centered at the solar plexus, that does not know how to talk. This is why all the gibberish comes out of their mouths; they literally become like animals.

This is really a form of psychic driving that can also open and activate programming as well as provide the gateway for astral entities to take over and/or astral attachments to happen

## Philosophy

Some people consider themselves philosophers; they regurgitate the thought, ideas, and ideals of others. This means that all of their answers come from others rather than from within. This is another example of people who have no Self-identity so they take their identity from others.

## Meditation

Meditation as commonly understood is about opening your mind to make it blank so you can then wait for information.

When meditation is practiced as it is outlined in ***Healer's Handbook*** or ***Decoding Your Life***, it is done in a balanced way.

When you meditate for hours upon hours, you are addicted; this is another way of escaping reality and not taking responsibility. This can also open up and activate programming as well as make you available for programming downloads, which some people misinterpret as "enlightened experiences."

## Astral Travel

Many people think that it is a positive to leave their bodies to astral travel so they spend many hours trying to accomplish this. The astral is an extremely dangerous neighborhood; it is not a great place to wander around. The astral is filled with such things as demonic entities, those who have passed on, Illuminati technology, and alien technology. People try to leave their bodies because they have programming, trauma, pain, and other issues from which they want to escape rather than face.

## Paranormal

Paranormal means "beyond normal"; not conventionally understood. Paranormal is actually "normal" rather than "beyond normal." The mind-pattern for the addiction to the paranormal is a need to disassociate from the conventional world and live in the nonconventional world.

## Psychic Phenomena

People become addicted to the "show" of psychic phenomena, which includes channeling, psychics, mediums, table-tapping, Ouija boards, astral realm, and anything else where they think they will find answers outside of Self instead of from within.

## Death

There are people who want to die and/or see people or anything die; they are addicted to anything to do with death, including cemeteries.

"Snuff films" involve murder and/or suicide for sexual enhancement. There is an actual programming technique where the programmer brings a person to the brink of death, then saves the person thus becoming the person's "savior."

People who have had this programming technique used on them can in this way become preoccupied/addicted to anything to do with death; that person is constantly looking to be "saved."

## Violence

Violence makes some people feel happy and strong when they watch or participate in it. Those who are addicted to violence often have been violated so they feel like they need to be blown up or injured in some way; these violent actions either toward others or themselves, or even just watching it, give them relief from whatever they feel inside.

## Reincarnation

Reincarnation addicts want to know who they were, where they lived, what they did, how many lifetimes they had, how many were male or female, how important they were, and so forth. Some people dress up like who they think they were, join re-enactments from that era, decorate their homes from a specific time period, and even become performers so they can "be" the person from that era.

This is another form of escapism. The reality is that whatever was not corrected in alternate timelines still plays out in your life today. All lifelines exist simultaneously, meaning all your lives happen in the Eternal Now.

## Kundalini

Premature kundalini activation happens when all of your chakras open simultaneously in sequence. This causes disassociation from the physical body because you become aware of many realities at the same time without the ability to focus in any one of them. Energy leaks into many locations so most people to whom this happens wind up in mental institutions.

The ones that survive commonly take alcohol or drugs to block the memories. Even if they do not consciously remember the occurrence, subconsciously they will. There is fear that the memories will resurface thus the need for alcohol or drugs to suppress the memories.

Eventually the alcohol and drugs become a physical addiction, which then allows astral influences on top of the kundalini activation. This becomes a convoluted cycle.

Astral attachments tell them to do harmful/hurtful things from taking drugs to murder. The addicts hear voices because they are possessed. If the person is put in a mental institution they may be given even more drugs, which may enhance the astral attachments and possessions instead of thwart them.

## Programming

Some people purposely look for triggers because they are addicted to their programming. When programming is activated they think they are special; they seek attention and even though it may be perceived as negative, they will take negative attention over neglect or anonymity.

They do not want to give up their programming because then how will they feel special and important without it? This also allows them to avoid responsibility because they can say "my programming made me do it."

All programming is hooked into an original mind-pattern. You cannot be programmed with something unless there is a foundational mind-pattern to begin with.

If, for example, you do not have a mind-pattern to be a murderer, you cannot be programmed to be a murderer. A mind-pattern cannot be manufactured; programming can only be added to or hooked onto a mind-pattern that already exists within.

## Specifically Targeted Individuals

These people believe that the whole world is about them. For example, a newsperson reports a story but the individuals believe it is about them. They may think the newsperson is in love with them or sending them a secret message that only they know.

These people often think they are continually watched, monitored, and tampered with. No one is this important, even a high-ranking political figure. There is not enough money or time in the world to target people in this way. Every time these people call their Self a "targeted individual," they are really resetting their own programming.

## Deprogramming

If you spend hours and hours deprogramming, you have an addiction. You cannot keep doing the exercises over and over in a row; you must take time to reset, analyze, ground, and balance. Without taking time to incorporate these steps, deprogramming cannot really happen; you can only go through the motions.

As an analogy, people need to eat, take a break, and allow the food to digest before they eat again.

Some people want to spend so much time deprogramming because they think this puts them ahead of others. Every person must deprogram at his/her own unique pace. You cannot be ahead or behind anyone when it comes to deprogramming.

If you deprogram incorrectly you do more damage to Self than good. You actually create a new program called "Deprogramming," which is another destructive loop.

## Pornography

Many people who are addicted to pornography know that they are addicted and this is not correct behavior but they do it anyway. The power of pornography is strong because sex is based upon the Original Mind-Pattern of Creation. Please read ***True Reality of Sexuality***.

This is why people frequent websites that can then escalate into sex with strangers as well as other abnormal and deviant sexual behaviors.

Pornography addictions can also be tied into programming.

## Alien Abduction

People who think that they are always abducted by aliens are addicted to the attention that they receive because they want to be "special" as well as abused. They have low Self-worth so this addiction gives them Self-importance and a sense of identity garnered from without rather than from within.

These people have no sense of identity because they were never allowed to be who they really are, so they try to find something that gives them a sense of belonging as well as a reason for being. They grasp at straws because "something is better than nothing."

## Specific Place in Life

Too many people are addicted to exactly where they are in life as well as how they live. They think they find a way that works for them and they do not want to rock the boat in any way, shape, or form. This mind-pattern is one of fear as well as stagnation.

## Extremes

Swinging from one end of the spectrum to the other end is one way of gaining balance. Like a pendulum, you eventually find your balance in the middle.

Some people become addicted to the extremes, never finding a balance because part of them likes the drama/trauma that extremes can bring.

## Addictive and/or Obsessive Relationships

Everyone has relationships, with the primary relationship always with Self. Everyone has some type of relationship with whatever their perception is of a Greater Power than Self. This means that even when you may think or feel alone, you are really never alone.

Any relationship can be addictive or obsessive. Often this stems from a mind-pattern of fear of loss or separation.

As you read through the following checklist, decide if this describes one or more relationships in your life.

## Checklist for Evaluating Addictive Relationships

- ☐ Do you assume responsibility for the feelings and behaviors of the other person?
- ☐ Do you have difficulty identifying your own feelings?
- ☐ If you are angry, lonely, sad, scared, joyful, or ashamed, do you know how you feel in the relationship?
- ☐ Do you have difficulty appropriately expressing your feelings, especially to the other person?
- ☐ Do you worry about how the other person may respond to your feelings or behaviors?
- ☐ Are you worried about how he/she will react to your feelings and what you do?

- ☐ Are you afraid of being hurt or rejected by the other person?
- ☐ Do you place too many expectations on yourself and therefore have difficulty making decisions so you are glad that the other person makes the relationship decisions?
- ☐ Do you minimize, alter, or even deny the truth about how you really feel?
- ☐ Does the other person's actions or attitudes determine how you respond?
- ☐ Do you put the other person's wants or needs first because you think they are more important than yours?
- ☐ Are you afraid of the other person's feelings because that determines what you say and do?
- ☐ Do you fear what the other person thinks or feels because it affects how you think and feel?
- ☐ Do you question or ignore your own values to stay in the relationship?
- ☐ Do you value the other person's opinions more than your own?
- ☐ Do you harshly judge everything you do, think, or say by the other person's standards?
- ☐ Do you believe or think it is not okay to talk about your problems outside of your relationship?
- ☐ Are you loyal to the person even if it is harmful to you?
- ☐ Do you believe the other person knows what is best for you?
- ☐ Do you believe the relationship with this person is more important than your own family and friends?
- ☐ Do you believe the other person in your relationship cares about you more than your own family or friends?
- ☐ Do you believe that everything that is good or right is due to the other person?

- ☐ Do you believe that everything that is wrong or bad is your fault?
- ☐ Do you have feelings of isolation or alternating kindness with threats, such as "kiss me, smack me"?
- ☐ Do you feel indecisive, not knowing what to do much of the time because you fear being "wrong" and the potential consequences thereof?
- ☐ Does the other person use their own language between you and them with terms and expressions?
- ☐ Does the other person make you feel like there is nothing that you can do that is correct?
- ☐ Are you told that you have a bad memory?
- ☐ Do you feel like you are constantly being judged?
- ☐ Does the other person focus on your weaknesses or make you think you have weaknesses where none exist?
- ☐ Is there violence in the relationship toward you, themselves, others, things?

After reading through this checklist, think about your current relationships to determine if any of these questions apply. Even if only one of these questions applies, you have a potentially addictive relationship.

You must have a strong sense of Self-identity to have healthy relationships. Otherwise, you are always looking for another person to tell you who you are. Remember, this does not have to be a significant other or spouse. This can be a friend, acquaintance, neighbor, roommate, peer, colleague, supervisor, client, religious figure, medical professional, and so forth.

In the beginning, your parents tell you who you are, then your teachers, caregivers, and perhaps religious figures. Because this is your initial imprinting you continue to extrapolate this need for others to define you. Who you are gets lost in this process.

Regardless of how strong or intelligent you are, if abuse is all you know then you think this kind of relationship is normal. Your mind-pattern draws these qualities and characteristics out of all your relationships in one way or another. You may think that something is wrong with you but you cannot figure out what. Trying to fix relationships by pleasing others does not change your basic foundational mind-pattern upon which these types of relationships are built.

If you are in any addictive relationships answer these questions:

- Why do you stay in these types of relationships?
- What is your justification for not leaving? Fear of being alone? Not being able to function by your Self? Finances?
- What do you gain from your addiction to this type of relationship? How do you benefit?
- Are you addicted to "hope" that makes you "hope" that the other person will change?
- Are you addicted to emotional pain, thus receiving pain of some kind on a regular/semi-regular basis fulfills this addiction?
- Are you becoming the very person that you do not like, because what you focus on grows?
- Do you feel loved by being hurt?
- Did your parents or someone you loved hurt you in your childhood so you associate pain and hurt with being loved?
- If someone poured gasoline on you and set you on fire, you would leave. Why would you stay in an emotionally and often physically inflammatory relationship?

When you do not know your own Self-identity it is challenging to get past your internal doubt and confusion, low Self-worth and victimization mind-patterns.

If you are addicted to others telling you who and what you are as well as relying on them to make decisions for you, disconnecting from what you know takes tremendous strength and Self-discipline.

Sometimes you do not know you are addicted until you become uncomfortable enough to leave. Ultimately all abuse originates from within. Anyone who outpictures your internal abuse does this as a result of what your mind-pattern pulls out of them.

This is why if you have one abusive relationship, you have multiple abusive relationships, albeit the degree of abuse may vary from extreme to minor.

This is why your abusers can be super nice to everyone but you. Ending your own Self-abuse/victimization mind-pattern is the realization that finally stops and releases you from this addiction.

## Contributing Addiction Factors

### Mind-pattern

The most important contributing addiction factor is always mind-pattern. An addictive mind-pattern needs repetition and consistency in something, whatever that may be, and you cannot live without it.

### Emotions

Your emotional composition creates addictive behavior. If you always emotionally react in a specific way, you need to ask why. Are your reactions what you feel or what you think you are supposed to feel? Are you trying to live up to the expectations of others? You can become addicted to whatever behavior your emotions enforce.

## GENETICS

You may have addictive genetics; after three generations the addiction is in your family lineage. This means that your genetics may not have been manipulated, but rather your addictions are genetically induced.

Take the time to determine the addictions of your parents to help understand your own. It is possible that you could be addicted to something different than your parents but the same basic addictive mind-pattern is in place. See how many generations back you can trace the addictive mind-pattern.

## PROGRAMMING

Programming is a major addiction factor. Programming has to hook onto the original DNA or mind-pattern. Many addictions can be programming. This means that you may have one or more alters with the addictions but when those alters are not active, neither are those addictions.

Knowing this, when you deprogram you must stay in your center, anchored into Source, so none of these alters can activate. In this way you can effectively remove these addiction alters from your mind-pattern.

## TRAUMA

Most people who have experienced some kind of trauma have addictive mind-patterns. Trauma usually means that something horrific happened out of your control and you want to escape the memory. For this reason people often resort to alcohol or drugs or do something else to block the memory.

## Physical Brain Disorder

A physical brain disorder can create addictions. Pica, for example, is a condition where the person is addicted to eating inedible objects. Tourette's Syndrome is another such condition with inappropriate verbalizations due to a physical brain disorder.

## Environment

If you live in a hot, humid environment where you must drink plenty of water, for example, you may become addicted to drinking water. Even when you leave the environment you are so conditioned to this behavior that you continue to drink water all the time whether your body needs it or not.

Some people who are used to warm weather put on hats, gloves, and scarves in temperatures that others would not find cold.

Other people may become addicted to wearing sunglasses; when it is foggy they say sunglasses help them see through the fog; when it is snowy they say it minimizes the glare of the snow.

Think about your environment and if it has created any addictive behaviors within you.

## Information

You can be addicted to accumulating information or information that triggers addictive behavior. Some people accumulate stacks of unread magazines, books, and newspapers; they may spend hours on their computers addicted to the plethora of information to which they have access. Hidden among all of this is information that can trigger addictive behavior.

## Alternate Realities & Simultaneous Existences

When an alternate version of you in another reality has an addiction, this can bleed through to influence addictive behavior in this reality.

Now that the Hadron Collider is collapsing alternate realities into this one, people could be even more influenced into addictive behaviors from an alternate Self with specific predilections. Should the Hadron Collider stop functioning, this would benefit all people with addictions that are influenced by alternate realities.

## Reptilian Brainstem & Addictions

The Reptilian brainstem is about fight or flight. This is where your real core personality is located. This is why the Reptilian brainstem is used in programming and so ignored by the scientific community, which considers it to be primitive.

In the womb, your Reptilian layer is the first to develop, followed by your Mammalian layer. This is why the Reptilian brainstem is targeted to hold programming and therefore your addictions. By holding you in your addictions you do not realize, nor can you actualize, your full potential.

In this way, approximately 90% of the brain is not used. Without use, this part of the brain atrophies so you always believe that you are 90% less than you really are; without access to this part of the brain you never realize your true potential in this reality.

Robotic nanotechnology can create organic and inorganic implants to control functions so that the person's inherent mind-pattern cannot directly control the body.

Organic implants are genetically manufactured by the body to be used as beacons to track individuals or to connect to the sympathetic nervous system. These organic implants can look like cartilage, bone spurs, or moles, for example.

These implants can be used to artificially bring specific alters forward. The body then subtly changes to accommodate each specific alter's mind-pattern. For example, different alters may have different patterns of speech or tone of voice; even medical conditions in the body change depending on which alter is forward.

If society does not break away from mind-control and programming, each individual will have increasingly less free will. These types of bodies attract Soul-Personalities that are first-level humans, animalistic, and more group-minded. These are all easier to control with a flick of a switch than people with strong Self-identities.

Addictions are easy ways to control people who do not know who they are. This is why it is important that you do your Hyperspace/Oversoul work so you are in control of your Self under the guidance of your Source. When no person, place, or thing can control you, then all control is Self-control from within.

# Part IV
# Articles by Janet

# Body Follows Mind

Many people want to build the body without considering the essential element of Mind and the role that it plays in the process. Every diet and health advertisement talks about this pill and that pill, and what it can do for your body. You can carefully read and research all you want, but without the missing element of Mind, be prepared to be stuck wherever you are.

Working on the body can begin to force the mind-pattern into a change, but until you recognize this factor there can only be a small change in the overall picture of your lifestyle. Without acknowledgement of Mind, you easily become reliant on a pill for every function of your physical body. There are pills to boost every part of your body and to regulate every part of your brain. When these fail, go to a surgeon and you can simply cut out whatever bothers you.

What if, one day, your supply of pills simply ended? How would you or your body function? These are scary thoughts.

You must go back to most basic building block of all, the one to which you have easy access without costing even one penny. Your Mind. This is the most undervalued and underrated tool you have, but by far the most important. You have given up your power, your Self-control, your ability to Self-empower by listening to "the experts." Who are these experts, anyway?

Most are faceless and unknown to you, but because they are quoted or highlighted in the media, you "assume" they know what they are talking about. With the bombardment of external opinions you forget about your own. Or your opinion is built upon someone else's. A house built upon sand cannot stand.

How did the indigenous peoples function without technology?

How did they know what they know?

Why were/are they purposefully studied, their information usurped/stolen, and the peoples exterminated, imprisoned, and/or relocated?

Knowledge is power. Money is not power. Money is a tool of power. But knowledge is the ultimate power. If you are sick and dying, and you give me all your money to cure you, what are you really buying? You are buying **knowledge.**

"Secret" knowledge is hidden in plain sight. People have lost the ability to use their own minds to determine what they need. The mind is quickly becoming a lazy, useless tool, continuing to expand into dormancy as people become more and more accustomed to others doing the thinking for them.

Why should I think if you will do it for me?

Why should I strive to attain my goals if you tell me what my goals are and how to attain them?

Why should I think about the creative possibilities of my mind when I believe the limitations that you place upon me?

If you believe that you are a microcosm of the macrocosm, and you believe that God-Mind is limitless, then remove your blinders to your own Self-imposed limitations.

Allow true recognition of Mind as the builder. Pull yourself into center; work with what you have. Use the outer accoutrements as boosters into your own Mind as necessary, remembering that these are crutches to use while you work toward the final goal of total Mind-dependency.

Know that at some point within the Eternal Now you cast off the crutches and stand solely within Self, Oversoul, and God-Mind. You are limitless in every capacity. Move outside the box, take control, and go within your own Mind.

# Mind Builds Body

When I first developed the idea for "Creating Your Ideal Weight" in August, I was a bit taken aback. I think of addressing weight in January after the holidays or in the spring to get ready for summer. But end of summer?

My Oversoul showed me that people who wanted to get in shape for the summer most likely did not and now they are looking at going into fall and winter with the same issue that began in the summer…or before. Continuing on that train of thought, few people realize how much the mind affects the shape and condition of the body.

It always surprises me how few people who study metaphysics associate mental strength with physical strength. I think in the past few years there has been some change. But even so, I still see most people focusing more on the food that goes into their body than the food that goes into their mind without making a connection between the two.

Even those who study these subjects may not realize that Mind not only builds your life, but Mind builds your body. Everything is built of the basic atoms and molecules. It is only their arrangement that determines if you have a table, an apple, or a human body.

Mind determines how or even if your food is assimilated. As I mentioned in the "Creating Your Ideal Weight" Webinar, I see people all the time with "water weight." If you follow conventional nutritionists, they talk calories and exercise…and drinking tons of water…then how can you put weight on with something that has zero calories?

To me, this is a testament to the strength of the Mind. It can build weight with something that has no calories…or, looking at it another way, Mind builds something with "nothing."

Every mind-pattern you have comes through in the physical body in one way or another. Every thought you think shapes your body. And, "thin" does not equal "healthy." I see people of all shapes and sizes in various stages of health. Conventional standards of health do not apply to what I see.

I look inside you. Inside your body. Inside your Mind. This is what I want you to explore this month. What is inside your body. What is inside your Mind that created the shape and health of your body. With awareness, you can make decisions about what you put in your mind and what you put into your body.

But, Mind always comes first. Mind builds your body. Or destroys it. We will explore both sides of the coin so you can understand YOU.

If you are ready to dig into your mind, you do it. Cycles are meant to be broken. This is the only way you can move along. What Mental or Physical Cycles are you ready to break?

Few people associate boundaries with weight, but it is definitely something that you need to think about. Boundaries cause people to gain weight. It can come at you from several directions.

Sexual boundaries—if your sexual boundaries were encroached upon at any time in your life, you may have a tendency to gain weight. First, you cushion your body against the outer world that hurt you. Your body also wants to protect the genitalia from further intrusion so it builds barriers around cells that were physically hurt.

Emotional boundaries—you cushion your inner Self against the outer world, which you learned can hurt you. Your weight is your boundary telling the world that they can see you but they cannot get too close to you.

Mental boundaries—if you find that you cannot say "no" to people who insist on taking more than you can give, you start fighting back with barriers in the form of excess weight. Your unspoken words are pushing out horizontally vs. going vertically to your Oversoul. This horizontal push spreads your psychic energy outwards and your flesh builds around it.

Out of center boundaries—do you allow others to pull your energy out of your center, creating a pull on your psychic, or personal, energy? Do you allow others to pull you into their world vs. staying aligned with Oversoul and God-Mind? Have you done the exercise in *Decoding Your Life* about releasing the psychic energy of others via the Oversoul level and vice versa?

Nurturing boundaries—if you are a natural caregiver and you want to take care of everyone, you bring them to you; you hold, hug, and take on their issues so they do not have to. After all, you reason, you are older, wiser, stronger and have more tools and experience and you want them to feel better. So you take their "stuff"—they leave happier than ever and you are burdened. You pull in their psychic energy, which flows horizontally, and the horizontal pull of their energy pulls your own psychic energy horizontally around and causes your flesh to build.

Do you have a boundary issue?

One or more of the above, or another one not listed?

Are you working horizontally or vertically?

Your emotions are extremely powerful. This is why the Global Handlers pull you this way or that way. They coldly observe you and calculate exactly what kind of reaction this or that will illicit to get the type of response they are looking for so they can sway the public mind.

The emotions that you feel move your body around, outpicturing absolutely everything. This may be expressed in your face, how you hold your shoulders, how you walk…and this is only the visible part of you.

What about your insides that only You know and can see?

What is the first part of the body to seize up when you are upset or distraught? The gut.

If believe it is a different body part, it means that you are so accustomed to your gut being tense that you do not even recognize the tension there. I know this to be true…but of course, YOU have to know this to be true!

When your gut seizes up you cannot possibly digest food. You are tense. You are upset. You are distraught. Your Mind says, "I am rejecting this life experience. I don't want to participate in it. I want to be anywhere but here. I will not absorb it. I want it to go away."

Your body responds by seizing up the gut—this is where this mind-pattern is outpictured. The gut absorbs physical food, which is only an outpicturing of the mental food, or life experience that your mind refuses to accept.

When the gut seizes up it is telling you not to put any food in. If you do not, you may wind up too thin. If you do, your body cannot absorb or digest the food, so it becomes weight that sits on your body.

Go back to your childhood. Think about your body and how you felt about it at that time. Find your earliest memory of being upset. As you go into that memory, feel your gut.

What was your memory and what was your very first physical response?

If you find another body part that seizes up instead of or in addition to the gut, what is it and what mind-pattern does it represent?

You are doing excellent work. You understand that you may have various parts of your body that seize up under stress, but the first area is always the gut.

I will tell you why. When you are a baby and you get upset, the stomach muscles clench up in order to scream and cry. This is a natural reaction as full force goes into the lungs and mouth as you are screaming and crying. If your needs are not met, the reaction in the body lasts long after the emotional anguish dissipates.

This is still true in adulthood. As the emotional anguish diminishes, the body is still reacting. It takes it a while to calm down. But if you are under stress or living a harried lifestyle (welcome to the world!), your gut is clenched more often than not.

Yet, you still continue to stuff food into the gut because you are still trying to make your Self feel better.

As a baby your needs are basic: food, water, shelter. When you need something, you scream. When you get what you want, you calm down.

As an adult, you have the cellular memory that "food makes me feel better." You can easily get water. You have shelter. The last thing on the list…food!

So even if you are upset, you revert to the "first in, first out" method of deduction on how to live your life. Your first imprinting was food makes you feel better so you shovel it in, not paying attention to what the gut is going through.

When you are upset, the gut is shut down, not functioning properly, not doing its job, yet you still expect it to…or you do not even think about it.

If you are a shrinking violet who wants to leave this planet, then no matter what you force in, your inactive gut is going to let it pass through because it responds to this mind-pattern.

If you are grudgingly here and know that you are not going to leave any time soon, the body still does not absorb, instead it turns everything into padding/protection/fat…don't worry, your gut says, you can save for a rainy day.

Survival instinct is strong. You know how to be upset. You know how to get food into your mouth because this is the way instinct tells you that you (or more accurately, your body) can survive.

So do you live your life in survival mode?

How does this affect your eating patterns?

Are you truly happy to be here or only here because…well, what is the alternative?

Is your mind building a body that is too heavy, too thin, or something else?

Now that you are aware of your absorption issues in the gut due to the various traumas and upsets in life, what are you going to do about it?

What can you do with your mind so that the body responds in a happier, healthier way?

If you can start unwinding the tension of the gut, the rest of the body has a fighting chance. Think about the internal organs that are affected by the twisting of the gut. If you are not ingesting your food properly, doesn't it make sense that the rest of the body follow with ill health?

To relax the gut, I highly suggest that you drink ginger tea. It is one of the best relaxants for the gut.

To feed a tight system, stay away from raw foods. Lightly steamed foods that are already partially broken down are easier for the system to assimilate.

Light soups from beef, buffalo, chicken, etc. are rich in nutrients that feed the body and are easily assimilated.

You can make the broth and store it in your freezer. If you cook the broth for a long time the water will evaporate leaving a very rich stock. When it is time to use the broth, you can "rehydrate" it by simply adding more water along with vegetable of your choice. You can add some small pieces of meat for protein. As an added bonus you can grate some fresh organic ginger root in if you like this flavor.

Add a small portion of brown rice, millet, quinoa, or amaranth if you want a heartier stock. These are all more easily digestible than other grains.

Releasing the Mind from turmoil releases the gut from turmoil. As you realize that every experience is an important one for you to digest…note that I did not say "easy"…you begin to take your power back from those experiences that hold YOUR power.

"Face" your experiences. Why do you think people have such an issue with their "faces"?

It does not matter what you eat, where you go, or who you see if you do not change your Mind-pattern.

Mind Builds Body.

Where has your Mind built your body that you do not like?

How has your Mind built your body in ways that it does not function properly?

And, can you give me the mind-pattern for what you are experiencing? Or make a guess at it?

As you ingest your food, the waste should be eliminated after every meal and at minimum one time per day. Easily. Without outside help.

I have heard people say that their doctors tell them that eliminating only one time per week is NORMAL!

No, no, no. Yes, every body is different, but once a week?

What do you think happens to the waste in your body when it is not eliminated?

If you hold onto it what does this mean about your mind-pattern?

How is your elimination process?

Are you releasing your old used up material or holding onto it? What is your mind-pattern?

What toxic mind-patterns do you hold onto that prevents proper physical release "out the back door" of your body?

What in your life do you dislike?

On a scale from 1-10, with 1 being "mildly dislike" to 10 being "Hate," where is it on the scale?

First, stop: find out where inside of you this quality exists.

Go back to your list and review it.

Now, think about what you are giving out into all these life streams, starting with dislike to hate.

What are you giving out?

What do you expect to come back?

You have to take the dislike/hate down to the base. If this is what you are giving out in ANY area of life, this is what is going to come back to you.

Every single negative thought that you have destroys your cellular structure.

In fact, when my boys were little and started yelling or screaming for any reason that was beyond what they "should" have been doing, I would simply observe them and say, "Well, if you want to destroy your cellular structure, that is your choice."

Negative thoughts destroy.

What negative thoughts have destroyed your body?

When you look at your body, what do you not like? Or, what does not work the way you think it "should"?

What is the mind-pattern behind it?

What do you do when you find your Self with a negative emotion toward anything, knowing that negativity destroys your cellular structure?

How is your communication process? Do you adequately express your Self? And to whom?

What about the thoughts in your head? How do these affect your physical body?

What kind of body are you molding and shaping with your thoughts?

How do you communicate with your Self?

Are you kind and gentle?

Do you observe or do you judge and criticize?

What kinds of words do you use that build your body?

What kinds of words do you use that destroy your body?

How can you re-shape your body through your thoughts, words, and actions?

Do you have thoughts like, "Every fall/change of seasons I get a cold/allergies"?

Do you belittle and berate your Self with words throughout the day?

Do you appreciate who you are and how far you have come?

What kind of Self-talk goes through your head every day that eventually solidifies in the physical body?

All the Self-talk that you do creates everything within the physical structure. Every thought that you have is busy creating something. Even destruction is a form of creation. Your mind is always so busy that you do not have time to stop and observe your own thought process.

This is why I am slowing you down this month. Bit by bit it is important that you watch your thoughts and understand where they come from.

In **Decoding Your Life** I talk about how your mind actually sits above your head. This is where your thoughts go "round and round" sometimes rather than up to your Oversoul for discussion. Re-read this portion of the book if you haven't for a while.

How can your body be harmonious if your thoughts are not harmonious?

Discordant thoughts produce discordant body cells. This is why I teach the toning work. Toning helps harmonize your cellular structure, opening up locked DNA, and harmonizing the physical body.

Spoken words ARE Tone.

How does YOUR voice sound when you speak?

What emotions do you express through your VOICE regardless of the words you speak?

Can you separate the two?

Your voice is your physical body's tuning fork. Do you speak with clarity?

Or do you send mixed messages?

Listen to the mind-patterns in your voice when you speak.

Do you have more than one tone going at the same time?

Do you say one thing when you mean something else?

How do your words convey one thought while you are thinking or feeling another one?

What is going on in your physical body as you speak?

How does your body react to the tones that you project?

I want you to understand how much your tone of voice affects your physical body. When you are imbued with negatives: sadness, depression, anxiety, fear, etc., it is in the tone that you speak. Every time you speak these tones, what happens to the body?

According to the www.usgs.gov info about water:

> Up to 60% of the human body is water, the brain is composed of 70% water, and the lungs are nearly 90% water. Lean muscle tissue contains about 75% water by weight, as is the brain; body fat contains 10% water and bone has 22% water. About 83% of our blood is water, which helps digest our food, transport waste, and control body temperature. Each day humans must replace 2.4 liters of water, some through drinking and the rest taken by the body from the foods eaten.

Really listen to the mind-patterns that come through in your tones.

The tones/mind-patterns that you do not care for, release up to your Oversoul and into God-Mind.

What happens to water when it is imprinted with tone?

Review the book ***The Healing Power of Water*** by Masaru Emoto.

What is happening to your own body when you speak?

Are you healing and regenerating it? Or destroying it?

Stress and tension…a BIG issue.

What happens when your body holds stress and tension; WHERE in your body do you hold it?

How much energy does it take for you to hold tension in your body?

Most people do not have a clue as to how much tension is held in the body. I used to be an insomniac for a variety of reasons. But during my farming days, I used to be up all night long to bale hay, then rake hay, then go to work—I was the Director of an Art Gallery at the time—come home, change irrigation lines, do my other chores, prepare the balers for another night of baling, and so forth. I had so little sleep that I just simply fell asleep when I sat down.

There were four cuttings of hay every season and sometimes a small fifth cutting, so this happened many times all through the harvest months.

Once I dreamed that one of my neighbors called to tell me that his wife was in the hospital. Except, I later learned, that I was so tired that I really did speak to him via phone and she really was in the hospital! It was not a dream.

At one time I used to hold my thumb inside my fist—standing, walking, even while sleeping. My nose used to run all the time (internal tears) and I always needed to have a facial tissue handy, so at night I simply stuck the tissue into this "thumb/fist" arrangement so I always had a tissue whenever I needed it! You try making a fist with your thumb stuck into it. Now sit, stand, walk, sleep with it and you tell me how much tension it takes to hold these very few muscles in this position. I had to make a conscious effort not to hold my hands this way.

When I did my vision therapy, I was taught about how much tension are held in the eyes…why? Because what do you see that makes you tense?

Working with my voice lessons I am learning how much tension I hold in my throat, neck, voice box, etc. because of all the words that I have never spoken but are still there needing release.

So while you are consciously acknowledging this or that body part, I want you to really *look* where you hold tension.

We started with the obvious—which some of you identified and some of you did not—which is the gut.

Now I want you to go even deeper into other areas of your body where you have not looked before to find out where else you hold the tension. I want you to feel it, release it, and consciously make an effort to relax that body part.

Often individuals think that something is "wrong" with they speak to other people. You concern yourself with what others say and think about you rather than what YOU say and think about You. How do you hear other people? This is an important question and also relates to what happens to the hearing of many people as they gather chronological years.

Inner and outer communication is really the same—when you speak to others, you really speak to your Self. What do you say to others that YOU need to pay attention to?

Recently I slipped on water and hit my head on the edge of a door. It left me with a headache and nausea for three weeks. However, this "shaking up" definitely helped me let go of more of what I no longer need to hold onto.

Have you had this issue—an accident or illness that "shook you up" enough to make life changes?

What issues do you want addressed?

Why won't you let your Self sleep?

Many people fall into this category for one reason or another. Often it is from programming experiences, nightmares, night terrors, stress of the day, and not living in the present moment—yesterday or tomorrow. Insomnia is a major issue in developing countries. Do you sleep? If not, which of the above categories describe you?

What do you know now that you did not know at the beginning of the month?

What have you specifically accomplished this month?

# Increasing Your Frequency

When a soul-personality enters into the Earth plane, only the smallest fraction of it can operate in the tiny baby's body that is first born. As the physical body increases in size, so does the amount of soul-personality that can function in and through it. Your Oversoul pours in more soul-personality as the body grows. Eventually, the physical body ceases to grow.

At this point, the amount of soul-personality operating in and expressing through the physical body also comes to a stop. This does not mean that there is no more soul-personality to put into your physical body. This simply means that your physical body cannot hold any more of "you."

Most people remain at this level. From here, for most people, it is all downhill as the process simply reverses. The physical structure becomes stagnant, the amount of space available to the soul-personality decreases.

As available space decreases, the soul-personality returns to the nonphysical. When all the soul-personality is gathered into the nonphysical, the physical body ceases to function, thus creating the condition known as "death."

If more of your soul-personality tries to enter into the physical body than the cellular structure can comfortably hold, the body literally "burns up." This is because your soul-personality is comprised of an energy frequency. The physical body is also comprised of an energy frequency. In order for the soul-personality to comfortably operate symbiotically with the physical body consciousness, the two frequencies must match.

You can increase the amount of soul-personality that your physical body can hold. This is accomplished by emptying out anything that you have accumulated in your cellular structure that you no longer need.

As the cellular structure becomes less dense, room is created for more soul-personality energy to pour in from the Oversoul level. At the same time, it is important to strengthen the cellular structure so that the physical body continues to match the frequency of the entering soul-personality energy.

This is sometimes accomplished through illness and/or accidents. Illness and/or accidents often shake up the cellular structure enough so that old, unnecessary mind-patterns are physically released.

This creates space for more soul-personality to flow into and function through the body. This is why that sometimes after a major illness or accident you hear that a person experiences some kind of sudden change. This may be acquiring new abilities, attributes, personality traits, liking different foods, etc.

Illness and/or accidents are "reactive" situations—this means the method of correction, or balance, seeks you out in such a way that you have no choice but to change.

The easiest way to increase your frequency is a proactive one. This means that you search out the experience before it finds you.

The correction at this point may not be pleasant or easy, but at least you are in control of it rather than vice versa. Usually this is less uncomfortable than being in a reactive position. This can be accomplished in two ways. First, release all old, unnecessary vibratory imprints up to your Oversoul. Watch them flow and flow and flow out the top of your head. Remember that these all have color, tone, archetype, weight, form, and consistency.

All of these vibratory imprints built up slowly over time and take up space in the physical structure, as well as in the auric field. In this way, you consciously cleanse the auric/energetic fields before the energy settles further into your physical body. This is why an "illness" can be detected before it physically manifests. Illness exists in your energetic field first, gradually becoming heavier and denser until it matches some part of your physical body.

Once the nonphysical frequency matches the physical frequency, the frequencies merge, settling into the more dense physical body.

When this happens, your physical body becomes "sick" or "ill." This is really an outpicturing of your mind-pattern. You can consciously cleanse the physical body in preparation for it to hold more of your soul-personality energy. This is the equivalent of cleaning an electronic device.

The cleaner the device, the clearer the communication and transmission of information. To develop clear, clean communication between Self, Oversoul, and God-Mind in this realty, it is important that your device, or body, and your energetic field, are as clean and clear as possible. The outside world does not support a clear, clean body. In fact, just the opposite. The powers that be want your physical body only healthy enough to be a productive worker, nothing more.

If you keep your body clean with too much inner communication, you just may be able to determine how to circumvent their plans for you and society.

If you want to become master of your own fate, one of the primary steps you can take is to become master of your own body. This is your vehicle through which your soul-personality operates. Your vehicle has its own consciousness and will follow the group programming if you allow it.

Establish who is in charge. For most people, the physical body is in charge. Whether it is hungry or not, it gets fed. Whatever it craves, from chocolate to sex, the body gets what it wants.

Most people usually follow the dictate of the body consciousness. Most people have a relationship with their bodies that is out of balance.

If you do gain control of your body, there are plenty of disinformation programs to continue to throw you off-track, such as vegetarianism, breatharianism, macrobiotics, raw foods, low/no-carbohydrates, etc.

Some may be appropriate as a healing diet. But, too much of any one thing can throw your body out of balance.

The real goal is to gain control over the body only long enough so that you can learn what your specific body consciousness needs. Then, you can work together to support the vehicle in the most efficient, effective, consciousness-evolving plan for all intelligences involved.

If your own body, the one organism with which you have the closest symbiotic relationship, can control you, then what leads you to believe that an external force cannot easily control you as well?

If you do not take the time to know your own body and mind, someone else will. Someone else will gladly run your body and mind for you. The more "minions" the powers that be have, the happier they are.

Controlling your body is an important step to controlling your mind.

Gaining control over your own body is another way to imprint the mind-pattern that you have control over your life. Setting the imprint for "successful self-control" definitely aids every aspect of your entire life.

Consciously cleansing the body tells the body consciousness that you are in control, not vice versa. The basic mind-pattern of cleansing says that you are finished with all mind-patterns that hold you down or anchor you to parts of your past that you no longer need.

Releasing the old, stored up heavy toxins from your physical body is symbolic of releasing old, stored, heavy toxic mind-patterns that you no longer need. As the cleansing occurs, your cellular structure becomes lighter, cleaner, more flexible and resilient, indicative of what is happening in the mind-pattern of your mental house.

There are several ways to cleanse the physical body. Before you start any cleansing program, it is always advisable to discuss it with your primary healthcare practitioner. If you are on any kind of medication, this is particularly advisable and even necessary, as the old stored medications will begin pouring into your bloodstream.

This can be toxic, and a slow, gentle cleanse is much better than an intense, aggressive cleanse. There are many gentle methods, ways that are much stronger and more forceful, to clean out the physical body. You can choose one way, or a combination of approaches.

During a cleanse, the less water you drink, the more vigorous the cleanse, although a minimum of four cups of liquid is suggested. During cleansing, you may experience headaches—this is the release of old toxins moving from the deep tissues into the bloodstream.

Tiredness and crankiness is also to be expected for the same reason. Prepare yourself. Make a decision that you will be comfortable in the midst of any discomfort that your physical body may experience.

A thick coating on your tongue is indicative of the toxins moving out of your system. A tongue scraper, found in many health food stores, is a great addition to your personal hygiene routine.

You may even want to incorporate a colonic, a deep cleansing of the bowels. The bowels can be a source of undesirable bacteria. This is particularly useful for anyone with a life-threatening illness, or a body that is highly out of balance. If you decide to incorporate this into your cleansing, take care to choose a reputable practitioner. Gravity flow tanks are better than machines or "do-it-yourself" colonics.

Since the liver dumps directly into the large intestine, once the large intestine is cleaned out the liver can cleanse on an extremely deep level. Every point within the colon reflexes to other organs. A colonic is like having an internal reflexology massage.

Be wary of the lubricant used on the colonics scope, as Crisco is often the oil of choice. Crisco is soy-based and should not be absorbed. You can choose to bring your own lubricant, such as organic palm oil. The oil should be taken out of the main container and applied to the scope. The scope should never be taken out and re-used on the same person. Always insist on a new scope if this is necessary. The scope should never be "double-dipped" in the same lubricant holder. If you observe this happening, question the cleanliness practices and find someone else.

Fasting promotes a quicker, more vigorous cleanse. If you decide to fast, your body will probably try to tell you that it is starving and needs food. Most likely, the body will not starve to death from skipping a few meals.

Talk to your body before you begin, let it know your plans, and then put yourself in charge. Even when you follow this preliminary routine, there is a strong possibility that your body will rebel. If this happens, remind yourself and your body consciousness that you are in control. What you are doing is the best for all involved.

While fasting may sound difficult, remember most people fast every night from after dinner until breakfast the next morning. A 12-hour fast is not unusual. Some people skip breakfast (break-fast), and do not eat until lunch or perhaps dinner, thus a 15- to 24-hour fast for many people is not abnormal.

If this is your routine, just extend what you are already doing. Go one more night—any easy 12 hours, for a total of 36 hours. If you are doing well, you may want to extend this for another 12 to 24 hours, continuing to take advantage of the night hours when you are sleeping.

Suspend taking herbs, vitamins, minerals, etc. during the fast to give your digestive system a rest.

If you feel like going on a long fast, the first three days may be the most difficult. Seven to ten days are the longest that you should attempt without direct supervision from your healthcare provider. During a lengthy or vigorous fast, you may even vomit toxins from the gallbladder, pancreas, and/or liver.

During the fast, while your digestive system is resting, the toxins are coming up from the deep tissues. They may sit in your digestive tract until you start it moving again. A minimum of two cups of raw, shredded cabbage plus one cup of raw grated carrot dressed with two to three tablespoons of fresh lemon juice is a good way to start your bowels moving again.

If they do not evacuate after two to three hours, eat the same combination again. Repeat this every two to three hours until your system is moving on its own.

Several cleansing suggestions follow. You can choose one, or combine two or three ways that work for you. Rather than wait for "the right time," pick one and get started. Even if you do not follow it "perfectly," it is still a start. Doing something counts for a lot. It means movement and growth.

## VEGETABLE CLEANSING SOUP

Using cooked, low-carbohydrate, non-starchy vegetables, this is a great cleansing soup. Eat as much as you want for three days, without adding any other foods. Once the bowels are moving, follow with intense red meat protein, such as steak, to replenish and maintain iron and amino acid levels. Or, use the soup to replace a regular meal or two.

## DISTILLED WATER/FRESH LEMON JUICE

If you cannot find steam-distilled water in the bottled water section of your supermarket, look in the ironing section. Steam-distilled water is used to prevent the build-up of mineral deposits in irons. Fresh lemon juice cuts the mucous build-up in the cellular structure and intestinal tract. You can add this into your daily routine, or use it as a fast. Because lemon juice alkalizes the system, it is best to drink between meals. Sweeten with stevia if desired.

## DISTILLED WATER/LEMON JUICE/MAPLE SYRUP/CAYENNE PEPPER

To steam-distilled water and fresh lemon juice, you can add a tablespoon of pure maple syrup. Many maple syrups in the United States use formaldehyde in processing, so either purchase Canadian or ask at your health food store. The maple syrup gives your body some natural, easily assimilated sugar along with some trace minerals. Cayenne pepper capsules boost body metabolism. Add this into your daily routine, or use as a fast.

## SUGAR/WHEAT/DAIRY FAST

Simply eliminate refined sugar, wheat, and/or cow dairy from your diet. These weaken and inflame the cellular structure, often resulting in swelling, aches, and pains. Formaldehyde is often used in the processing of white sugar.

## CAFFEINE/ALCOHOL/TOBACCO FAST

If caffeine, alcohol, and/or tobacco control you, then eliminate it long enough so you know that you are controlling it. Use Brown around your auric field to ground yourself. Visualize Pale Yellow in your nervous system. Add Omega-3 fish oil tablets to your diet, as well as greens—steamed greens with olive oil and garlic—and/or liquid chlorophyll.

## APPLE JUICE/CIDER FAST

A home juicer is a good investment. There are many good brands on the market for under $100. While they take a few extra minutes to clean, the fresh juice retains the best nutrients available. Organic produce contains less pesticides/herbicides than non-organic, but nothing these days is totally pesticide/herbicide free. Drink as much apple juice/cider as you desire for 24 to 72 hours to pull toxins from your system. Use a reputable colon cleanse product, such as the one sold by www.blessedherbs.com—let them know when ordering that you are an Expansions referral.

## Vegetable Juice Fast

Two raw carrots for skin toning, inside and out; two raw ribs of celery for your nervous system; one 2"x3" cube of raw beet for iron; raw beet tops for calcium and iron: and a raw fresh apple if desired to pull out toxins and make the drink more palatable. Add in any other kind of leafy greens you desire. You can drink this with or without a good protein powder, depending upon your requirements.

## Vegetable/Juice Fast

Drink fresh vegetable juice in the morning and fresh fruit juice throughout the day.

## Liquid Chlorophyll

Add liquid chlorophyll to steam-distilled water. This is great for toning and strengthening the cellular structure, either while fasting or drank daily.

## Milk Thistle Herb Liver Cleanse

Support your other cleansing work by using this herb for 7-10 days only. Follow the directions on the bottle.

Whatever you drink and/or eat, ask that it be blessed and cleansed by your Oversoul and God-Mind for the most effective and efficient use by all levels of your cellular structure. Ask that the body keep what it needs while allowing what it does not require to pass right on through.

A byproduct of a cleanse may be weight loss. This means that you are shedding old mind-patterns that you were holding onto. The mind-pattern behind excess weight is needing to insulate against the outside world.

Specific places of weight gain represent the part of your life that you are insulating against. For example:

- Excess weight on the stomach represents not digesting what your life is giving you;

- Weight gain on the hips are childhood issues;

- Weight gain on the buttocks represents carrying your past with you.

Some people eat very little, yet still cannot lose weight. This is a perfect example of how strong the mind is—it can create weight from virtually nothing!

Weight gain from water retention is a perfect example of this. Water has absolutely zero calories, yet many people retain excess water as a way of insulating against life. Of course, cutting down on food does not reduce weight, because the excess weight is not from food—it is from water—and the strong mind-pattern that holds it there!

See how powerful you are?

Water weight may also be the result of suppressed, unshed tears. Sometimes water weight represents issues of others that you hold onto yourself. So now, your strong mind-pattern is creating weight from other people's stuff!

Pretty incredible how strong you really are.

A thin body is not necessarily a healthy body. You must look at the cellular structure to make this determination. Often a body is thin, or too thin, because the mind-pattern of the soul-personality operating within it says that it does not deserve to live. People who are bulimic and/or anorexic have this mind-pattern. A part of them does not feel like it deserves to have a body and live here on the Earth.

People with bodies that are too thin have bodies that are underfed and/or undernourished. Your stomach can be full while the body is actually hungry. White flour and white sugar will make you feel full, but neither contains enough nourishment to adequately maintain a healthy cellular structure.

Or you can eat foods that are mismatched for your frequency. They may be nourishing foods, but not nourishing to your specific body.

Or, you may have an absorption issue–something that is all too common these days.

You may want to use one or more of the following affirmations to help you in the process:

*I easily cleanse and release all, old unnecessary mind-patterns from all levels of my Being.*

*I easily cleanse and release the need to insulate.*

*I deserve to exist.*

*I create a healthy relationship with the physical consciousness of my physical body.*

*I increase the frequency of my soul-personality operating in and through my body consciousness.*

Personalize any of the above affirmations in a way that works for you. Write them and place them around your home or office so they emanate throughout your living space. Carry cards with your affirmations written on them, or place them under your pillow while you sleep. Or, simply write them in a journal or notebook.

Using all these techniques help you know yourself on all levels, gain self-control, and increase the amount of frequency, or soul-personality, that can function through your physical body.

In turn, this increases and deepens your Oversoul and God-Mind connection. The more that you clean out your physical structure of old debris on all levels, the more room you create for more of the nonphysical portion of your soul-personality to function in this reality.

This increased frequency gives you access to new information that propels you into new layers of personal growth. Opening the body to hold more of "you" changes your life in ways that you will never know until you start the process. So, take a deep breath and begin!

# Free Permanent Weight Loss— No Gimmicks!

There is only ONE thing you need to know about permanent weight loss, and it is FREE! You already own it! No one wants you to use this because then they cannot sell you everything else. Tips are rampant throughout the media, from Internet to television to magazines, touting how to eat less and lose weight so you look better for the New Year, vacations, and the upcoming spring and summer. In addition they tell you to exercise more, harder, longer, etc.

They want you to buy their weight-loss products, from pre-packaged meals to pills to exercise equipment. You are constantly bombarded as they rope you in with constant media pressure, filling you with guilt and tension as you try to live up to these artificially implemented standards. None of this works! AND it is expensive and time-consuming!

What do you already own that no one can take away from you? Your OWN MIND filled with all the mind-patterns that you have already created! Mind-pattern is everything. If you are eating too much, then you are trying to fill the empty holes in your life. If you are too heavy, then you are insulating against the life you have. If you need more physical exercise, you need more mental exercise—a strong, well-exercised mind is outpictured in a strong, well-exercised physical body. Strong mind = strong body.

Really delve into the mind-pattern behind your physical issues. The physical is simply another reminder that your mental house needs to be put in order. Release the need for fancy diets and complicated exercise programs that eventually fall by the wayside as the strength of the old mind-pattern takes over your new resolve. Take the simple, easy road.

Use your mind to release the tension of eating, which in turn releases the mind-pattern that holds onto the food in an incorrect way within your physical body. Create a new mind-pattern that lets the food nourish and flow through the body in appropriate proportions for you.

Your mind is now in control of the food, rather than vice versa. As you learn more about your mind and emotions, you release the need to overindulge. Eating becomes a natural part of life instead of one more thing that you can use to feel bad about yourself. Develop a new attitude for the New Year and enjoy wonderful new beginnings filled with everything you love, including good food.

Do not let the powers-that-be continue to strip away your self-esteem and ability to feel good about yourself. Every body outpictures the owner—you do not have to look like the pictures in magazines and television. Be who you are and the body follows. Be proud to be YOU!

Release your negative self-talk with this affirmation :

*I now have a magnificently healthy, well-nourished, strong body and mind!*

**Now reap the physical benefits of your own mental work within your own mind—FOR FREE!**

# Parasites

According to Dr. Hazel Parcels, "85% of adult North Americans are infected with parasites." Dr. Frank Nova, Chief of the Laboratory for Parasitic Diseases at the National Institute of Health says, "In terms of numbers, there are more parasitic infections acquired in this country than in Africa." This is thought to be true because of the highly processed food, stressful living conditions, lack of exercise, and overuse of antibiotics routinely prescribed for such things as a common cold.

Parasites can inhabit the bloodstream, muscle tissue, digestive tract, brain, heart, liver, kidneys, and other body parts. Parasites embedded in their hosts are very difficult to eliminate. Many bacteria and viruses feed off parasites. In fact, parasites, viruses, and bacteria have an extremely low frequency. You can research to find videos that demonstrate the killing of parasites with frequency, such as the Rife machine.

I have a Rife and have used it for many years with amazing results. The man who builds these machines is a genius, living right here in Michigan. He is a researcher and does not diagnose. A fascinating website to peruse. His research has positively impacted thousands.

When your physical structure becomes weakened in any way, it vibrates at low frequencies. When this happens, your "tone" matches the "tone" of the parasite and it thrives within you. Depression, unhappiness, sadness, fear, you name it; any negative emotion vibrates at low rates, setting the stage for these parasites to not only take hold, but to infest your physical body.

Some people are even diagnosed with brain tumors that turn out to be parasite nests. I personally know someone who had eye surgery after vision issues only to be told by a surgeon that he found a parasite previously dormant that had been triggered and was wrapped around her optic nerve.

Tapeworm eggs can live in formaldehyde up to three months. This is why you must do parasite cleanses for a minimum of three months. Parasites can be embedded in so many places throughout the body that it is a challenge to pull them all out.

People are filled with parasites because this has become a parasitic society. People live off the energy of others without giving back. Not a "win/win" but a "win/lose," as evidenced in almost all aspects of life, from sports to business to daily living to crime.

This nonphysical activity has to have a physical representation. Holding parasites in the physical body is a way for the Illuminati to hook into the parasitic frequency in you and use it for their own benefit.

I have done layers of parasitic cleanses since I was in my 20s and did not realize I was even doing a parasite cleanse! I did rigorous fasting for three years. My fasts consisted of only steam-distilled water from 36 hours to periods of 10 days. During this time many parasites came out of me.

Since then I have used a variety of products through the years. I believe the results, each time, go into deeper layers of my physical body as I shed the parasitic conditions I host in my mind-pattern.

### Physical Parasite Symptoms

Too skinny—Yes, you can be too thin. This can be the result of parasites robbing your physical body of nourishment.

Too heavy—you can be the host of numerous parasite nests that literally take over your body.

Depression—you feel the die-off and death of the parasites as they go through their life cycles. You react to hosting their dead carcasses on their way out of your body.

Sugar cravings—your body needs sugar/carbohydrates; your body craves sugar because the sugar/carbohydrates you ingest go to feeding the parasites while your body starves.

Physical weakness—parasites feed off of your life blood.

### MENTAL PARASITE SYMPTOMS

No boundaries—you let people in who are not mutually beneficial

Nourishing others without nourishing self—you do for others without doing for your Self.

Allowing your past to suck the joy out of your present—past memories prevent you from pursuing or enjoying current joy.

Allowing clutter to rob you of peace of mind and calmness—your environment is cluttered just as your mind and body are cluttered.

Over-cleaning—you feel the physical dirt of parasites and try to clean up by over-cleaning your environment or sometimes even your Self, such as OCD.

As you understand how you allow parasitic activity in your life, or how you participate in it, you are then able to release the physical representation of the nonphysical mind-pattern. I have learned about parasitic activity in my Self and others via Expansions' blogs: "December's Daily Discard" and "January Jumpstart."

You and I are re-setting our mind-patterns by physically "doing something." This is another trick the Illuminati use—subliminal imprinting the subconscious.

You are moving your muscles differently, thus forcing your current thoughts to re-route themselves in your neuro-network to create a new avenue of action. As you move your body while "doing something different," your mind has to move differently.

Is your mind following your body or your body your mind? Where on the wheel are you starting? Does it matter?

You are told one thing while shown another. Your focus is continually on the negative. Don't do this, don't do that; isn't this awful; terrible; murder; mayhem; fighting; disagreements; death; destruction; and so forth.

Don't eat this; don't eat that; don't go here; don't be this way; don't be that way; don't take anything for your Self and, and, and…

Your focus continually is on the negative. And where you focus is what you eventually become. A perfect example: I am sure you have read or maybe even know, someone who was in an auto incident where the car left the road and struck a lone tree in the middle of a field. Why the lone tree when there were so many other places to go? Because the focus becomes "Don't hit the tree, don't hit the tree" and because this is the focus, the car goes into the tree.

The more you are told and/or shown "don't," the more you focus there, drawing out and eventually manifesting this aspect of the God-Mind.

You react to their subliminals by quiet acquiescence. Consciously, you may not like what you see but you still see it. It is there. It becomes embedded in your subconscious mind. You learn to overlook it, but you become accustomed to it. Your "non-protest" means that on some level you "accept" it.

It takes just 15% of a population to firmly believe/accept something to imprint the rest of the population into accepting and believing it. Because we are all connected, we are All One. You and I want to use this as a positive enhancement. The Illuminati use it as a negative enhancer.

They use the mental/emotional/spiritual connection Law of All One to move negativity through the masses. Like the trees do through the forest. Your subconscious negatively feeds off these subconscious imprints—unless you are using self-protection tools and techniques shared in our publications.

This means that the masses become parasitic, living off your energy. You may not like crowds or you may even dream of living off on a mountain by your Self. These thoughts and feelings push you into isolation programming.

Or, you may love crowds and activity because you may be feeding off the energy of others without conscious awareness. You may love feeding others your life blood because then you do not have to look at you. It is easy to hide in a crowd and let others suck your life blood. Think about it.

We are All One.

Do you use this for or against you?

Do you allow others to do this for or against you?

## Unhook Parasite Frequency

Where are you parasitic in your life?

Where is your life parasitic in you?

I have listed numerous examples that I want you to think about. As I move into deeper levels, I am amazed at what I have allowed to be parasitic in my life. What I have allowed to take my joy. What I have subconsciously and at times consciously handed over to others. In retrospect, I can more clearly see the patterns and I even ask my Self, "Why did I allow this to go on for so long?" Do you ask the same question?

It is time to stop the parasitic "whatever" that exists within you. Do your flushing and clearing. Continue to raise your frequency. Use the maple syrup and baking soda recipe shared in my podcast.

I am unhooking the parasite frequency within my Self. I am doing everything that I can to release the physical representation of the nonphysical mind-pattern.

It is time that you know Universal Law as well as the Illuminati knows it. This is why they use sexual ritual for everything. As I wrote in ***True Reality of Sexuality*** and discussed in the ***Sexuality, Ritual***

***and Relationship*** DVD series, the joining of male and female is to manifest.

The male is the "key" and the female is the "door" through which manifestations occur. Female to female sex opens the door wider. Male to male sex creates a bigger key. Extrapolate this into group sex and you begin to more clearly see the bigger picture.

You must understand Universal Law and its working at minimum at least as well as the Illuminati. It is time for you to know this information and then learn Universal Law BETTER than the Illuminati if you want to protect your Self and truly unhook its parasitic frequency within you.

Learn as much as you can as fast as you can. The Illuminati is stepping up its agenda and closing the net. You need the tools so that you are not caught within the net.

Refuse to be the host for anyone's or anything's parasitic frequency. Learn how you perpetuate the parasitic frequency. Understand how YOU are parasitic in your life and mind-patterns.

YOU are still the key.

Know who and what you are so that you know who and what is out there.

They are waiting to ensnare you with wonderful traps to en-trance you.

Do you want to be a host to Parasites?

Do you want to be a Parasite?

Think about it. The choice is yours.

# Victim Mentality

This planet primarily attracts two types of beings–those with a victim mentality and those with an oppressor mentality. In order to be a victim, you must have oppressors. In order to be an oppressor, you must have victims. Together, this creates balance in God-Mind.

This planet is designed as a place where beings with a victim mentality can learn to overcome it. Therefore, any "higher-level" being will not become involved because it is necessary for those here to have the opportunity to work through their victim mentalities. To become involved would mean interfering or taking away the lessons of those with victim mentalities. Higher-level beings will be objective observers who will guide and instruct you through your victim mentality once you reach them, but that is all. They are not here to "save" you or this planet.

Any being who says that they are here to "save" you is interfering in your soul growth. Only you can "save" yourself from a victim mentality. Only you and the lessons you self-design will teach you about victim mentality. Only you can move through these lessons that will allow you to make a final release of your victim mentality. No one is waiting to help you–do not be fooled by any being making such promises.

When you learn to move through your victim mentality, your mind-pattern will no longer attract oppressors. The more stubborn you are in your determination to hang onto your victim mentality habits, the more intense the lessons that you attract to encourage you to release those ways. This means, metaphorically speaking, a bigger, meaner, stronger stick until you finally "get it."

You have to become hurt, belittled, and finally, angry enough to stand up for yourself and declare that you will no longer be a victim to anyone, anywhere, anymore! Perhaps when you finally have had enough, you release your victim mentality by saying, "I just don't give a damn anymore what anybody thinks! I am speaking my mind regardless! I am taking care of myself, regardless!"

Sometimes, people are beaten up so much that instead of releasing the victim mentality, they decide to become the oppressor when the opportunity presents itself. This is why cycles repeat themselves. People who were oppressed find other victims; this gives them a sense of control. In doing so, they relive their earlier experiences when they felt like they had no control. They become the perpetrator, just so they can be the "winner" for a change. Of course, this is another imbalance, or extreme flip–from victim to oppressor.

The ideal is to find a happy medium, or balance, between victim and oppressor. Victim and oppressor are opposite sides of the same coin in the Mind of God. In this case, two individual soul-personalities are needed to maintain equilibrium in God-Mind. One carries the weight of a victim; one carries the weight of an oppressor. You need to find the balance within yourself, so that equilibrium within the Mind of God is maintained within one soul-personality instead of two.

Yes, you must learn to speak your mind and not allow anyone to walk on you. Yes, you must sometimes be harsh and cruel with words, and sometimes even actions. But when this must happen, it must be done in an objective manner–what is best for everyone involved to get the point across while causing the least amount of pain. Boundaries must be set.

What are your boundaries? Who crosses them and how? Who is a belligerent person in your life that you try to avoid because of their bullish, pushy ways? Why do you avoid this person? Why not practice letting go of your victim mentality and speak your mind? So what if your heart races and palpitates, and your palms grow sweaty? So what if your knees shake so hard that you think you will fall down, and your voice is shaky, squeaky, or barely audible? Somewhere along the way, you must stop your victim mentality before it stops you. Learn to be proactive instead of reactive.

When you allow others to push you around, you become angry, sullen, and introverted. Then, you lash out at the undeserving with misdirected frustration and anger. Sometimes your body becomes ill because of all that you suppress, or you insulate your body, or perhaps stop eating. One way or the other, you suffer.

There is a part of you that feels that you deserve to suffer. There is a part of you that enjoys this pain and self-punishment. It feels good to some part of yourself, or you would not do it. Some people create others to give them pain, sometimes physical, sometimes emotional, sometimes both. Some people do it for themselves–a self-contained, fully functional, victim mentality unit. Some people are extremely successful at this.

Why do you feel so bad about yourself that you believe you are meant to suffer, to be alone, to feel guilty, to have ill health, to be overweight or underweight? Did it start in this lifetime, or did it start before? Follow those feelings, and allow yourself to release it. This physical reality is your chance to overcome it. The more you ignore this situation, the harder and more intense lesson you will attract to beat it out of yourself. You came here to learn–now do it. Quit whining, moaning, and complaining–because there is a part of you that enjoys that too.

Aches and pains can create a great deal of entertainment. You can run from doctor to doctor, trying to find a cure for something that will never be cured as long as you maintain your current mind-pattern.

"Bad luck" can attract attention and sympathy from others. Dire circumstances will force someone to pay attention to you. Never getting a raise or a promotion is an excuse not to climb higher in your career or company. You can moan all you want about being alone, with a partner who does not understand you, or without one at all. But this self-imposed isolation also gives you time to selfishly take care of yourself without any interference. The same for saying you want children but are unable to have them. A part of you does not want a spouse, or a caring spouse, or children, because if ALL of you wanted this and it was truly in your mind-pattern, you would have it!

Victim, victim, victim! Let us count the ways...refuse to be a victim. Find a new source of entertainment. Release yourself from this mind-pattern so you can move into new vistas of growth—ones so vast that you cannot even imagine or comprehend them. You must let go of the old to make room for the new. No one can do it for you. No one can "save" you from yourself. No one is waiting to help this planet. Only you can make a difference. Only you can save this planet. Do it!

# Can Money Buy Happiness?

How many times have you thought, "If I only had money for this or that, everything would be okay. I could pay my bills, go where I want to go, take care of my friends and family, have money in the bank, etc., etc."? Dreaming of having "enough" money is a fantasy world where many people live.

Dreaming of financial success is a wonderful place to put your energies. What most people do not realize is that if $100 million fell in their laps, they would still be the same people that they are today with the same mind-pattern.

This means that if some part of you does not feel that you deserve a windfall, you will sabotage the outcome. One way or another, you will lose the money, fall prey to predators, open your heart up to the "wrong" people, fund projects that will fail, and attract people who will use you and throw you away. All this and more can be yours! Then you will wonder why you ever had the money in the first place and you will dream about how much happier you were before you received the windfall!

If you manage to hold onto your money long enough to pay off all your debts, put money in the bank, and buy all the toys you want, you are going to find that you are bored.

What is your incentive now to get up and get going?

Would you become selfish, inconsiderate, and demanding?

Who would be your friends?

Would people be your friends because you have money or because they genuinely like you?

Would they give you their real opinions or would you be surrounded by "yes men"?

You *can* buy your "friends," you know. Throw your money around and all kinds of people come running. After a while, this gets boring, too.

Would you help people?

How would this happen?

How would you know whom to help and why?

If the people you choose to help have self-worth and sabotage issues, they are going to lose what you give them. So, what have you accomplished?

If you "bail" people out of their life circumstances that on some level of awareness they set up in the first place, you take their lessons away. Then *you* are responsible for their learning —do you want this on your shoulders?

When you have lived financially from day to day and suddenly you have enough funding to last a lifetime and beyond, how do you make this leap?

For most people, it is more than they can handle. They do not have time to build the mind-pattern that allows them to keep the money, discern their friends, make correct investment decisions, or help the people who are able to accept help.

Most people see money as the answer to their prayers. Like anything, money is an adjunct to the mind-pattern. Mind first, then money— not vice versa. You always take *you* with you wherever you go. You take all your current issues—past, current, and the future issues that you are now creating. "You" do not change just because you have money. "You" are the same; "you" just now have money. "You" in your current state would spend it according to your current mind-pattern.

If you cannot hold onto the little bit of money you have now, what makes you think you can hold onto *more* money? If you lose what you now have, your mind-pattern dictates that you are just going to lose more if you suddenly gain more. Then you are going to be even more depressed and upset because you will think about all the "could haves, would haves, and what ifs."

If you cannot draw supportive friends to you now, why do you think that money would attract supportive friends?

If you do not have a functional relationship now, how would money change this?

Yes, you might meet more people, but of what caliber and character?

Money does not change "YOU." "YOU" are still the same, only with more funds. Simply because people already have more money than you can imagine does not make them scrupulous, trustworthy, intelligent, and wonderful friends. Material wealth does not equate with anything else except material wealth. The bottom line is still, "So?"

Rather than focus on getting more money, focus on creating a better "YOU." As you develop a mind-pattern of high self-worth, release sabotage, and develop discernment, you automatically change the recipe of your auric field and mind-pattern. As the energy shifts and changes, it automatically develops into a money magnet. Money cannot NOT come to you. Your own internal recipe now automatically emits: "I now have lots and lots of money."

When money does come to you, you have high self-worth without sabotage, so you keep what comes to you. You have discernment in place, so you know how to spend and invest. A solid support structure with people whom you can trust automatically moves to you. Friends who are supports and not takers rally to you. Personal relationships change and improve because of WHO you are, not because of what you can buy.

You know who to help and who not to help. As with all things, money is a result of your inner work. When YOU are in order, the money comes to you in the correct way for the correct reasons in the correct timing.

The more you work on YOU, the greater your chances of easily improving finances, automatically attracting money to you, and KEEPING and MULTIPLYING the funds that come your way.

Slow down, balance out yourself and your life. Pave the way for money to flow to you like water. Abundance of all things exists within God-Mind. It is up to you to decide in what area of your life you want abundance and then create the recipe to attract it. You have many choices. Make the correct choice for the correct reason in the correct way, and watch your life automatically change for the better.

Do you want more money right now? Do you have the mind-pattern to attract it? This is the key that only the wealthy know! They always have plenty because their mind-patterns only know wealth. There is not a doubt in their minds of who they are, what they have, and what they will have.

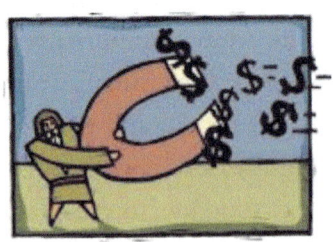

Do you live with a mind-pattern of scarcity and lack?

What did your parents tell you when you were a child?

Things like, "Money doesn't grow on trees, we cannot afford it, it is too expensive"?

These kinds of words imprint you with scarcity and lack.

Do you have abandonment issues?

While this may seem entirely unrelated, be aware that "money" can abandon you as easily as people. Working through any abandonment issues with people strengthens the mind-pattern that holds onto money and all that money buys.

People can abandon you emotionally as well as physically. If you felt emotionally abandoned by either parent, there is a good chance that your financial wealth abandons you also, leaving you feeling stranded in life.

Do you deserve to have everything you need?

How is your self-worth?

What does your internal self-talk say?

Do you judge and criticize yourself?

Do you denigrate and downplay your abilities?

To pull money to you, and retain it, you must know in the deepest levels of your being that you deserve to have it! Otherwise, you create more issues for yourself.

Sometimes you create money, but cannot seem to hold onto it. This is the low self-worth mind-pattern that does not allow you to keep it. There is a part of you thinking, "Who am I to have all this wealth? I don't deserve it."

Whenever thoughts of scarcity and lack enter into your mind, release them up to whatever you consider to be your higher power. Replace with these words:

*I now have more money than I need.*

When you feel as though your finances leave you stranded, release those thoughts and replace with:

*I now have a flow of more money coming in than going out.*

When negative self-talk enters your head, release those thoughts, replacing with:

*I now deserve and accept more money than I ever thought possible.*

As you address old mind-patterns and re-imprint new ones, you, too, can attract money and wealth into your life. Use these simple tips to find out for yourself!

# Appendices

# Complete Body Scan

Did you know that your health concerns show up in your mind-patterns and energy field before they manifest in your physical body? That conditions you have yet to be treated for in the future are visible in your energy field right now?

The Complete Body Scan allows you to correct any potential health problems —both known and unknown —before they manifest in physical form.

Stewart uses his tremendous mental abilities to scan each Chakra Band of your body and determine your areas of concern. "Chakras" are groups of nerve cells that come together in the body called "ganglions," which emit light throughout specific sectors of the body. These chakras are actually bands of colored light that permeate through the body and when viewed from a distance look like a cylindrical tube. When the body is in balance, each band of the body emits a specific color.

After Stewart scans all your Chakra Bands, he explains the mind-pattern that created the issue in the first place and suggests a variety of mental and physical exercises along with dietary and supplemental nutrients to improve those areas.

Use your Complete Body Scan to answer your health questions and help direct your body into a state of optimal physical balance.

# A Compilation of Interesting Notes Through the Years

### Abuse

First, it is important to understand objectively why these thoughts are in your head. Learn Object Observation techniques (***Decoding Your Life***). If something is within you, ignoring it does not make it go away. Sometimes focusing on it helps it to come out, but you must learn to proactively release it in the least uncomfortable way that does not harm you or others.

Often people are abusers because they have been abused, either in this lifeline or another. They perpetuate this because the person they harm is really "themselves" and what the abuser feels he/she deserves. There are a variety of mind-patterns behind this type of behavior and each case would need to be looked at individually.

The body is a representation of all mind-patterns. All disease is from a mind-pattern.

The drugs only mask the symptoms.

A long-term health issue requires a detailed protocol. This could be accomplished via a one hour Email Consultation where you email a complete birth name and date of birth with this request. AND you would have to be willing to follow the protocol.

## Acid Reflux

Mind-pattern:

*I cannot stomach my life and it burns me
to analyze it or speak about it.*

First use Ice Blue in the area to "cool" it off. Use Pale Yellow daily in that chakra to normalize it. Take horsetail herb and Omega-3 fish oils and drink chamomile and licorice tea. Work on the mind-pattern behind all of this.

## ADD AND ADHD

ADD and ADHD are "manufactured" diagnoses in order to prescribe drugs forever. Perform daily chakra spinning and T-Bar archetype balancing as delineated in **Healer's Handbook** and **Hyperspace Helper**, with emphasis at the Royal Blue pineal area. Use Ice Blue and Brown around the body when excited. Use Pale Yellow to help with studies and understanding. Also use Shiny Copper at the skull. Take Omega-3 fish oil and kava kava daily.

## Addictions

### Drugs, Alcohol and Addictive Behaviors

Anyone who is an addict of any kind is trying to escape life. It is not your place to judge his/her experiences. When he/she is ready to move out of the addiction, better to be there to lend a helping hand. In the meantime, communicate with this person via the Oversoul level as described in **Decoding Your Life**. Whenever the person is ready for help, then he/she has to face the life issues that caused this to happen in the first place, plus build up a stronger body to hold a stronger mind-pattern, as most likely the physical structure is severely depleted. Not an easy scenario, but you have to love people enough to allow them to go through their experiences without making their experiences yours. It is a tough job.

Many substitute one addiction for another. It is not the item itself, but the mind-pattern of needing to blot out reality with whatever it takes to do that. This stems from trauma and abuse of one type or another. These people need release work and deprogramming.

## AGING

Change the mind-patterns that create aging. Human DNA is designed for immortality.

## ALLERGIES

Allergies involve things that irritate you in physical reality. Pollen develops into the male reproductive cell, so allergies mean a male or spirituality, something small, or a grouping of many small things, are coming together to irritate you in a large way. Ice Blue can help relieve the pain and irritation. Flush with Violet and then hold the eyes in Royal Blue. See what works best for your system.

## ALZHEIMER'S

The soul-personality is not affected, only the brain. It is the result of a mind-pattern of a fear of death. So parts of the mind leave while parts remain to hold the body. It is like a foot in both worlds. They are leaving their bodies head first instead of the other way around, which is normal.

Proper chakra spinning, T-Bar balancing, and correcting pertinent mind-patterns is needed.

You can do color therapy to enhance the color Violet. Comfrey is a good heavy metal detox. It is off the market now in the U.S., but you can grow it yourself. Do not buy comfrey, grow it. It is abundant in the woods. Gold and silver are good heavy metal detoxes; take only homeopathic or elixir versions. It is best to start when you just notice the symptoms because otherwise it gets harder to do.

## Anemia

The mind-pattern is one of feeling weak in the current world situation, also giving away one's power.

Do not take iron supplements, as they are toxic over time. Do color therapy with Medium Green, take CoQ10, and eat organic liver, spinach, and red meats.

Asians typically have more copper-based blood so therefore have more anemia. See **Blue Blood True Blood** for details.

## Anorexia

The mind-pattern behind anorexia is one of extremely low self-worth and feeling like one does not deserve to exist and cannot digest any life experiences. Anorexia is a slow form of suicide. Typically anorexic individuals have many emotional issues that they need to deal with, not "shrink" away from.

## Anti-Depressants

Most anti-depressants are really mind-control drugs or chemical outgrowths of the Montauk mind-control experiments. Prozac was one of the first of these medications that had a direct link to Montauk.

## ANXIETY AND PANIC ATTACKS

The mind-pattern of anxiety and panic attacks is deep fear.

There are many psychological causes of panic attacks, depending upon the individual. There are ELF pulses, especially at night, which can cause some people to react with panic feelings. Use the Violet bubble with the external mirror to block these transmissions.

Take Kava kava and/or valerian if feelings persist.

Use the affirmation, "I release the need for deep fear."

Generally use Ice Blue and/or Brown.


## APPENDIX

Everyone has an appendix, both male and female. The appendix serves a purpose that involves your intuitive abilities. Because it is on the right-hand side it connects with spirituality or a male figure. It is considered to be part of the immune system, which protects the body, and it concerns your ideas about being protected by either a male figure or your spiritual ideas/concepts.

Explosions (ruptures) involve anger issues. So the overall mind-pattern involves anger toward a male figure that you perceive did not/is not protecting you (this could even be yourself) or anger about your spiritual ideas, concepts that did not/are not protecting you. It also concerns digesting ancient foods (ideas) that "no longer exist," at least not consciously in the minds of most people.

An appendix that has ruptured is serious and the individual may need the allopathic meds to save their life. Remember that all things come from God-Mind and there is a place for everything. The individual can ask their Oversoul to bless and clean up the meds so that they do what they are supposed to do and anything excess leaves the body.

Take sea salt baths, 1-2 cups per bath plus 1/2 -1 cup of aluminum-free baking soda. This will help detoxify and draw out infection.

Flush the body with Medium Green to oxygenate and use Violet to kill the infection. You can use the Logos Christos Healing Archetype as well as the "N" Archetype for overall healing.

Work on the mind-pattern that caused this to happen in the first place. There is much you can do, but as with so many events in every person's life, you have to put yourself in a reactive vs. proactive position. You must deal with "what was" so you can create a new path for yourself.

## Arthritis

The mind-pattern of arthritis concerns self-criticism and anger towards Self. Are you criticizing yourself? If so, these mind-patterns have to be released.

The mind-pattern behind rheumatoid arthritis is a painful support structure in life, deep self-criticism and may involve self-hate.

Use warm castor oil packs and soak hands in warm sea salt with aluminum-free baking soda. Work on detoxing the entire body to be free of calcium deposits. Increase your levels of Vitamin D to help absorb calcium. Deep tissue massage therapy can help to break up the crystals that create arthritis. Sometimes adding fresh lemon or lime juice to the diet can help. Do what you can to support the change of mind-pattern. These steps will get you started.

Visualize Shiny Copper surrounded by Ice Blue in the affected bones for 45 seconds, three times daily. Ice Blue may help stop the pain, but it is important for you to understand the mind-pattern that you are trying to "ice" so that you can permanently release your issues.

## Asthma

The mind-pattern of asthma is being emotionally overwhelmed in childhood, usually by a parent.

Asthma concerns deeply suppressing your emotions and feeling smothered in life. It can also involve a fungal infection. Many people get asthma or allergies when they move, which is caused by becoming emotional about moving away from your friends and family. That is called reactive asthma. It also occurs when the seasons or temperature change. It develops and can be triggered when there is a change from warm weather to cold weather or when individuals go from being outside in the heat to air-conditioning.

What does that mean? Let us bring that temperature change into an emotion, which provides a clue as to what is going on in the mind. If you move from a warm environment to one that is cold and distant, you can translate that to what will happen anytime you go from warm to cold. What was the issue where you felt warm and happy emotionally and what made you feel cold and took your breath away?

That means something so traumatic literally took your breath away and made you react where you cannot breath and your lungs close up. Anything that triggers that from then on, whatever associates in the mind with that issue, will trigger an asthmatic attack. So here is the key for this type of situation: Look at the issue where there was that emotional coldness, isolation, or distance that literally takes your breath away.

Sports-induced asthma physiologically means the alveoli and lungs are closing down due to excess exertion. It would imply that during the exercise, you are not breathing properly and it is causing the oxygen levels in the lungs to drop. The lung tries to overcompensate by breathing quickly and then causes an asthmatic attack. You have to look at what the trigger is for that. See if you can find the age where it began. Males have it more commonly and it concerns some parent or coach or authority figure who tried to push them beyond their real limits. So, they always feel anxious in a similar situation even if that person is not there anymore; that makes them feel they cannot achieve the goal and they are being punished or put down for it. It is an emotional stress, which is another clue. Usually it involves another person in their childhood who was too pressuring on them to achieve something they could not achieve.

Use the Green Spiral Staircase exercise in ***Hyperspace Helper***. You should go down it while holding the word "asthma" in your mind to see when the issue developed in your lifetime and imprinted as a pattern. Go back to the point where you did not have it, then move forward until it began. When you get to the point where it began, what was going on? What was overwhelming you emotionally that was creating it? That is what you have to examine, then do the release work. Release the emotional experiences up to your Oversoul by using the techniques described in ***Decoding your Life***.

Usually there is Red in the lungs; breathe that out. Using the breath as a tool, push the vibratory imprints, which are comprised of energy, out the top of the head and up into your Oversoul. Review the experiences as they pass before your inner eye. After releasing, breathe in and fill the lungs with Medium Green from your Oversoul to oxygenate the body and for emotional healing. If you do not replace what you have just released, it will either bring the old experiences back in, or recreate similar ones that will complicate the process.

Be mindful of eliminating mucous producing foods in your diet. Rye Grass Extract and Marshmallow Herb can be helpful as well.

## Autonomic Functions

All autonomic functions are connected to baseline God-Mind patterns. Everything else is a result of individual mind-patterns.

## BIPOLAR ISSUES

In order to address this properly, you need a reading to learn the causes and what is going on mentally. I used to be a Developmental Specialist in a clinic for dually diagnosed patients. I have dealt with this type of issue many times.

There are techniques and herbs that can be done and taken to remove you from those harmful meds. However, I am not allowed to tell anyone to stop taking their medications. Everyone must make their own decisions based on their comfort zone.

## BIRTHMARKS

Birthmarks all mean something related to the mind-pattern of the individual who has it. The meaning depends on the shape, color, location, and size.

## BLADDER

Anything that involves bladder issues has a mind-pattern of anger.

## BLOOD

### Hardening of the Arteries

Anything to do with blood/blood veins involves joy in life. In general, a person with this symptom has the mind-pattern that life does not carry joy for him/her. Diet follows the mind-pattern to build the body this way. Correcting diet without correcting the mind-pattern only means the issue will come back or surface in another way, perhaps even worse.

Omega-3 fish oil capsules are one of the best supplements to prevent this, while there are others depending upon the finer nuances of the person's mind-pattern. Mind-pattern is key to any physical, mental, emotional correction.

## Blood Clots

Blood clots represent clogs in the joy of your life.

There are alternatives to the medication Coumadin, but you need to find a medical professional who can appropriately advise you. If you need an allopathic drug to get you through, then ask that it be blessed and cleaned up via the Oversoul level to do what it is supposed to do and reject what the body does not need. In the meantime, do the mental work to correct and balance the mind-pattern so the outpicturing in the physical body can change to match the "new you."

Use Medium Green to help unclog the physical, and also to help unclog the mental/emotional aspects of your life that created this outpicturing of your thoughts.

Flush with Violet to push the blood clot out of the artery or vein. If the blood clot is in the legs, use Brown after flushing in Violet. Take Lecithin and Omega-3 fish oils to loosen the clot.

## Blood Transfusions

Blood transfusions absolutely have an effect on the body. The recipient picks up the vibrational energy of the donor. This gets imprinted on your cellular structure even after you start making your own blood cells. However, this is not an accident. Your mind-pattern attracted it in the first place.

Blood is one of the most intimate frequencies that a person has. When you receive the blood of another, you receive their frequencies and the associated mind-patterns that created it.

Flush the blood with Violet energy and then eat red meat to build back your own blood.

### Fear of Blood Test/Donation

The mind-pattern is fear of losing your joy in life. There may be other contributing factors that need to be addressed, such as, is this something that you are supposed to be doing?

### High Blood Pressure

High blood pressure is about feeling stressed and overwhelmed in life. The remedies will depend on that person's issues and body type, which requires a scan. There are different reasons for high blood pressure that require different remedies. Mentally, staying in Ice Blue for a few moments will help.

### Low Blood Pressure

Low of blood pressure means that the person does not feel like there is much joy flowing through his/her life.

### Hughes Syndrome

The "sticky blood" issue comes from the viscosity of the blood, meaning that you are dehydrated and need more water/fluids. It is also beneficial to take Omega-3 fish oils and eat more red meats.

## BOWELS / DIGESTIVE TRACT / SMALL AND LARGE INTESTINES

### Colitis

Anything that involves the colon relates to a mind-pattern of releasing. Colitis is related to the nervous system as well as to the digestive system. Digestive issues, both mentally and physically, need to be balanced; the nervous system needs to be strengthened, and there needs to be intense release work around the issues that created the physical symptoms in the first place.

### Constipation

The mind-pattern of constipation is a refusal to release the past.

### Diarrhea

Evacuating your bowels represents releasing the past. Diarrhea is usually watery, and water represents your emotions. So, watery discharge involves releasing your emotions. This could even be considered "tears," as in crying for your past. Release your emotions via the Oversoul level and examine your digestive system, which is most likely involved as well, and the foods you are eating. This could also concern a bacteria or virus that may need to be addressed. You can mentally flush the system with Violet as an aid.

### Irritable Bowel Syndrome

Irritable bowel syndrome is needing to rapidly release the past and present and not holding on to anything of value.

### Stomach

The mind-pattern is not being able to "stomach" what the outer or inner world is trying to "feed" you.

For stress in general and to relax the digestive system, drink ginger and/or peppermint tea.

Burning concerns anger issues, even if your anger is "justified." Anger is anger and will destroy.

## BUGS

The mind-pattern is that something in your home is "bugging" you and annoying you. What insignificant thing is bothering you? Physically, it could be from many things. Spray apple cider vinegar is a good preventative to block them.

### Bed Bugs

You have a rough time relaxing and resting. Something bugs you on many levels.

Literally–what is bugging you at night? What is a bother in sleep? Look at your dream state.

To kill them, prepare a mixture if distilled water, organic powdered garlic, food-grade hydrogen peroxide, and agrisept. Mix well and douse all over your mattress. Let it soak in. You may need to sleep on a rubber pad until it dries. That will get the little buggers organically. Sprinkling bay leaves and cayenne pepper on your mattress keeps the little buggers away.

## BURNS

Burns result from anger. For example, if you burn your left leg it involves moving through physical reality and/or a woman, which could be yourself or someone else. The basic mind-patterns concern anger at physical reality, a woman, or a woman in physical reality. You have to look at your life to see which one makes sense for your situation.

Use Brown in the legs to help that area return to its natural color; Ice Blue for any pain; Green to oxygenate and regenerate; Pale Yellow in the muscle and nerves; and flush with Violet to avoid infections.

## BULIMIA

The basic mind-pattern behind bulimia (vomiting ingested food to prevent absorption) is low-self worth, which says you do not deserve to assimilate the learning of your life's experiences. It also involves rejecting all that you are taking in, or ingesting, from life. Anyone who "denies" anything about their life has a mind-pattern of self-denial.

Bulimia is usually coupled with anorexia, which has the low-self worth pattern of not feeling like you deserve to live, literally shrinking out of existence. People with these mind-patterns actually are in the process of a slow suicide.

Do release work and visualize all that you no longer need going right out the top of your head and up to your Oversoul. Replace it with Pale Pink unconditional love from your Oversoul.

Fresh pineapple and papaya are full of good digestive enzymes; probiotics such as acidophilus and whole milk yogurts with these cultures are helpful. Fermented rice drinks are also especially beneficial options for probiotics.

## Cacao

Cacao inhibits digestion of proteins. Most low-end chocolate is primarily white sugar with enough chocolate to color it. The processing often leaves the candy with a myriad of other by-products, including lead. Yes, it can be addictive, like anything else. Knowing all this, I still like chocolate, buy high-end organic dark chocolate, and only eat it on occasion.

## Cancer

All cancers are initially caused by a mind-pattern of held resentment. Cancer is caused by viruses that enter the cells and alter the genetic material and mutate cells. Diet and lifestyle changes alone do not cure anything unless one changes the mind-pattern. If you kill the virus, no new cancer will form. If you correct the mind-pattern, the disease will reverse. If you want to prevent cancer, remove all your resentments.

Sugar feeds parasites and cancer. The best diet has no sugar, wheat, or processed foods.

### Breast Cancer

Those who get it have one common mind-pattern—what is eating away at you? The area of the body where it exists tells you about your issue. Notice how Breast Cancer is the latest popular cause. At my supermarket, upon checkout, I was asked, "Do you want to give $1 for breast cancer?" To me, this means if I give $1, I am helping to create breast cancer. Breasts involve nurturing, so people who have breast cancer do not feel nurtured. What are women doing these days to prevent breast cancer? Cutting them off! No breasts, no breast cancer…another step toward androgyny and "equalizing" males and females. Finally, notice the pink ribbon alters that are the symbol for breast cancer awareness. What happens when you give something energy? It grows! It does not diminish. The Illuminati are merely following Universal Law. You see it in action. You learn Universal Law and you do not have to succumb to the path that they are leading people down, whether it be cancer or financial downfall. Always remember: MIND-PATTERN!

Breast cancer usually involves a lack of nurturing by parental figures or self.

Breast Cancer is now in the public eye to help aid in the denigration of females. The more energy and attention is given to any matter increases its growth. This also means that many women with histories of breast cancer are choosing to remove healthy breasts so they will avoid breast cancer in the future. Plus, no breasts, no way to feed naturally feed babies–another plus for the artificial womb!

Ultimately, this is leading to the artificial androgyny of human race–where you cannot tell male from female.

### Lung Cancer

This is from held resentment emotionally for what is taken from life.

### Stomach Cancer

This is from held resentment from what is learned and assimilated in life.

## Uterine Cancer

The mind-pattern behind uterine cancer is resentment for having one's creativity blocked/repressed, but there could be other factors. I would have to scan the person to see what is going on before recommending treatment. Wild Yam root capsules should help. I only recommend Dead Sea salt; it is the most powerful.

## Canker Sores

The mind-pattern is suppressing a hurtful issue that needs to be verbally expressed but has been held back.

There could be many causes for this manifestation from bacteria to viruses to heavy metal toxins.

Put tea tree oil on the sores and follow up with aloe vera gel. Mentally place them in Ice Blue after a Violet Flush.

## Cartilage

Cartilage involves what holds your support structure together.

Knees are your flexibility in the future, so if they are sore, you feel like your future flexibility is torn out from underneath you. Work on the mind-pattern to correct this.

Use Pale Yellow in the cartilage, warm castor oil packs on the affected area, and take Glucosomine Chondroitin and shark cartilage. Cartilage can take a long time to heal because of low blood flow to the area, so also use Medium Green to aid this process. Of course, stay off of it as much as possible, but that is easier said than done.

## Cellulite

The mind-pattern depends on where the cellulite appears on the body. If on the legs, the mind-pattern concerns fear of the future and insulating against it.

It is all part of an insulation mind-pattern, especially if there was childhood trauma. Release work is in order.

Work on the mind-pattern that creates this in the first place and correct it. In the meantime, you can use organic mudpacks to cleanse the face and break down cellulite and feed your skin with castor oil and/or coconut oil. Also do your detox work—the Internal Cleanse, ginger flavor, from www.blessedherbs.com is great. Remember that this did not happen overnight and most likely will take some time to rectify. The more detox/release work that you do, the more opportunity that these tissues can replicate healthier cells. You should consider a ph-balancing diet.

## Chicken

It is the "symbolism energy" of chicken that represents fear issues. You are what you eat. However, changing mind-patterns and releasing fear issues removes the negative affects.

All food is contaminated in some way. The additives like MSG, soy, corn syrup, flavorings and colorings, etc. all serve to destroy the body and later DNA. Organic foods are not pure either, but are still better than the commercial types.

The Illuminati eat whatever they want because they have a mind-pattern that does not consider pain or suffering. Plus, they have access to all cures and reversals of illnesses.

## CHIROPRACTIC AND ACUPUNCTURE

Chiropractic and Acupuncture work can alleviate painful symptoms so that the person has the presence of mind to work on the mind-patterns that caused them. When a person is in pain, they may not be able to concentrate enough to do the mental work. It would not be a crutch unless that was all you relied upon.

## CHLORINE

Technically, it is your mind-pattern that determines what your physical body does with chlorine. Chlorine can help kill bacteria in the body (both good and bad!) so it does have a positive function as well as a negative one.

Do your mental work; this is the best protection.

## CHRONIC FATIGUE SYNDROME

The mind-pattern of chronic fatigue syndrome is feeling weakened by the world, being overwhelmed by experience and unable to handle it.

## CROHN'S DISEASE

The mind-pattern is not being able to assimilate experiences in life and being angry at it. It is an extreme unhappiness and loss of joy about what you get out of life and learn about life. It is from nerve action, not viruses.

I was once diagnosed with it and now it is gone. The mind-pattern is extreme irritation and pain from what you are learning about yourself.

Use Pale Yellow on the solar plexus daily. Eat organic foods only and include red meats. Drink aloe vera juice in the morning and evening. Do release work on the past. Drink ginger tea.

I had success with Raw Tienchi Powder tea. This was an amazing cure.

## Cysts

Whether cysts are internal or external, anything that "bursts" usually involves angers that are welling up inside and then instead of "bursting" out mentally (as in release work to your Oversoul), these outpicture via your physical body into bursting cysts.

When there is a history of abuse, these will develop in the same area as the abuse occurred.

## DNA

Mind-pattern creates DNA. It attracts experience via frequencies like a magnet. There is no destiny or fate, other than knowing oneself.

Everything we experience and everyone we meet, we attract with our mind-patterns. They represent something inside of us that we are reflecting out.

When someone has a disease at a young age, they entered life with this mind-pattern from other lifetimes where it went unresolved.

There is no physical way for DNA to have 12 helixes or strands. It is always a double helix, no matter what the species. There are 12 groupings of DNA components that may open up depending upon the person's mind-pattern.

Remember, the mind-pattern creates the DNA. So, whatever you become, the DNA will reflect and express.

Ultimately, you need to look at the mind-pattern that created this condition in the first place and the contributing mind-pattern. Consider a Personal Consultation at some point to put yourself on a healing path specific to you.

A Personal Consultation will also suggest a diet and supplements to help balance the mind-pattern as well as the physical body.

We cure nothing. We help guide you into the mind-pattern that created your situation in the first place, how to correct the mind-pattern and what you can do on a mental/physical level to boost/support a new mind-pattern that allows you to heal yourself.

You may choose a Personal Consultation (90 Minutes) either by phone or email; this also includes a written report. We particularly recommend the following books and DVDs as supplement and further reference: **Hyperspace Helper, Decoding Your Life, Healers Handbook.**

A part of you knows what you did to create your life experience, therefore, you know how to "uncreate" it and build something differently. You may also want to consider attending a seminar intensive in St. Joseph Michigan.

## Deafness

Deafness is from a mind-pattern of not wanting to hear. The genetics are created by the mind. All can be corrected if there is a willingness to do so.

## Depression

Mind-patterns and experiences from childhood are usually the cause of depression. These need to be released. There is ELF (extreme low frequencies) that can cause depression, but that is not the only cause.

## DIABETES

The mind-pattern for diabetes concerns feeling like you cannot process or digest the sweetness in life. It is there, but you cannot take it in. You have to return to the point of origin and release it, with the supportive nutrients.

The type of diabetes (Type I or Type II) is important in the "cure" process and its origin in your body. There can be underlying infections/heavy metal conditions that can be traced back to immunizations. You have to rebuild the entire system to help the pancreas come back online, as well as doing the mental work. The physical cure is meaningless unless the mind leads.

Chiropractic care and perhaps massage therapy are also beneficial.

Diabetes is not a bacterium. It is a general diagnosis when the pancreas is malfunctioning. Once you know it is malfunctioning you must trace down the mental beginning so it can be corrected in the mind-pattern as well as find the correct mix of nutrients to boost the physical structure.

If you have diabetes, you should be drinking peppermint tea daily because it helps regulate insulin production as does the flowers of the ginseng plant.

## DRUGS

Legal drugs can be equally dangerous to the physical and energetic system. The physical structure can be purged of these medications over time, which then allows the energetic structure to mend itself. In the meantime, use heavy Violet Flushes (mentally), sea salt baths, and general detoxification–this is usually a process and does not happen overnight. The length of time to correct this depends upon the residual drugs in the physical body as well as the determination of the mind-pattern.

# Ears

Hearing difficulties depend on the cause, however you could be using Pale Yellow to regenerate nerve tissue in that area.

## Ear Wax

Try using castor oil, mulein oil, hydrogen peroxide, and ear candling.

Look at the mind-pattern: What are you trying not to hear?

## Eustation Tube

You can use this experience as blessing in disguise to study one aspect of hearing. The positive side is to be able to hear. Use heavy Royal Blue in the ear, along with some hydrogen peroxide. This is a GENERAL answer. You need to find the mind-pattern and do a full body scan (which you can do yourself) as the physical structure functions as a unit.

There is something you do not like hearing in life.

## Tinnitus

What is happening in your life that you do not want to hear? Use Royal Blue in this chakra band, balance your T-Bar, use high quality castor oil drops in the ear, and work on the mind-pattern that originally created this situation.

## Ear Piercing

I have them because they enhance the eye/vision meridian. As a mind-pattern, it means I place double value on what I hear from females.

# Elbows (see Joints)

## Epstein Barr Virus

The Epstein Barr mind-pattern is one of feeling like life is too much trouble and the person is not willing to be a full participant.

## Eyes

Mind-patterns of eyes involve how you see the world. Anything concerning the eyes affects what you see and how you react to it.

Suggestions on eliminating specific eye conditions require a personal consultation to look at your specific mind-pattern.

### Conjunctivitis

The left side of the body involves a female figure, logic, or physical reality. This could be anything from you, if you are a female, to the world around you. This is an infection that indicates anger at someone, or more than someone, that you are seeing–this could include you.

Natural remedies–load up on Standard Process Immuplex, Vitamin C, and Echinacea, as well as put pure quality castor oil (such as PRL brand from www.healthwarriorblog.com). Keep your T-Bar balanced, keep your chakras in proper sequence, keep Royal Blue in the eyes, and do your release work!

### Corrective Eye Surgery

Corrective eye surgery is certainly a fast route, if you find a competent doctor to perform the operation. My research has shown that generally speaking, if you correct for near-sightedness, then your far-sighted vision may need help via corrective lenses, or vice versa. Contacts/glasses create barriers between you and the outside world.

Personally, I opted for vision therapy after using corrective lenses for over 40 years. For me, it was some of the most satisfying mental work I have ever done. This is a slower process and my eyes are still not 100% "perfect" all the time, but they continue to improve steadily and I no longer require corrective lenses. I do not believe in laser eye surgery. Vision therapy is a slower process, but it has helped me deal with my mind-patterns. I still work at it on and off as I can. However, I do know that many people are happy with their laser surgery, so you must make the best choice for you.

For anyone thinking about this route, I highly suggest viewing our DVD *Health Intensive: A YOU Makeover*; vision is far beyond the far/near sightedness that most people associate with vision disorders. I learned so much through my process, it was incredible, and I discuss vision therapy in greater detail in this DVD.

My goal is to correct the mind-pattern that created my issues in the first place so that I NEVER need corrective lenses–regardless of what the stats say!

Corrective lenses require people to be dependent on the outside world rather than on their own internal Self.

Lasik surgery depends upon the individual, his/her goals and health issues but I strongly recommend vision therapy.

Correct the mind-pattern and the body follows.

## Eye Color

Eyes represent how individuals mirror what is in their mind-pattern.

When one's eye color changes from dark brown to amber, gray, or hazel. What are the mind patterns that cause it?

This could anything from programming to genetic activations to health issues.

## Teary Eyes

This is a form of crying. The mind-pattern is one of constant sadness. You should be doing release work and Growing Up the Child Within.

## FEET

### Athlete's Foot

The mind-pattern is about feeling that the future support in life is contaminated and annoying/painful.

Soak the foot in distilled water mixed with hydrogen peroxide. Take MMS. Take sea salt baths. Stop putting your feet in dirty places!

### Infected Toenails

This means you feel your future protective abilities are weak and compromised.

First soak the foot in Dead Sea salt water. Then apply the tea tree oil. Use castor oil overnight.

### Toenails

Toenails that are too long mean "I'm protecting myself from the future; I don't want to go there."

### Toes

Pain here is a mind-pattern of fear of stepping into the future, as related to female energy or daily living.

In general the left side of the body concerns female figures (including yourself) and physical reality. Toes involve balance as you walk forward.

### Foot Warts and Corns

Your mind-pattern is letting these viruses in. It involves future support structure.

## Fibroids

Generally, the mind-pattern for this is blocked creativity causing unhappiness. Not being able to be productive in life.

You may need wild yam root, warm castor oil packs and pituitary homeopathics.

## Fibromyalgia

Fibromyalgia comes from a microplasma that can be killed with the use of hyssop and golden seal. The general mind-pattern is being pained by life in every way. It will be specific, depending on the person.

I cannot say without a reading, but it may be associated with being out of balance in the future.

It may be a mind-pattern of self-abuse and self-punishment. The treatment varies by individual depending on intensities, specific abuse issues, and damage to the nervous system.

## Food

Eating represents understanding new information and digesting what you learn.

## Genitals

### Circumcision

It is supposed to be a "sign" that you are one of God's chosen–clean and wholesome. It was originally to identify the Hebrews from the "goyim."

The mind-pattern for circumcised males is that you do not protect your most private creations and sexuality.

It is a form of mutilation as almost 30% of sensitivity is removed. Read ***Template of God-Mind*** for what circumcision really means.

### Erectile Dysfunction and Impotency

The mind-pattern behind erectile dysfunction is feeling like you have lost your creative power in life. If this happens when you are engaging in sexual acts with a female, then you have to think about which female in your life causes you to feel like this. It could be the woman you are with, or she may represent someone else. Does this happen when you are not with a female? Is it a specific female? Release work will help and of course you need to look at the physical side to see what is going on there as well.

Also see ***True Reality of Sexuality***, Basic Sexual Archetypes section, pages 108-110. To support the male reproductive system, read the information on page 42 of ***Hyperspace Helper***.

### Feminine Dryness

The mind-pattern behind this is a fear of creativity on some level. Use the following affirmation: "I allow my deepest creative desires to fully express in physicality."

Taking supplements for the female system such as wild yam root (850-1200 mg), aloe vera gel capsules, and black cohosh should help. Take the wild yam root when you are not bleeding. Once you start bleeding, stop it, and then start again when the bleeding stops. Take the aloe vera and black cohosh continuously.

### Itching

Mind-pattern of itching the genitals:

*Annoyance in creative issues and sexual activity.*

### Testicular Pain

Physically this shows that the hormones are backing up in this location and not flowing out properly. It can be a blockage in the seminal vesicles.

The mind-pattern is that you are blocking your creative flow with females and suppressing creative urges by using logic instead of emotion.

Treat the area with warm castor oil packs daily. Take extra Vitamin D and at least 50 mg of zinc. Use a Violet vacuum hose to remove the cysts.

Think to yourself, "I NOW have perfect relationships with females."

### Varicocele

The testicles concern the male's creative energy. If the veins are abnormally large, then the male has the mind-pattern of draining away his creative energy.

## GUMS

### Gingivitis and Periodontal Disease

The mind-pattern for gum diseases is being unable to adjust to certain circumstances in your life. It also may involve saying damaging or foul language frequently.

Gum issues are related to your ability to adjust to your life circumstances. You might want to try tea tree oil on the gums, or a tea tree oil mouthwash. You also might want to use hyssop tea and capsules for latent infection. A product our dentist recommends and we use is by Dental Herb Company called "Tooth and Gums Tonic." It is a great herbal mouthwash.

## HAIR

The general mind-pattern or energy behind what hair represents on the body is personal strengths. It depends where on the body the hair is located; this means there is strength in that part of the body.

## Shaving

Hair represents strength, so shaving it off means you feel like you are "cut off" from your strength.

## Shaving Legs

Females are called "the weaker sex." It is one of society's ways of maintaining this mind-pattern. In many countries women do not shave these body parts.

## Grey Hair

Grey means doubt and confusion, so look at that within yourself.

There are many organic hair dyes out there. They are not as effective as the commercial kinds.

## Hair Thinning

The mind-pattern is not speaking up properly and feeling a loss of personal strength. The mind-pattern is that you feel your personal strength is unsure and tenuous.

## Hair Loss

The mind-pattern is that you feel that you are losing your personal power and strength. Stop that!

Try using jojoba oil and shampoo on the scalp. Get cranio-sacral massage. Take Omega-3 fish oils. Use the Power Archetype template.

You may need more proteins in the diet. There may be heavy metals that need detoxing. Do not wear hats. Take folic acid and biotin.

Inversion of the physical body means more blood flow to the head, which in turn feeds the scalp; this in turn MAY assist in the growth and thickening of the hair. Like all things, your mind-pattern determines if you can hold the effects or not.

Hair represents your strength–when you feel in a weakened position, your hair is apt to respond accordingly.

Hair falling out is most often due to stress. The tension in the body cuts off circulation to the scalp/hair follicles and then the hair dies from lack of blood supply and falls out, unable to reproduce new hair.

Hair loss is often attributed to poor diet and heavy metal buildup, among other things.

Eat well, take your supplements, massage your scalp and/or brush it, inversion tables MAY help (standing on your head may adversely effect the neck vertebrae), and above all else, do your mental work.

**Heavy Hair Gel**

The heavy hair gel means holding your power in place–no progress.

**Dandruff**

Dandruff represents annoyances that need to be removed from whatever is "covering" your life. You also feel that your surface thoughts are "dirty" or bad.

Use jojoba oil shampoo and conditioner. Increase Omega-3 fish oils and eat more organic red meats.

## HANDS

The mind-pattern for nails is protection. For example, when you see someone with long, claw-like nails, the mind-pattern is saying, "Stay away from me; I'm protecting myself from you."

**Biting Nails**

If someone bites their nails and there is almost nothing left of them, it means the person is vulnerable and allows others to hurt or abuse them without defenses. Nails on the hands also represent what you grasp in life right now. They also represent what you are currently protecting in your life.

### Broken Fingers

The mind-pattern depends upon what finger is broken:

index finger—direction in life

middle finger—sexuality

ring finger—relationships

small finger–family.

The finger tells you what is not healing in your life, and is remaining the way that it is.

### Cracking and Popping Fingers

This is a release of gases that are built up in the joints–so it is detoxification of the hands, which hold and grasp what you hold onto in life. This can also be the mind-pattern of a nervous or anxious person.

### Cold Hands

Emotionally scared about what you are grasping in life right now. This shows extreme fear about current issues.

### Numb Fingers

Your left hand concerns what you grasp in physical reality. If it is numb, it is because you are numbing yourself to what it is you think you have to grasp. This will spread if you do not fix the mind-pattern. In the meantime, rub the area with castor oil or coconut oil to wake up the nerves in this area and do your release work!

## HEART

### Fibrillation and Palpitations

Your heart chakra is the seat of your emotions. Generally, something is happening or has happened to unsettle your emotions. You need to find out what that is and correct the mind-pattern.

These mind-patterns can result in a nutritional deficiency. Some people find that taking Hawthorne Berry strengthens the heart muscle. Flush with Medium Green and do your forgiveness and release work, as well as develop compassion for Self and what you have been through.

**Heart Attack**

The mind-pattern is being overwhelmed emotionally, literally creating an overwhelming sensation in stress and emotions and creating a blockage in the heart. A section of the heart muscle dies; it just does not get any more oxygen or nutrients. That is what a heart attack really is.

It is also important to note if other symptoms were present before the heart attack. These are clues before it ever happens but unfortunately you do not know until the attack occurs. We also have to look at the other symptoms. I know a runner who had a heart attack and now has kidney problems from processing past experiences.

The colors in the heart chakra for a person who is about to have a heart attack are either a deep Navy Blue and/or a Bright Red, depending on the type of heart attack. This represents lack of oxygenation, irritation to the heart muscle, and heavy emotional stress to the point they cannot sustain that emotional state any longer. This happens to people who do not work on their emotional issues and who suppress, hold in, and do not express or release.

First the person must be stabilized with the color codes to fix the heart. Medium Green must be put back in the heart chakra to oxygenate it and to assist with breathing properly. Surround that with a layer of Violet to protect and a layer of Brown over that to seal it in. There have been remarkable results by using Pale Pink for nurturing the heart if the issue is with the parents.

Next, work on the mind-pattern, the issue. You must determine what it is you are feeling stressed out about emotionally that you do not want to deal with. That is critical. It usually involves one person or a group of people very closely related. The people around you are important, but many times there exists a lack of self-esteem and issues within yourself as well. You might identify by looking at who is around you and what is being reflected back, because you do not want to see it in you. That is why a heart attack can happen. You might be blaming everyone around you for causing the emotional distress and upheaval.

A protocol with releasing techniques must be done in order to move the pressure and strain from the heart tissue so that there would be no further problem. Use the Golden Altar release technique and daily affirmations.

At least 100 mg or more of CoQ10 is helpful. It is actually made in the liver and it helps to oxygenate and energize the body, particularly in the heart/chest area. When we have a problem and the liver does not produce enough CoQ10 we need to add it into our daily minerals, vitamins, and supplements. It is expensive, but very important for someone for this issue.

Take folic acid daily to help the heart tissue. If the heart attack is due to plaque building up, then also take niacin. Also Vitamin E, which you should be taking daily anyway. Hawthorne berry is important as well. In fact, the drug Digitalis is a derivative of this.

## Height

Height concerns self-image ideas. You can grow taller. It is based on releasing low self-worth images and feeling "less than."

Visualize Copper in the skeletal structure, Pale Yellow in the muscular structure and nervous system. Release the mind-pattern of low self-worth. Review your genetics and why you chose this specific energy stream for this lifeline. If you do not correct the mind-pattern for feeling small, you will still feel small regardless of the size of the physical structure.

## Hemorrhoids

Soak in sea salt, then put tea tree oil on them. Overnight, you can use castor oil and/or aloe vera gel.

The mind-pattern is that you feel pain from releasing the past.

## Herbs

Herbs are a science unto themselves. Anyone's overall healing has to first start with correcting the mind-pattern. The herbs, or any other healing modality, is simply a boost to the mind-pattern. When the mind-pattern is corrected or open to correction, the healing modality comes to the person.

## Hormones

Use Perimenopause & Bioidentical Hormone Replacement Therapy; we highly recommend the fresh royal jelly for both male and female hormone balancing.

## Hurt and Pain

Hurt and pain are an illusion. It is not real, so no one can really hurt anyone. You can create a situation where you "think" you are hurt and blame others, but you do it to yourself with your own mind-patterns.

## Implants

Implants are considered to be an anomaly; there is usually no scar tissue found around them. They are predominately found on the pineal gland and elsewhere in the body. Some of these implants are crystalline, metallic, and some look organic. Nevertheless, they are not natural to the body and do not belong there. Physical implants are impossible to remove with the science available on this planet. There have been cadavers dissected in medical school where there are implants found when students cut open the brain. They do not have an explanation for these implants and are not allowed to talk about them.

What about the future of human bodies? If we are under mind-control and programming, how will it effect our mind/body correlation? What is the obvious answer? Robotic, nano-technology, which will create organic and inorganic implants in our body to control functions naturally so the mind-patterns cannot control the body directly. To enhance that, it will bring forth alters in the body that will create different cellular structures. As you know, when different alters come forward, the body changes in subtle ways to accommodate that alter's mind-pattern. So, if they want a specific type to come forward and stay forward, that is where the programming and mind-control comes in.

What is an organic implant?

An organic implant is one the body manufactures genetically that can be used as a tracking device, as a beacon of some sort. It can look like cartilage, bone spurs, or some kind of stone naturally developed by the body, but it is organic. The body is manifesting it for the purpose of connecting to the sympathetic nervous system of the implants.

What kind of soul personality would go into that body?

What kind of mentality would associate with a group mind? First level humans, animalistic-type, hive-mind, no free will, no independence, like the Borg. Yes, they want little Borgs.

## Glands

### Swollen Glands

Anything swollen represents something that someone is holding onto and not releasing. Glands are throughout the body and usually concern detoxification. So individuals are holding onto some kind of toxic mind-pattern that is making them ill.

### Swollen Glands along the Jaw (left side)

You are holding back something deep that you want to say to a female.

## Heavy Metals

Heavy metals can be purged via chelation, sulfur, comfrey, silver elixir, ionic foot baths, and of course, the mind.

## Hepatitis

Generally, anything concerning the liver involves a mind-pattern of holding anger and resentment.

## Hives/Urticaria

The mind-pattern behind hives involves something "getting under your skin" and irritating you. You can use anything you want, from traditional to nontraditional medicines, but until you find the mind-pattern creating the situation, it will continue to recur, or you will create new body issues.

## HUNTINGTON'S DISEASE

The mind-pattern is fear of losing your mind.

## INFLAMMATION

It can be caused by anger about what you are learning in life and hurting about releasing the past.

## INSECTS/BUGS

These concern suppressing/burying old emotions that bug you until you cannot hold it in anymore.

## INSOMNIA

Insomnia can be from fear of dying, avoiding rest due to self-sabotage/ punishment, or it could be a programming issue. The cure depends on the cause.

Try using the Dolphin Frequency work and taking valerian, kava kava, and/ or St. Johns Wort.

## INCURABLE DISEASE

There is no such thing as an "incurable disease." All dis-ease starts in the mind-pattern. Correct the mind-pattern and the physical body follows. Frequency medicine is the physical antidote to every dis-ease. With a powerful enough machine, the cure can be forced or the ailment created when the mind-pattern allows one or the other.

Mind-pattern is still the key. What does your mind-pattern pull to you and why?

No matter what the condition, mental, emotional or physical, the cause is a mind-pattern. Programming is based on the person's original mind-pattern so that it has a foundation to hook into. Even if an illness or condition is from programming, the mind-pattern had to exist in the person first. The health care industry is designed to keep you sick as long as possible. That is how they make money and create repetitive business. If you are well permanently, they lose.

All healing takes place in the mind, first. The physical always follows the mind. We have helped people with HIV move through this health issue and we know one medical doctor who also can do this. Using the word "cure" would get us in a lot of trouble! Where there's a will, there's a way; there is no greater strength than your mind.

First it was smallpox, then bird flu, now a flu pandemic and tuberculosis. One way or the other, you are being imprinted with the fear of illness and possibly death. Refuse to allow these news reports to gain any hold within your mind-pattern. Continue your quest to strengthen body, mind, and soul. You know what to do!

All healing takes place in the mind, first. The physical always follows the mind. Healing of any kind is a process of moving through the layers of the "condition," be it mental, physical, emotional, or spiritual.

## ITCHING

Itching can arise from many causes, from eczema to parasites to raw nerves. In general, you could try sea salt baths and castor oil rubs. Without a scan it is difficult to determine.

### Itching in the Genitals

The mind-pattern is annoyance in creative issues and sexual activity.

## JOINTS

### Elbows/Tennis Elbow

Problems with the elbow represent a mind-pattern of being inflexible with a current life situation. If it is in the tendons or ligaments, use warm castor oil packs and Omega-3 fish oil.

## KARMA

Karma is an illusion. It is based on cause and effect. However, if you realize the mind-pattern and change it, no further action is necessary.

I address the balance of life in my ***Decoding Your Life*** book. All of our work is about balance, which is really what "karma" is. If you balance your own mind-pattern, then you do not need the outside world to balance it for you. Be proactive rather than reactive.

## KIDNEYS

The kidneys are processing past experiences.

### Chronic Renal Failure

Chronic renal failure is related to the kidneys.

Everything can be cured. You can vacuum them out with Violet, flush in Pale Orange, use cranberry products, and drink pure grapefruit juice to help clean them out. The mind-pattern involves processing life experiences.

Kidney cleansing can be good without animal protein if your body can sustain this kind of a cleanse. If you do go off of animal protein for so long, introduce it easily back into your diet. If you keep eating animal proteins, you might want to reduce your intake and see how you feel. If you feel like you need protein, then it could be that you are cleansing too vigorously.

## KNEES

Knees represent flexibility in the future. Pains in the knees show that you are feeling hurt by having to change future plans and you refuse to be flexible.

### Knee Pain

Problems in the right knee are a mind-pattern of not being flexible with a male figure into your future. You could be worried about your support structure with this person. Do your releasing work, the Golden Altar. Put castor oil on the knee every night. Use Ice Blue to stop the pain. Visualize Shiny Copper on the bone daily for 45 seconds.

### Swelling in the Joints

Any swelling in the joints is a result of self-criticism. You could be criticizing yourself about what you are stepping into in the future.

Work on the mind-pattern and support your mind-pattern by soaking the afflicted area in warm sea salt water http://www.deadseawarehouse.com/ (please mention you are an Expansions referral) and use warm castor oil packs when you can. Flush in Medium Green and do your affirmations.

## LAMELLAR ICHTYOSIS

Ichtyosis is a skin disorder; individuals afflicted may be 50/50 Reptilian-human hybrids who were born in their Reptilian form. These babies were born with yellow eyes and vertical, slit-like pupils. I have never seen anyone with a genuine case of ichtyosis who had Reptilian eyes! Also, I think that actual icthyosis might have something to do with a Reptilian mind-pattern.

## Leaky Gut

Leaky gut is a mind-pattern of wasting or not utilizing what is important in life–such as nourishment for the body.

## Left Brain/Right Brain

The left brain is logic, earth-based, and feminine. The right brain is creative, emotional, and spiritual and relates to the non-physical.

The cross-over occurs past the brain, not within it. This is due to the mirror imaging of the non-physical into the physical.

When we look at physical symbolism, we must go to the area where the mind-pattern is centered, not the physical mirror image.

## Leukemia

Leukemia involves feeling like the joy of life (if in the blood) is tainted, or the support structure of life (if in the bone) is tainted. Leukemia is really an infection of the physical structure and with proper mind-pattern analysis and nutritional support, like all physical issues, it can go away.

## Limbs Upper/Lower

### Calf Muscles (Right Side)

The pain would symbolize hurt regarding a male figure, creative issues, or spiritual issues that affect future support structure and balance in life.

### Numb Limbs

If your limbs are numb, you need to check with a physician as you could have a serious health issue. The mind-pattern is that you are numb to life.

The mind-pattern is about feeling that the future support in life is contaminated and annoying/ painful.

Soak it in distilled water mixed with hydrogen peroxide. Take MMS. Take sea salt baths. Stop putting your feet in dirty places!

## Lips

### Biting your Lips

If you are biting your lips, then you are not speaking up with what you need to say. This person has communication issues coupled with low self-worth.

### Dry Lips

Dry Lips basically represent that you are fearful of what you said recently–or may not believe what you say.

## Liver

Usually for a liver cleanse we recommend milk thistle herb for 7-10 days, but it all depends upon your body system and what is going on with it.

Whatever you do with the physical body, be sure you work on the mind-pattern that created the situation in the first place.

### Chronic Liver Failure/Cirrhosis

Liver failure is a mind-pattern of being unable to handle present life events or not processing what you are learning.

Rife treatments can be a part of the treatment, but not the entire protocol.

## Loneliness and Isolation

The mind-pattern is emotional isolation and abandonment with low self-worth and self-punishment.

## Lungs

### Bronchitis

It is a strong need for emotional attention.

## Lyme Disease

There is a victim mentality mind-pattern; take hyssop and/or Cat's Claw.

## Lymph Glands

### Kawasaki Disease

Kawasaki Disease involves swollen lymph glands and unexplained rashes.

Lymph nodes filter out bacteria, and the blood filters through the lymph nodes as well.

Use a good detoxification program, including colonics and the far-infrared sauna like the one that my family uses:

http://www.hightechhealth.com/index.htm?ref=808

Try MMS and color therapy, along with archetype and sound. A mind-pattern analysis will also be beneficial.

If they are open to these types of protocols then I highly suggest a Personal Consultation.

## Lymphodema

The mind-pattern involves exaggerated fear of the future.

## Mad Cow Disease

The brain begins to liquefy and the brain tissues deteriorate. Mind-pattern:

*My mind is turning to jelly, I cannot think properly.*

## Melanoma

The shoulder concerns carrying objects. The left side involves either physical reality or a woman. An issue here means he is carrying resentment toward either physical reality or a woman that was not properly expressed, so it rose to the surface into his left shoulder. Without proper mental work, it can happen again. You can keep cutting out the physical all you want, but until you address the mind-pattern that created it, it will continue to recur in one form or another.

## Microplasma

This may be associated with being out of balance in the future.

## Migraines & Cluster Headaches

The mind-pattern is deep self-denigration. Migraines are a common effect of programming–especially when there is an overload.

Consider doing the deprogramming techniques. Try peppermint oil for the pain. For prevention, daily take feverfew herb, spin chakras every morning, balance T-Bar daily. Migraines represent severe self-denigration. Work on this mind-pattern.

Treatment: Use Ice Blue in the area of pain, put peppermint essential oil over pained area, visit a chiropractor for spinal/neck adjustment, cranial-sacral massage, reflexology on hands and feet. Masturbation also reduces symptoms.

Take Omega-3 fish oils, eat fresh pineapple, and use Ice Blue to reduce and stop pain.

Most likely you are getting into some programming areas where your Internal Programmer does not want you to venture. This is self-sabotage and not an unusual reaction to true Self-growth. Be sure to keep chakras and T-Bar balanced, protection around yourself, and the Brown Merger Archetype (Self-Integration) at the pineal gland.

## Mold Allergies

Mold can cause all kinds of havoc in the body and home. Unfortunately, usually the only way to get rid of a mold infestation is to rip up the area. You also may need to contact a professional to see if there are other places in your home where mold has grown that you cannot see.

Visualize Violet within your home and body. This will help to kill off the molds. Work on the mind-pattern that manifested the mold. What "moldy" mind-patterns do you have?

## Moles and Warts

Moles and warts on the face indicate a mind-pattern of a need to "face" all of your negative qualities and present to the world all of these issues as well. Basically, these are characteristics you do not like about yourself that should be aired and eliminated.

Use tea tree oil, castor oil and mudpacks.

## Mononucleosis

There is a mind-pattern of rejecting sustenance in life. Energize yourself with a little Bright Red, but do not over-utilize or you will find yourself in an aggressive, hostile, and agitated state. Vacuum the system with Violet. Oxygenate with Medium Green.

## Mucus

Use citrus, marshmallow herb, and hyssop to remove mucus. You can also use warm castor oil packs on the chest.

## Multiple Sclerosis

The general mind-pattern behind MS is not wanting to move through life. If you have attracted this, then there is a part of you that feels like this as well.

## Myelin Sheathing

Supplement with folic acid and Vitamin B12. These two vitamins are required by the body for the protection of the nervous system and the proper repair of myelin sheaths. In a study published in the Russian medical journal "Vrachebnoe Delo" in 1990, researchers found that patients suffering from Multiple Sclerosis who were treated with folic acid had significantly improved symptoms and myelin repair. Folic acid and B12 may help to prevent and repair myelin damage.

Vitamins B-12, choline, and inositol protect the myelin sheath from damage, according to nutritionist Phyllis A. Balch, author of **Prescription for Nutritional Healing**. Specifically, the methylcobalamin form of vitamin B-12 could increase the production of proteins that regenerate nerve cells, which is particularly useful for the myelin sheath. The recommended dose of vitamin B-12 is 1,000 mcg, taken two times per day.

Glycine is an amino acid necessary to build muscle and tissue. The amino acid is typically used for repairing connective tissues that have been damaged, including the myelin sheath. Glycine is particularly effective for treating the central nervous system function. Excessive consumption of glycine can cause fatigue, and an appropriate amount will improve energy levels. The recommended dose is 500 mg two times per day on an empty stomach.

Omega-3 fatty acids may repair the myelin sheath because it nourishes the protective coating's fat content, according to Balch. Omega-3 oils can be found in flaxseed oil, walnut oil, and fish oil supplements. Balch recommends consuming the oil three times per day with meals and following the supplement's dosage instructions. However, flaxseed oil is extremely delicate and turns rancid almost as soon as it is harvested. For this reason, we do not recommend it.

## Nasal Polyps

Keep the area in Royal Blue, visualize a Violet hose vacuuming them out, and think about what mind-pattern within you blocks your ability to comfortably and cleanly inhale your life breath.

Warm castor oil packs will help, as will a neti pot–cleaning your nose out with warm salt water.

## Nerve Damage

Nerves concern your emotional state. So, what kinds of future emotional concerns about a female (if on the left side; male on the right) or physical reality involving stepping forward into the future do you have? Remember that until you have a firm foundation, void of past issues that you no longer need, you are going to have problems.

## Nipples

Third nipples are much more common than most people think. It is estimated that up to 10% of people are born with a third nipple, sometimes in the chest area, sometimes in the groin, and sometimes only resembling a freckle. Most people have these removed during childhood. These can be the result of Lemurian/Atlantean genetic experiments or other genetic anomalies.

The mind-pattern is that this person needs extra nurturing.

## Obsessive Compulsive Disorder/OCD

It can be from experience or programming. The type of OCD varies depending on the mind-pattern. There is no standard answer.

## Organ Donation

To save a life, it is appropriate. However, the energy/frequency must match or troubles will ensue.

Ideally, preventive mind-patterns should be used to remove the physical issue. If transplant is necessary, cloning organs from the same individual is best so that they are really getting their own body part.

## Organic Red Meat

If you cannot get organic red meat, then take what you have, flush in Violet and know that what you need stays in the body and what you do not need leaves the body. Ultimately it is the mind-pattern that determines what happens with your food, whether it is chocolate, red meat, or the poison that is in small increments in all our food.

## Ovaries

The mind-pattern is creative energy or power for physical and non-physical experience. That is why doctors like plucking them out of women; it keeps women non-creative and enhances their negative mind-pattern of themselves.

## Paratid Gland (blockage on the left side)

The mind-pattern is holding back expression toward a female. Release work is in order. Also, try using warm castor oil packs over the area and gargling with tea tree oil mouthwash.

## Parkinson's Disease

For any situation, you need to look at the mind-pattern that creates it. Why is the person shaking, what is the fear caused from?

To support the nervous system, use Pale Yellow in the nervous system, and Brown around the entire auric field for grounding. Take fish oil capsules, cell salts and minerals, a good multiple vitamin, and olive oil.

## Personal Affirmations

The correct affirmations can bring amazing results. They adjust the mind-pattern to create, allow, and accept all that is for your higher good. You might want to choose our Personalized Affirmation Service to help with your personal issues. Many people find this helps give them an extra boost along their path.

## Petechia

The mind-pattern is wanting the world to see how unhappy you are.

## Plantar Fascitis

The mind-pattern is feeling a need to block the future support system and feeling like you cannot go forward in life.

Steroids are VERY bad. You should be using mudpacks, tea tree oil, castor oil, and aloe vera gel.

## Plastic Surgery

I do not believe in any such procedures. If you change the mind-patterns that cause the issues in the body, then they will be naturally corrected.

## Polio

The basic mind-pattern is feeling restricted by the world and being overwhelmed with fear of participating in life.

## Poison Ivy

It is a mind-pattern of being so angry at the world that you feel irritated by the very nature of it.

First soak the afflicted area in sea salt. Then put tea tree oil on it–it might burn for a bit. Then place castor oil over it. You can even use aloe vera gel or apple cider vinegar directly on the irritation.

## Protein

Protein needs are different for each person depending on their configuration and mind-patterns. That is why I scan people to see what they require. There is such a thing as too much protein.

## Prostate

### Enlarged Prostate

The mind-pattern is feeling frustrated creatively and stifled. You may no longer feel productive in life.

Take saw palmetto, Siberian ginseng, pumpkin seed oil, selenium, nettles, zinc, and sarsaparilla. That should make you all better!

### Prostate Cancer

Prostate cancer has the mind-pattern from males that they are no longer productive and creative in life. Given the circumstances in today's world, it is no wonder. Physically, many cancer-causing viruses have been released into the public to eliminate people with certain mind-patterns.

## Psychological Testing

These psychological tests are not only for sports figures, but are now common in the average workplace, even as part of the interview process. These tests are an outgrowth of the mind-control experiments of the 1960s, '70s, and '80s. They are actually quite accurate in determining the type of mind-patterns a person has, and then the type of programming to be entered is known.

## Puberty & Masturbation

Hormones can kick in anytime between the ages of 9 and 14. This is due to the hormones placed in commercial foods. Puberty really should not start until around 12 or 13. Puberty can cause secondary characteristics to appear as the hormones and sexual urges begin to increase. The mind-pattern would be one of a heightened need to create in order to feel powerful. It could also indicate a desire to grow up fast due to the home situation.

## Running

Running is not healthy and destroys the joints. It depletes calcium and other vital elements from the body. It is a mind-pattern of running away from life.

## Scoliosis

The mind-pattern is a lack of support in life.

## Sexually Transmitted Diseases

The mind-pattern would be feeling that sexual activity is incorrect and dirty and needing to be punished for it. Sea salt baths, hyssop herb, and flushing the body with Medium Green and Violet will help. Obviously, there is a relationship issue that needs to be addressed as well.

### Herpes

This might be a bit borderline for some, but there have been many clients who have issues with the herpes virus, both 1 and 2. This is nothing to be ashamed of, as it is very common—more than you think.

The mind-pattern comes from feeling that sexual activity should be hurtful and punished.

The mind-pattern is hurt and anger about sexual union, which comes from a mind-pattern that promotes: I am a bad person because of my sexual ideas. Usually that mind-pattern is formulated in childhood. This may come from some sort of sexual abuse in childhood, from strictly religious parents, or from parents who dominate by trying to control the child and make them think anything they do sexual is bad and requiring punishment. So, they allow the virus to enter the body to prevent them from enjoying that aspect of their life.

Work on the issue of shame, particularly with sexuality, using Golden Altar. There are also frequency machines that help with these issues.

The mind-pattern promotes: I am a bad person because of my sexual ideas.

Affirmation: I am a wonderful person who deserves wonderful sexual experiences.

Releasing that mind-pattern is the main cure.

As you work on the issue, there are physical remedies; take hyssop herb to kill the virus within and daily soak in a Dead Sea salt bath.

Take hyssop and Larreastat tablets, which are made from cactus and have been shown to kill the herpes virus. Take several thousand units of Vitamin C daily and use goldenseal herb for five days in a row. This is a body purge.

When an outbreak occurs, and it will with this protocol, which brings the virus up to kill it, use tea tree oil on the sores the moment they appear. Oral chelation will remove any dormant viruses in your system.

Try www.lauricidin.com for a new product reporting excellent results. Some people find results with rife treatments. As with all chronic health issues, detox and rebuild.

Work on detoxing the physical structure and the mind as well; rebuild both the body and the mind-pattern.

Things may look worse before they get better, so be patient and consistent. Don't give up! Yes, you CAN get rid of the virus!

## HIV

HIV takes the entire immune system down. The immune system is what protects you from "outside intruders."

People who have HIV have the mind-pattern of being too open, unprotected, and vulnerable to outside influences.

## SCIATICA

The mind-pattern is feeling fear about moving forward in the future. Do releasing work and apply castor oil nightly.

## SHOULDERS

A right shoulder injury indicates issues with females from the past that burden you.

## Sinuses

Sinus problems involve dealing with problems that are "right under your nose." The mind-pattern is that you are being severely annoyed and irritated.

You can start by using a Violet vacuum hose to mentally vacuum it out. You can also put castor oil over the sinuses daily and stop all dairy products and increase citrus. Keep the area in Royal Blue.

## Skin

The skin concerns what you show the world. Breakouts involve what is going on in your inner world. Usually they are about inner angers that are breaking and are too intense to hold inside, so they literally are popping out of your skin.

These can also be symptoms of parasites.

Detoxification is a great way to start. You most likely need to clean up the gut; www.blessedherbs.com has a great colon and internal cleanse. Soak in Dead Sea salts. Remember that the skin is the largest eliminative organ of the body.

Since Brown is grounding energy, people with brown skin tones are more grounded and connected to Earth's energies, which is why the Illuminati wants to eliminate them.

### Acne and Pimples

Pimples are a mind-pattern that something you are suppressing needs to be faced and cannot be held back.

Often acne is caused by subcutaneous infections as well as hormonal imbalances, with the mind-pattern of feeling like you are "facing" the world with little inner beauty to offer. Self-esteem work and affirmations are crucial to help.

Adequate rest is important, good nutrition, Vitamin C for cellular integrity and to fight infection, B vitamins, and A vitamins are great for skin (along with pumpkin and squash).

Mudpacks are good physical boosts, available at www.deadseawarehouse.com.

Acne often originates in the gut. It can also be a result of infection.

The wonderful colon cleanse products available at www.blessedherbs.com will help clean up the colon, which in turn helps clean up the gut.

**Boils**

The mind-pattern is that the individual holds on to the past in anger and refuses to let things go.

Use tea tree oil on the area followed by warm castor oil packs. That will dissipate the boils within days.

**Biting Skin**

The mind-pattern of biting skin around fingernails is that you are trying to get to the core of what protects you. It can mean that you are trying to undermine your protection support as a side-effect of low self-worth.

An affirmation is said/thought until it takes hold. It is different for each person.

**Bruising**

The mind-pattern relates to self-punishment.

**Cold Sores**

The mind-pattern behind them is anger that you are not speaking out, and you must work on this issue to permanently relieve yourself of the cold sores.

**Cold Sores Left Side**

Something you have held in saying from the past regarding a female or logical issue is coming out and you can no longer hold back negative words.

Use Ice Blue, then Violet.

**Eczema**

Eczema involves "what is getting under your skin." This is caused by the disintegration of the myelin sheathing around the nerves. It comes from a mind-pattern of being scared, nervous, and worried about life experiences.

Use Omega-3 and cod liver fish oils, pure coconut oil, and B-Complex.

Use castor oil, sea salt baths, and aloe vera gel as topicals.

Ultimately, the individual needs to calm down. Use Brown in and around the body.

**Hidradenitis Suppurativa**

Anything concerning Red, sores, and boils has a mind-pattern of deep angers. Even righteous anger is anger.

Detox is always recommended for any chronic condition. Generally, I would suggest sea salt baths (even though these might be uncomfortable with open sores) mixed with aluminum-free baking soda; coconut oil both internally and externally applied; far-infrared sauna: http://www.hightechhealth.com/;

MMS; lauricidin (www.lauricidin.com); colonics; watching your diet; and alkalizing the system.

There a great deal you CAN do, but it is a process. When you detox and cleanse, rather than suppress, symptoms can appear to become worse before they get better. This is likely to happen, so you have to detox slowly, and then build up, then do more detox, etc. To really work on this, you may want to consider a Personal Consultation via email so everything can be written down, or even a Body Scan.

**Itching**

Itching can have several causes, from eczema to parasites to raw nerves. In general, try sea salt baths and castor oil rubs. Without a scan it is difficult to determine the source of the problem.

Itching can mean that something in life is irritating you and needs to be released.

**Moles**

Moles are like tumors that metastasize on the skin. Moles are wild cellular growth. Very often, warts and moles are caused by viruses. Red moles indicate angers that you are allowing on whatever you try to grasp in life.

Put high quality castor oil on them and work on releasing the mind-pattern that created them in the first place.

**Morgellon's Disease**

These people have life experiences that "get under their skin." Morgellons are tiny filaments that seem to protrude from their skin and skin rashes that do not heal. These tiny filaments originate from chemtrails. To aid healing, use sea salt baths and warm castor oil packs, as well as work on the mind-pattern that originally attracted the situation.

**Piercings**

Why would you want to put holes in ANY part of your body? That said, if you insist on filling yourself with holes, use the color Ice Blue for pain, Medium Green for healing, and Violet for flushing out infection. Check that chakra band every second to make sure nothing is infiltrating it. Also examine the body part to see what it represents so you know what part of your mind-pattern has a hole embedded in it so deeply that you are now going to such lengths to outpicture those holes!

**Psoriasis**

Mind-pattern:

*What in the world is annoying you?*

Castor oil will pull debris from the skin, which ultimately makes the condition look worse, but is actually part of the healing process.

There are different qualities of castor oil, including the carrying agent.

If you are looking for alternative oils, coconut oil is good and so are the Winged White Dragon products: www.wingedwhitedragon.com.

You may have other issues; MMS will help the cure from the inside out, as will far-infrared sauna: http://www.hightechhealth.com.

**Rosacea**

Use a combination of hyssop, Echinacea, and goldenseal in tablet form. For topical, use pure Vitamin C cream in the day and calendula cream at night. There is a mind pattern involved that concerns facing the world with your subconscious negativity.

Rosacea involves blood vessels in the face that are really popping open and bursting. Blood concerns your joy in life. What joy is popping in your life that you do not want to face? This is the mind-pattern behind Rosacea.

You must first deal with the issues that created it, and balance the entire body and mind. While it looks like an easy answer, it is not. In the meantime, raise your dosage of Omega-3 fish oils and use castor oil at night. Flush with Medium Green and perhaps even check your blood sugar levels. Our basic books **Hyperspace Helper** and **Decoding Your Life** will help.

**Scars**

Most conventional medical personnel will not support alternative healing techniques. Personally, I believe in the combination of the two modalities as everything has a place and purpose, and everything comes from God-Mind.

You should try sea salt baths—½ to 1 cup per bath for many days (www.deadseawarehouse.com). Mudpacks mixed with Heavy Metal Nano Detox and or DHLA for trauma (made by PRL and available from Robert at www.healthwarriorblog.com) that you mix and apply yourself to the surgery scars once you have doctor's approval may also be helpful.

Applying castor oil topically can help remove scar tissue, but it is a long process; it does not happen overnight.

**Shingles (Facial)**

First take sea salt baths to purge the anti-virals. Then take 4000 mg of Omega-3 fish oil daily. Use warm castor oil packs on the area daily. Also use aloe vera gel and Vitamin C cream.

The mind-pattern is about something traumatic you are facing that makes you very nervous.

**Tattoos**

Whatever you permanently embed on your body will constantly create an energy of that image. So, choose carefully what you tattoo.

The arms represent what we hold in our current life. That means tattooing arms shows a need for support from whatever image you place on there. Many tattoos imply a weakness in life and a need for support and help.

The part of the body tattooed gives a clue to the mind-patterns involved in the need to embed energy.

Tattoos of any archetype, symbol, or pictogram anchor this frequency into the physical body.

Some images invoke astral energies and attachments. People who get them are most likely programmed for ritual and even sacrifice.

Tattoos boost mind-patterns, so whatever you have on your body is going to do that—either positively or negatively. Be mindful of anything that you permanently do to your body, because the mind-pattern you want to boost may change! The inks and ink carriers have extremely damaging heavy metals and other toxins that can accumulate in your internal organs. Some people with tattoos cannot use an MRI or other type of body-imaging machines because of the heavy metals; some tattoos create allergies so you cannot use commercial hair dyes.

**Vitiligo**

Vitiligo is where there are areas in the skin where pigmentation does not occur. The skin represents what you show the world. They are each trying to withdraw from the world and not show themselves. Hands and arms represent what you can grasp and hold.

The mind-pattern has to be reversed before this can be healed and there are many mental exercises that can help. There is body chemistry that is out of balance, so individuals should investigate a body scan for the most accurate information.

## SLEEP

**Insomnia**

Never sleeping is a mind-pattern related to fear of death and/or trauma.

You really SHOULD correct the mind-patterns. But as a sleeping aid, use organic valerian root capsules; they work well.

**Narcolepsy**

You sleep your life away. There are chemicals produces in the brain that cause it to go to sleep. Mind-pattern:

*I want to sleep away my life.*

What are the alternatives to developing this? Drink, take drugs. It is just another way to block out their life. Narcoleptic people are safety-conscious because they decided to sleep their life away instead of damaging their body with alcohol or drugs. It is just a milder form of the addiction.

Can there be a connection between a diabetic coma and narcolepsy?

All illnesses in which the brain goes dormant in the body are related. There is just a different mechanism to get there.

I have some clients who fall asleep after a meal, which is quite common after eating foods with tryptophan, like turkey.

The body also has difficulty assimilating heavy carbohydrates. It is like when you have too much blood sugar and your body cannot process it, the body shuts down so it is not overloaded by all the sugar. It is a safety mechanism. Just like when you have a heavy traumatic experience, you might faint; the body protects you from experiencing the full trauma.

If someone eats and falls asleep, then they should not be driving. They should adjust their schedule.

## Social Anxiety Disorder/Selective Mutism

The mind-pattern depends on the situation. It is based on fear and may have its origins either in childhood trauma, alternate lifetime experiences, or programming.

## Spontaneous Combustion

Spontaneous combustion is ancient. It occurs when a kundalini activation occurs prematurely and the nervous system cannot handle it. It literally creates a fire within the body.

## Stroke

The mind-pattern of a stroke is extreme mental unhappiness to the point of not wanting to participate in life.

Omega-3s are good, as is choline, inositol, and CoQ10. Specific needs are different for each person depending on their frequency.

## SUICIDE

It is the mind-pattern of the person who commits suicide that determines what happens to him/her. No one is "incarcerated forever" unless the mind-pattern of that person creates it. Once you say, "I'm coming to Earth to accomplish this and that!" and then you do not complete what you started, your lessons are more harsh on the other side than what they would have been here.

The more the soul-personality suffers, the harder it tries to extricate from the experience. This pushes the soul-personality deeper into the inner reserves to finally reach the resources to accomplish this goal. That is why it is better to proactively seek out the answers to life's challenges because then you are in control. If you wait, then your situation becomes reactive, and it feels like life is in control of you (read my book ***Decoding Your Life***).

The soul still exists within the Oversoul, the same as a drop of water still exists within the sea. It does "cease to exist"—this is why I put it in quotes—according to a human definition.

## TEETH

Teeth and gum issues are related to your ability to adjust to your life circumstances.

Teeth involve adjustments you make in life. The way that any of your teeth grow is a reflection of your mind-pattern.

You can take myrrh tablets as a preventative daily. It cannot harm you.

### Dental Fillings

The mind-pattern is victimization and needing artificial assistance to adjust to life.

### Wisdom Teeth

The left upper wisdom tooth is about old female issues coming to the surface again now that you refuse to adjust to at the moment.

## THROAT

The mind-pattern behind a sore throat involves being angry. It usually concerns words not spoken and suppressed, or too much anger emanating from your voice box. Release the Red to your Oversoul, flush with Violet, keep the throat in its natural color of Ice Blue. You can gargle with warm sea salt water, put castor oil on the outside of your throat, and of course take vitamins to boost your immune system. There are also homeopathic remedies that one can take, and it is important to make sure that you do not have a strep infection.

## THYROID ISSUES

The mind-pattern is one of feeling loss of personal strength.

### Hypothyroidism (T3 & T4)

Get thyroid glandulars, kelp, and blue-green algae. There could be a protein and/or hormonal issue not originally related to the thyroid. If so, eat more organic red meats and increase progesterone production via wild yam root.

There are natural supplements that you can take for the thyroid, including kelp, color therapy, and release work. There are natural iron supplements available, such as yellow dock and dark greens, as well as eating liver. Of course, you must also be able to absorb what you are eating.

Always look for the mind-pattern behind what is going on so that you can correct that and release the need for all the "stuff" you are taking.

## TOURETTE'S SYNDROME

This is the brain and nervous system connected. The symptoms are inappropriate verbalizations, facial tics, and an inability to focus or concentrate.

Mind-pattern:

*I do not think properly.*

Tourette's Syndrome is uncommon; individuals are typically heavily medicated and sent to special schools with others like them.

## UTERUS

The mind-pattern is creative support and development. As a female becomes older, she develops more problems here because she has issues of creative support and development.

### Endometriosis

The mind-pattern is blocking proper creative energy and spreading improper creativity.

### Hysterectomy

It is a mind-pattern where you no longer feel you can be creative in life. This will, of course, bring up feelings of sadness and loss.

But remember, creativity is of the mind. You will always have that!

## Varicose or Spider Veins

These are caused by unhappiness toward support structures in the future.

Put organic castor oil on them every night for three months. They will vanish.

The mind-pattern is feeling unhappy and stressed about future support and events.

## Vertigo

It could very well be related to stress. The mind-pattern is one of feeling unbalanced in life. Use heavy Royal Blue in the ears, and keep the T-Bar balanced at all times. Ground all in Brown.

If this is worse on the left side, your logical mind/female side is out of balance.

## Victimization & the Judicial System

If you release victimization, then the courts can become a tool that you use to gain what is yours. However, if you retain the victimization mind-pattern, you will lose the case.

DNA instructions can be manifested at any time as long as the correlating mind-pattern opens them.

There are many people with residual genetics from ancient Atlantean experimentation. Try some of my DNA techniques and see what comes up.

## Water

Human beings are designed to drink rain water, which is naturally distilled by the atmosphere. Now it is polluted. So, we make our own water in a distiller daily.

There is propaganda about distilled water. Water should be a coolant and flush, not a food. Distilled water can be imprinted with whatever thought-forms you want to project.

## Water retention

Water retention in the legs is a mind-pattern of fear of the future and insulating against it. Eliminating the mind-pattern is the best cure. Herbally, try astragalus or wild yam, and a good visualization is vacuuming out the legs with a Violet hose.

## Weight Issues

Weight is always from a mind-pattern of insulation. You are blocking the outside world and build a wall of fat between you and it. Removing the fear issues will allow the weight to drop off. When you release the mind-pattern that creates you to insulate against relationships, places, things, experience, then the weight will drop off. Letting go of the past is a challenge–but where there is a will there is a way–and it will reflect in your weight loss. Continue to work on any physical issues that might be sabotaging you, but mind is the builder–so keep at it!

Nothing can eliminate the insulation around your mid-section except watching what you eat, exercising, and correcting the mind-pattern that built the extra weight in the first place.

I suggest you start with a Personal Consultation so that you understand why you have the extra weight to start with. Then you need to examine how you can mitigate the mind-pattern that put on the extra weight.

Being thin does not mean vulnerable. Being skinny or emaciated may imply that. But even a heavy-set person can be vulnerable. The two issues are mutually exclusive. The aura would denote the mind-pattern no matter the weight.

**Over-Eating**

It is to insulate from mind-patterns of lack and a fear of being "less than."

**Starvation**

It comes from a mind-pattern of very low self-worth and wanting to be "less than." It leads to death, the ultimate avoidance of life and total abandonment.

## Wounds Not Healing

Loss of blood concerns loss of joy in your life. Hands involve grasping what is in front of you. The loss of joy in your life is creating a situation where you are unable to grasp what is in front of you. Think about what each item in your body represents, put it at your pineal gland, and explore. This is about YOU learning about YOU.

## Yeast & Antibiotics

Yeast are fungi that live off their host. Anyone with a yeast infection feels like someone/thing is living off of him/her and needs to set better boundaries. "Infection" implies being internally angry about this.

Many people develop yeast infections after taking antibiotics because they kill off the good bacteria that keeps fungi in check. A probiotic will help (www.blessedherbs.com; please mention that you are an Expansions referral), as well as eliminating sugars/carbohydrates from the diet. Using a far-infrared sauna will help, alkalizing the body helps, and using a product called MMS will help. There are many actions that either male or female can do, but usually yeast infections are stubborn so the mind-pattern must diligently be worked on.

**Yeast Infection**

You are allowing something to feed off of the sugar (or sweetness) in your life, thus weakening you and "vampirizing" your energy. Stop allowing others to feed off of you. Set up better boundaries and take care of Self.

Yeast live off the host in a parasitic way–if something is living in the vaginal area, then you might want to think about who/what is living off your personal/feminine energy. You need to determine how you feel about your sexuality and whom you are sharing it with (or not sharing it with). Use apple cider vinegar to balance the ph, take sea salt baths, use Pale Red to balance that area of the body, and Violet to eradicate the yeast (and of course, use MMS!). Read ***True Reality of Sexuality*** so you can learn to understand sexuality in its proper context, or view the *Sexuality, Ritual, & Relationships* DVD.

Because you are multidimensional, you can flush any way you like. Think about your goal and then the most appropriate way to accomplish that with the colors.

**Yeast Infection in the Mouth**

Most likely you are repeating words that come from others that are not elevating to your system.

# Glossary

## A

**ACTIVATION:** When a program is brought to full function.

**AFFIRMATION:** A statement that defines a course of action, or a state of inner being; repeating words many times by thinking, speaking, or writing it to bring new avenues of action into your conscious mind.

**ANIMAL MIND:** Located at the solar plexus and controlled by the Reptilian brain stem; controls the physical body; in charge of fight or flight.

**AURA:** Your personal energy field.

**ALIEN:** A physical being from another planet.

**ALTER:** Section or compartmentalized personality within a programming matrix.

**ANDROGYNOUS:** Male and female combined without sexual distinction.

**ARCHETYPE:** Symbol or glyph from hyperspace or mind-patterns.

**ASTRAL PLANE:** The border zone between physical reality and hyperspace.

## B

**BEAR FREQUENCY ARCHETYPE:** Increases protective nature; enhances introversion for self-study; best for males.

**BISEXUAL:** Sexually desiring both males and females.

**BREASTS ARCHETYPE:** Enhances healthy breasts for Men and Women.

## C

**CANCELLATION ARCHETYPE:** Removes anything unwanted.

**CENTER:** Your center is aligned along your spine, providing a safe space from which to work; you pull yourself into it by willing yourself into it.

**CEREMONY:** Gathering to celebrate or honor an entity or Illuminati holiday.

**CHAKRA BAND:** Energy center of the body and encompassing area.

**CHAKRAS:** Along the human spinal column there are main nerve bundles called ganglions, which are esoterically called "chakras," a word that means "wheels" in Sanskrit. They form along the "S" curve of the spine, which looks like a snake. For this reason the chakra system is referred to as "Kundalini," the Sanskrit word for snake.

**COLLECTIVE CONSCIOUS MIND:** The body of space that contains the accumulated known knowledge of humankind.

**COLLECTIVE UNCONSCIOUS:** The body of space that contains the accumulated thoughts of humankind; these established thought patterns directly affect what you move through today.

**COMMUNICATION ARCHETYPE:** Speaking up as appropriate.

**CONSCIOUS MIND:** Contains your present.

**CONSTRUCT:** Similar to a physical object created in the programming matrix to work with the alter in a specific function.

# D

**DEPROGRAMMING:** Techniques to block and/or remove mind-control/programming.

**DIRECT AWARENESS:** To know by experiencing the knowledge.

**DNA SEQUENCES:** This refers to the DNA sequences opening up in the body, which is a form of Kundalini activation. DNA codes are the instructions that tell your body what to do and be. Some instructions you are running at birth. These dictate that you will have blue eyes, two legs, two arms, etc. Others activate later in life, such as health conditions, ability to play music, sing, etc.

**DOLPHIN FREQUENCY ARCHETYPE:** Eases mental shifting into hyperspace.

# E

**EMOTIONAL BALANCE ARCHETYPE:** Obtains healthy emotional balance by balancing left and right hemispheres of the brain.

**ENERGY:** A physical substance consisting of shape, weight, consistency, and color.

**ELF:** Extra low frequency generally related to microwaves for mind-control purposes; energy.

**ET (EXTRATERRESTRIAL):** Borderline physical/non-physical beings not bound to our reality.

**EXPANSION ARCHETYPE:** Increases and expands goals and desires.

# F

**FEMALE ORGASM ARCHETYPE:** Removes female frigidity; increase sexual responsiveness.

**FREQUENCY:** A rate of vibration that distinguishes one flow of energy from all other flows.

# G

**GOD-MIND:** Neutral energy; All That Is.

**GOLEM:** Human animal created from mud; animated by a controller.

**GROUP-MIND:** Formed when vibrations band together.

# H

**HABIT RESPONSE:** An established pattern of behavior that allows you to react to any given situation without thinking, whether physical or mental. It can be positive, negative, or neutral.

**Happiness Archetype:** Establishes happiness.

**Horizontal Experience:** Pulls you out into similar growth.

**Hyperspace:** A region of consciousness that exists outside of linear space and time.

# I

**Illuminati:** Member or associate of one of the 13 ruling families on Earth.

**Illusion:** The way you perceive things to be.

**Individualized Consciousness Archetype:** Helps you rise out of the Group-Mind into Your Own connection with Mind and Personal yourOversoul and God-Mind.

# K

**Know by Knowing:** To understand through direct awareness; to understand the feeling of an experience.

**Knowledge:** Information.

# L

**Language of Hyperspace:** The Original Language that emanates from the Mind of God consisting of color, tone, and archetype (symbol).

**Leadership Archetype:** installs Self-Leadership.

**Lion Frequency Archetype:** Increases your direct awareness to God-Mind power.

**Logos Christos Archetype:** Healing generator on specific body locations.

**Love:** Neutral energy that emanates from God-Mind that does not discriminate.

**Lyrae:** Star system in the Milky Way Galaxy that is the origin point for all humans.

## M

**Macrocosm:** God-Mind; All That Is; the larger picture of everything.

**Male Orgasm Archetype:** Removes impotence; increases virility.

**Matrix, Programming:** The structure in the mind that facilitates mind-control; 13 x 13 x 13, which equals 2,197 compartments.

**Meditation:** A process that moves you beyond words and connects you with silence, the level of feeling; the listening from which information is gathered; centered in the right brain.

**Mental Balance Archetype:** Creates mental balance in all areas.

**Merging with Aspects of Alternative Selves Archetype:** Bring current goals to fruition by merging with your Self in the Eternal Now.

**Microcosm:** You; a world in miniature.

**Mind-Pattern:** Blueprint of a persons' thoughts.

## N

**Negative:** Negative is not "bad," but merely a condition that exists; the opposite of positive, which explains another part of the same experience.

**New Beginnings Archetype:** Start new projects, relationships, health, finances.

**New World Religion:** Global religion.

**New World Order (NWO):** Global government dictatorship being created by the Illuminati.

## O

**Objective Listening:** Listening and evaluating without judgment or criticism.

**Objective Observing:** Watching and evaluating without judgment or criticism.

**Overall Healing Archetype:** Heals body, mind, and soul.

**Oversoul:** Neutral energy that comes out of God-Mind; your Oversoul is to you what your Earth parents are to your body. Your Oversoul is your point of origin out of God-Mind.

**Oversoul Archetype:** Your Point of Origin out of the God-Mind.

# P

**Pineal Gland:** Organ at the center of the head.

**Positive:** Positive is not better than negative, but is merely a condition that exists; the opposite of negative, which explains another part of the same experience.

**Power Archetype:** Increases personal power via your mental abilities.

**Prayer:** Request that affects the results of meditation; centered in the left-brain.

**Pregnancy Archetype:** Increases fertility; maintain healthy pregnancy.

**Pregnancy Prevention Archetype:** Cancels your fertility.

**Proactive Learning:** Active learning; gathering knowledge before an experience occurs.

**Psychic Energy:** Your personal energy; it flows back and forth, and is horizontal.

# R

**Reactive Learning:** Passive learning; gathering knowledge after an experience occurs.

**Reality:** The way things really are; it may vary considerably from your perception of the way you think things are.

**Rejuvenation Archetype:** Enhances physical, mental, emotional, spiritual rejuvenation.

**Release & Resolve Past Issues Archetype:** Cleans out what you no longer need.

**Relationships Archetype:** Improves and enhances people connection.

**Reptilian:** A being with lizard-like characteristics from either the inner Earth or Draco star system; colonized Lemuria.

## S

**Self-Integration Archetype:** Brown Merger Archetype; merges all parts of Self into one; great deprogramming aid.

**Shapeshifter:** A person who physically changes from one species to another.

**Silence:** The deepest level of inner awareness; the level of feeling; you connect with your Oversoul and God-Mind within silence.

**Simultaneous Existence:** All lifelines occurring at the same moment in the Eternal Now.

**Spirituality:** A state of inner being.

**Spiritual & Intuition Connection Archetype:** Improves conscious connection with your Oversoul and God-Mind.

**Soul-Personality:** Individual strand of an Oversoul.

**Subconscious Mind:** Contains your memories, moment-by-moment, lifeline-by-lifeline.

**Sub-Personality:** A group of similar emotions that becomes strong enough to develop its own consciousness; a sub-personality is not you, but it is a part of you.

**Superconscious Mind:** Provides the direct link to your Oversoul and God-Mind.

## T

**T-Bar:** Archetype emanating from the pineal gland relating to balance.

**Trigger:** Sensory input that opens a program.

## U

**Ultimate Protection Archetype:** Protects whatever you desire.

**Universal Energy:** Energy that is available to everyone; using it allows you to keep your psychic energy; it flows up and down, and is vertical.

**Universal Law:** Rules and regulations that pervade all creation; emanates from God-Mind.

## V

**Vertical Experience:** Pulls you up into new growth.

**Vibration:** Frequency rate of an energy.

**Vibratory Imprint:** Accumulated feelings of like experiences; they cause you to react to your experiences of today through your accumulated feelings of yesterday.

**Visualization:** Creating a mental scenario that can be manifested either mentally or physically; centered at the pineal gland.

## W

**Wealth & Prosperity Archetype:** Increases finances.

**Wisdom:** Knowledge applied.

**Wisdom Archetype:** Enhances your correct use of knowledge.

**Wolf Frequency Archetype:** Enhances family relationships.

## Y

**You:** Individualized neutral energy.

# Index

## Symbols

7-Keto DHEA  229, 243

## A

Abandonment  369
Abdomen  37, 39
Abduction  111, 380
Abuse  365, 441
Acid reflux  179, 231, 442, 444
Acne  179, 495, 496
Activations  511
Acupressure  21
Acupuncture  21, 458
ADD  180, 442
Addictions  64, 181, 182, 341–389, 442, 443, 501
Addictive Relationships  381
Adduction  111
Adenine  16
Adenoids  85, 182
ADHD  183, 442
Adrenal failure  102
Adrenal glands  183, 184
Affirmations  178, 271, 272, 419, 473, 480, 490, 495, 511
Aging  288, 443
Agoraphobia  185
AIDS  187
Alcohol  354, 416, 442
Aliens  4, 511
Alimentary  32
All That Is  513, 515
Allergies  10, 185, 186, 443, 485
Aloe vera  179, 219, 232, 234, 236, 248, 263, 278, 286–288, 290, 297, 304, 317, 323, 456, 459, 467, 474, 490, 491, 497, 500
Alpha lipoic acid  182, 216, 223, 321, 323, 325
Alter groups  63
Alternate realities  388
Alters  63, 180, 286, 360, 386, 389, 455, 475, 511
Alzheimer's  58, 59, 60, 188, 221, 443
Amnesia  59
Amphiarthrosis  129
Amputation  188
Anal warts  203
Androgynous  511
Andropause  335
Anemia  444
Aneurisms  28, 100
Anger  54, 102, 367, 452
Anger issues  54
Animal mind  273, 352, 353, 357, 361, 362, 375, 511
Anorexia  10, 108, 189, 365, 444, 453
Anti-depressants  444
Antibiotics  508
Anxiety  445, 502
Appendicular skeleton  23
Appendix  101, 103, 104, 189, 190, 445
Apple cider vinegar  164, 207, 259, 264, 297, 323, 452, 491, 509
Archetypes  511, 518
Arms  142
Arnica  194, 262, 310, 323
Arrythmia  190
Arteries  28, 30, 31, 75, 88, 115, 116, 117, 120, 191, 200, 217, 325–328
Arthritis  135, 191, 192, 334, 446
Ashwagandha  230, 336
Asthma  86, 87, 192, 193, 327, 447, 448
Astragalus  263
Astral attachments  63, 375, 378
Astral plane  511
Athlete's foot  465
Attention Deficit Disorder  180, 442
Auditory system  74
Aura  511
Autism  193
Autonomic functions  448
Avena sativa  337
Axial skeleton  23

## B

B-complex  216, 237, 238, 266, 268, 275, 277, 286, 309, 497
Back  37, 42
Balance  518
Baldness  195
Barett Syndrome  195
Basil cell carcinoma  203
Bear Frequency  511
Bed bugs  452
Bed-wetting  197
Beet juice  245, 323
Berberine  179, 202, 208, 213, 220, 309
Betaine HCL  199
Biaxial  135
Biceps  152

Bile  98
Bile duct  203
Biological clock  65, 288
Biotin  195, 323
Bipolar disorder  196, 449
Birch  327, 328
Birch bark  262
Birth  512
Birthmarks  449
Bisexual  511
Biting nails  470
Biting skin  496
Black cherry  191, 245, 288
Black cohosh  243, 283, 323
Black pepper  330, 331
Bladder  54, 101, 102, 108, 120, 197, 203, 254, 324, 327, 449
Bloating  103, 198
Blood  4, 28, 198, 199, 200, 201, 245, 324, 326, 363, 444, 449, 450, 451, 499
Blood clots  450
Blood pressure  28, 29, 30, 31, 115–117, 245, 323, 327, 451
Blood system  85, 325
Blood transfusions  450
Blood vessels  28, 115, 325, 335
Blue Blood, True Blood  4
Blue cohosh  229, 283, 323
Blueberry  191, 241, 245, 288, 323
Body Scan  440, 497
Boils  496
Bone density  82, 110, 113, 135, 141, 253, 282
Bones  49, 78, 82, 101, 104, 109, 110, 113, 120, 135, 141, 142, 147, 150, 173, 202, 214, 253, 282, 298, 299, 310, 316, 321, 328, 332, 388, 404, 475, 480, 481
Boron  198, 247, 321
Boundaries  10, 78, 347, 348, 349, 350, 351, 369, 396, 397, 425, 430, 431, 508, 509
Bowels  451
Brachiali  152
Brachioradials  154
Brain  19, 26, 27, 57–63, 65, 67, 68, 94, 109, 120, 122, 128, 136, 144, 170–172, 188, 196, 221, 225, 235, 237, 244, 251, 269, 289, 292, 317, 324, 337, 341–344, 350, 355, 374, 387, 388, 393, 404, 423, 424, 443, 475, 481, 484, 501–505, 515, 516
Breast cancer  165, 454, 455
Breasts  89, 117, 201, 455, 511
Broken bones  471
Bronchitis  10, 483
Brown Merger Archetype  224, 485

Bruising  496
Bugs  452, 477
Bulimia  453
Bunions  141, 202
Burns  453
Butter  128, 189

# C

Cacao  454
Calcium  30, 82, 117, 127, 136, 141, 173, 192, 200, 214, 236, 253, 257, 264, 272, 277, 301, 302, 309, 328, 417, 446, 492
Calcium citrate  127, 257, 277
Calendula  211, 215, 287
Calf muscles  159, 481
Calories  110, 396, 418
Cancellation  511, 512
Cancer  28, 81, 91, 100, 103, 110, 116, 161–167, 169, 202–213, 342, 454, 455, 456, 491
Cancer cells  28, 161, 213
Canker sores  456
Capillaries  28, 115, 126
Cardiotrophin PMG  217
Cardiovascular system  28
Cartilage  25, 127, 129, 167, 213, 214, 234, 261, 301, 388, 456, 475
Castor oil  127, 141, 179, 186, 195, 211, 218, 219, 227, 229, 234, 236, 238, 239, 241–243, 246–248, 250, 253–255, 260, 263, 265, 280–283, 287, 290, 294, 295, 297, 301, 302, 311, 313, 314, 318, 319, 446, 456, 457, 462, 463, 465, 466, 468, 471, 474, 478–480, 486, 488–491, 494–500, 504, 506
Cat's Claw  483
Catuaba  337
Cayenne  31, 117, 195, 200, 239, 332, 416, 453
Cedar wood  195
Cellulite  109, 123, 124, 214, 215, 457
Celtic sea salt  255
Center  512
Cerebrum  57, 58
Ceremony  512
Cervical region  125, 126
Chaga mushroom  190, 215, 235, 250, 263, 295, 312
Chakra bands  9, 512
Chakra Mind-Pattern Correlations  51, 57
Chakra spinning  442, 443
Chakra system  9, 21, 49, 50, 51, 105
Chakras  53, 440, 512
Chamomile  333
Chapparel  166, 213, 261

Chelation  60, 188, 213, 221, 235, 256, 288, 299, 324
Chemotherapy  169
Chicken  457
Chicken Pox  215
Child Within  181, 182, 189, 197, 237, 246, 249, 271, 278, 286, 304, 321, 322, 464
Childhood  70, 83–87, 94, 109, 124, 126, 215, 255, 262, 268, 296, 303, 321, 346, 351, 352, 354, 365–367, 370, 373, 384, 398, 418, 447, 448, 457, 460, 488, 493, 502
Chiropractic  268, 301, 458, 461
Chlorella  199, 219, 324
Chlorine  458
Chlorophyll  417
Chocolate  268, 352, 411, 454, 489
Cholesterol  30, 31, 116, 117, 191, 200, 201, 236, 245, 249, 253, 325
Chondroitin  141, 253, 456
Chromosomes  63, 355
Chronic body pain  10
Chronic Fatigue Syndrome  216, 458
Cilantro  324
Cilia  97
Cinnamon  182, 223, 324
Circulation  217
Circulatory system  21, 28, 31, 34, 50, 117, 121, 161, 162, 199, 200, 245
Circumcision  466
Circumduction  111
Citrus  260
Clary sage  333
Cleansing  71, 164, 165, 207, 220, 249, 281, 288, 299, 411–415, 417–419, 424, 457, 479, 482, 495, 496, 497
Cleft palate  217
Clots  100, 199, 313, 450
Cluster Headaches  485
Coca  230
Cocoa powder  297
Coconut oil  190, 194, 216, 217, 219, 237, 238, 257, 266, 276, 287, 290, 291, 294, 297, 310, 312, 324, 326, 457, 471, 497, 499
Coconut water  199, 245, 278, 324
Coffee  165, 207, 259, 268, 271, 324, 353
Cold hands  471
Cold laser  290
Cold sores  496, 497
Colds  85, 218, 324
Colitis  218, 247, 318, 451
Collagen  192, 256, 265, 266, 275, 318
Collagen ointment  192
Collective conscious mind  512

Collective unconscious  512
Colon  95, 101, 103, 162–164, 205, 219, 220, 288, 413, 417, 451, 495, 496
Colonics  165, 207, 219, 321, 413, 414, 483, 497
Color  513, 514
Color code  30, 200
Color therapy  444, 484, 504
Color, tone, and archetype  514
Comfrey  213, 261, 279, 444
Communication  512
Concentric  148
Confusion  370
Congaplex  215, 218, 250, 263, 312, 324
Conjunctivitis  463
Connective tissues  25, 105, 332, 487
Conscious  511
Conscious mind  512
Constipation  95, 123, 451
Construct  512
COPD  216, 326, 346
CoQ10  166, 191, 213, 240, 249, 266, 309, 324, 444, 473, 503
Corn silk tea  236
Corns  465
Corpus callosum  68, 225
Corrective eye surgery  463
Coumadin  100, 450
Cramps  264
Cranberries  197, 252, 324, 479
Cranial nerves  37, 48
Cravings  352
Creation  4
Crohn's Disease  10, 247, 458
Crown Chakra  50, 53, 57, 59, 60, 180, 189, 299
Crowns  79
Crying  71, 220
Cryonic centers  170
Cryopreservation  169
Cumin  220
Cypress  328, 329, 332
Cysts  30, 117, 220, 282, 328, 459, 468
Cytosine  16

# D

Dairy  165, 183, 207, 279, 290, 297, 322, 416, 495
Dandelion root  164, 207, 259, 324
Dandruff  470
Dead Sea salt  63, 215, 312, 456, 465, 493
Deafness  460
Decoding Your Life  4, 178, 349, 350, 376, 397, 401, 441, 442, 448, 460, 479, 499, 503

Deltoids  151
Dementia  59, 221, 373
Dendrites  127
Dental fillings  504
Depression  111, 222, 368, 423, 425, 460
Deprogramming  5, 180, 181, 189, 224, 246, 268, 289, 294, 296, 317, 379, 380, 443, 485, 512
DHEA  229, 239, 243
Diabetes  222, 223, 461
Dial Visualization  199, 222, 223, 278, 279, 314
Diarrhea  92, 215, 218, 328, 452
Diastolic  28, 115
Diathrodial  135
Diet  356, 449, 454
Digestion  23, 54, 65, 94, 123, 265, 324, 325, 326, 454
Digestive enzymes  107, 224, 273, 454
Digestive system  32, 54, 91, 219, 238, 323, 414, 415, 451, 452
Digestive tract  451
Direct awareness  512
Disc degeneration  126
Dissociative Identity Disorder  224
DNA  15, 16, 17, 17–173, 266, 282, 284, 286, 320, 386, 403, 443, 457, 459, 506, 512
DNA sequences  512
Dolphin Frequency Archetype  225, 293, 513
Down Syndrome  225
Draco  517
Drug addiction  355
Drugs  355, 442, 458, 461
Dyslexia  225

### E

Ear piercing  227, 462
Ear wax  462
Earache  75, 226
Ears  70, 74, 75, 76, 226, 227, 462, 506
Earth  514, 516, 517
Eastern medicine  21
Eating  227, 228
Echinacea  218, 281, 295, 324, 463, 499
Eczema  10, 229, 497
Edema  10
Elbows  462, 479
Elderberry  288, 295
Eleuthero root  167, 210
Elevation  111
ELF  513
Elicina cream  211
Emotional addictions  366

Emotional balance  513
Endocrine system  21, 34
Endometriosis  505
Energetic systems  21
Energy  511, 513, 514, 516, 518
Energy field  63, 83, 289, 300, 440
Enlarged prostate  491
Epsom salts  331
Epstein Barr  216, 263, 463
Erectile dysfunction  230, 467
Esiak extract  167, 213, 261
Esophagitis  91
Esophagus  86, 91, 179, 230, 231, 232, 241
Essiac tea  213
Estrogen  107, 116, 165, 166, 209, 229, 243, 247, 283, 321, 323, 326
ET (Extraterrestrial)  513
Eternal Now  20, 360, 378, 394
Eucalyptus  329, 330, 333
Eustation tube  462
Exercise  3, 78, 107–110, 113, 161, 178, 222, 237, 253, 271, 338, 356, 396, 397, 421, 422, 423, 447, 448
Expansion  513
Extension  111
External rotation  112
Eye color  464
Eyebright  233
Eyes  10, 67, 68, 70, 71, 85, 232, 233, 254, 406, 443, 463, 464, 480

### F

Far-infrared treatment  177, 187, 188, 192, 199, 213, 216, 218, 220, 221, 235, 242, 256, 258, 260, 261, 263, 275, 281, 295, 305, 312, 313, 324
Faret syndrome  234
Fast  219, 271, 416, 417
Fat  77, 92, 95, 107–110, 113, 122, 123, 128, 201, 271, 321, 325, 399, 404, 487, 507
Fear  294, 367, 384, 451
Fear of Blood Test/Donation  451
Feet  56, 105, 234, 255, 465
Female orgasm  513
Feminine dryness  467
Fermented foods  279
Fertility Archetype  250
Feverfew  262
Fibrillation  471
Fibroids  30, 117, 323, 466
Fibromyalgia  235, 466
Flibroid tumors  234

Fillings  80, 144, 213, 326
Fish oil  190, 194, 237, 266, 276, 310, 313, 416, 442, 450, 479, 487, 490, 500
Flexion  112
Flexors  154
Flowchart of Creation/Existence  54
Flowchart of God-Mind  51
Flowchart of the Human Body and Digestive System  121
Fluoride  62, 63, 144, 235, 327
Folic acid  195, 217, 240, 249, 324, 469, 473, 487
Food  73, 76–79, 83, 91, 92, 94–98, 100, 104, 109, 122, 123, 173, 177, 187, 219, 227–229, 288, 315, 316, 326, 348, 354, 356, 365, 379, 395, 398–401, 404, 413, 414, 416, 418, 422, 423, 453, 457, 466, 489, 507
Frankincense  63, 196, 215, 235, 255, 261, 279, 291, 292, 328, 334
Frequency  193, 225, 288, 293, 299, 409, 427, 477, 513, 518
Fusciform  112, 113

## G

Gallbladder  92, 98, 206, 235, 236, 415
Gallstones  30, 98, 117, 236
Ganglions  9, 440
Garlic  30, 31, 117, 191, 200, 201, 242, 311, 416, 453
Gastric bypass surgery  92, 93
Gastrocnemius  159
Gastroesophageal Reflex Disease (GERD)  236
Generalized Anxiety Disorder  237
Genetic defects  63
Genital system  32
Genitalia  104, 237, 466
Geranium  330
Germs  85, 290
Ginger  234, 236, 248, 260, 264, 278, 324, 330, 334, 400, 452, 457, 459
Gingivitis  468
Gingko biloba  188, 221, 324
Glands  22, 34, 62–64, 76, 80, 82, 101, 102, 105, 161, 476, 483
Glandular treatments  60, 98, 164, 165, 166, 187, 196, 207, 209, 216, 223, 225, 233, 236, 239, 243–245, 247, 256, 258–260, 274, 275, 285, 292, 293, 299, 314, 317, 324, 504
Glucosamine  141, 253
Gluteal  155

God-Mind  4, 6, 51, 53, 54, 86, 178, 293, 350, 357, 359, 361, 369, 374, 394, 397, 405, 411, 417, 419, 426, 429, 430, 436, 445, 448, 467, 499, 513–518
Golden Alter  167, 181, 182, 189, 193, 213, 222, 237–240, 242, 246, 249, 260, 271, 286, 304, 321, 322, 473, 480, 493
Goldenseal  218, 325
Golems  513
Gonads  34
Gout  238
Governments  515
Gracilis  155
Grapefruit  252, 271, 479
Green Spiral Staircase  181, 183, 185, 189, 193, 195, 266, 283, 290, 317, 363, 448
Grey hair  469
Group-Mind  513
Guanine  16
Guilt  368
Gums  326, 468
Gymnema sylvestre  223
Gynoplastia  239

## H

Habit response  513
Hair  332, 468, 469, 470
Hair loss  239, 332, 469
Hair thinning  469
Hallucinogens  63
Hamstrings  159
Hands  470, 471, 501, 508
Happiness  514
Hardening of the arteries  449
Hashimoto Syndrome  239
Hawthorne berry  217, 240, 249, 325, 472, 473
HCL Betaine  265, 325
Head  37, 47
Healer's Handbook  4, 178, 369, 460, 499
Healing  4
Healing Archetypes  4, 63, 119, 178, 349
Health  513
Healthcare professionals  355
Heart  28, 30, 34, 49, 53, 54, 86, 88, 90, 98, 115, 116, 119, 120, 147, 199, 217, 240, 245, 249, 321, 324–327, 423, 431, 433, 471–473
Heart attack  472
Heart Chakra  49, 53, 54, 86, 90, 98, 119, 199, 217, 245, 471, 472
Heavy metals  58, 476
Height  172, 473
Helichrysum  328, 334

Hemorrhoids  241, 474
Hepatitis  476
Herbs  335, 474
Hernia  91
Herniated disc  126, 301
Herpes  242, 493
Hiatial Hernia  231, 241
Hidradenitis Suppurativa  497
High blood pressure  451
Hips  214, 242, 320
HIV  187, 478, 494
Hives  476
Homogenization  325
Honey  182, 186, 248, 290, 297, 325
Horizontal experience  514
Hormonal Imbalance  243
Hormones  34, 64, 102, 116, 169, 184, 243, 264, 283, 467, 474, 492
Horny goat weed  230
Horsetail herb  127, 301, 302, 327, 442
Hughes Syndrome  451
Huntington's Disease  60, 244, 245, 262, 276, 477
Hurt  367, 474
Hydrangea root  197, 252
Hydrogen peroxide  187, 227, 295, 311, 453, 462, 465, 482
Hydrotherapy Treatment  244
Hyperbaric treatment  180, 183, 188, 193, 201, 213, 221, 225, 244, 261, 266, 275, 281
Hyperspace  4, 19, 27, 58, 63, 64, 68, 83, 105, 119, 125, 178, 186, 213, 250, 289, 320, 345, 349, 350, 363, 389, 442, 448, 460, 467, 499, 514
Hyperspace Helper  4, 178, 349, 460, 499
Hypertension  30, 115, 245
Hyperthyroid  81, 246, 314
Hyperventilating  246
Hypothalamus  62, 65, 245
Hypothyroid  81, 247, 314, 504
Hyssop herb  166, 208, 213, 242, 260, 281, 325, 466, 468, 483, 486, 493, 494, 499
Hysterectomy  102, 505

## I

Iliacus  155
Illuminati  512, 514, 515
Illusion  514
Immune system  99, 324, 328, 445, 494, 504
Immuplex  215, 218, 250, 259, 263, 295, 312, 325, 463
Implants  79, 213, 249, 388, 389, 474, 475
Impotency  467
Imprintings  66
Incurable disease  477

Indigestion  103
Individualized Consciousness  514
Infected toenails  465
Infertility  250
Inflammation  477
Inflammatory Bowel Disease  247
Influenza  250
Insects  477
Insomnia  407, 477, 501
Insulin  97, 98, 223, 274, 326, 461
Integumentary  21, 22
Internal rotation  112
Intestines  54, 92, 96, 97, 101, 206, 218, 220, 237, 248, 251
Inulin powder  325
Inversion Therapy  251
Iodine  325
Irritable bowel syndrome  10, 248, 452
Ischemic Heart Disease (IHD)  249
Isokinetic  148
Isolation  349, 369, 483
Isometric  148
Isotonic  148
Itching  467, 478, 498

## J

Jade Machine  188, 192, 199, 220, 221, 262
Jaundice  90
Jaw  143, 145, 251, 476
Jerusalem artichokes  223, 325
Joints  23, 25, 129, 135, 136, 251, 326, 329, 332, 462, 471, 479, 480, 492
Jojoba oil  195, 239, 469, 470
Juniper  330, 331, 332, 334

## K

Karma  441, 479
Kava kava  185, 196, 222, 237, 292, 300, 442, 445, 477
Kawasaki disease  483
Kegel exercises  283
Kidney stones  30, 117, 253, 328
Kidneys  34, 101, 108, 116, 184, 252, 254, 423, 479
Knee pain  480
Kneecap deterioration  141
Kneecaps  253
Knees  17, 135, 141, 155, 254, 456, 480
Know by knowing  514
Knowledge  512, 514, 516
Krebs Cycle  108
Kundalini  378, 502

## L

L-Arginine  325
L-Carnitine  182, 223, 321, 325
L-Citrilline  325
L-Glutamine  321, 325
L-Lysine  245
L-Theanine  198
Lactic acid  108, 254
Lamellar Ichtyosis  480
Language of Hyperspace  514
Large intestine  95, 103, 451
Larynx  76, 83, 102, 184, 254, 255
Lasik  464
Latissimus Dorsi  150
Lavender  195, 330, 331, 332, 333
Leadership  514
Leaky gut  481
Left Brain/Right Brain  481
Left side  20, 497
Legs  56, 105, 140, 204, 234, 255, 313, 469
Lemon juice  294, 415, 416
Lemon water  164, 207
Lemongrass  195, 328, 332, 334
Leprosy  256
Leukemia  99, 100, 207, 256, 481
Leukoplakia  256, 257
Ligaments  25, 136, 147, 479
Lion Frequency  514
Lipoic acid  182, 321, 323, 325
Lips  482
Liquid oxygen  193
Live cell treatments  60, 173, 223, 225, 258, 265, 266, 275, 284
Liver  34, 63, 86, 89, 90, 92, 97, 116, 162, 164, 165, 169, 199, 207, 230, 248, 249, 257–259, 288, 323, 324, 326, 355, 413, 415, 417, 423, 444, 473, 476, 482, 483, 497, 504
Locomotor system  25
Logos Christos Archetype  260, 282, 514
Loneliness  483
Longitudinal  112, 113
Love  514
Low blood pressure  451
Low Self-worth  366
Lower back injury  11
Lower limb  37, 45
Lumbar region  125, 126
Lung cancer  455
Lungs  63, 86, 87, 193, 216, 259, 260, 281, 325, 399, 404, 447, 448, 483
Lupus  260
Lutein  233
Lycopene  285

Lyme disease  483
Lymph  28, 105, 161, 162, 483
Lymph glands  261, 483
Lymph nodes  28, 483
Lymph vessels  28
Lymphatic system  28, 85, 116, 161, 162
Lymphodema  484
Lymphoma  208, 261
Lyrae  514

## M

Maca root  198, 229, 234, 243, 247, 277, 282, 283, 321, 323, 326, 336
Macrocosm  515
Mad Cow Disease  262, 484
Magnesium  264
Male Orgasm  515
Mandible  145, 251
Marijuana  63, 355
Marjoram  329, 330–333
Marshmallow herb  208, 216, 260, 281, 326, 448, 486
Masturbation  262, 485, 492
Matrix, programming  515
Measles  215
Meditation  515, 516
Melanoma  484
Melatonin  61, 62
Memory  57, 65–67, 100, 104, 109, 123, 224, 283, 286, 311, 324, 329, 341, 343, 346, 354, 363, 378, 383, 386, 398, 399, 425
Mental Balance  515
Merging with Simultaneous Existences Archetype  515
Metabolism  34, 62, 80, 81, 219, 321, 325, 416
Methylene Blue  181, 187, 188, 199, 213, 215, 220, 221, 250, 256, 259, 279, 295, 297, 317, 320
Microcosm  515
Microcurrent treatments  256
Microplasma  484
Migraine headaches  10, 262, 485
Milk thistle  164, 207, 259, 326, 417, 482
Milky Way galaxy  514
Mind of God  514
Mind-control  512, 513, 515
Mind-Pattern analysis  9
Mind-patterns  9, 10, 11, 17, 20, 21, 51, 54, 60, 65, 75, 82, 185, 195, 268, 271, 273, 276, 304, 311, 353, 359, 366, 368, 384, 386, 401, 404, 405, 410, 412, 418, 419, 421, 425, 428, 436, 438, 440, 441, 443, 446, 448, 450, 453, 457, 458, 459, 464, 472, 474, 475, 485, 489–492, 500, 501, 508

Minerals  107, 414, 416, 473, 490
Missing link  9, 11
MMS  187, 250, 259, 295, 465, 482, 484, 497, 499, 509
Modifilan  213, 235, 288, 326
Mold allergies  485
Moles  263, 486, 498
Money addiction  357, 394, 433, 435, 436
Mononucleosis  10, 263, 486
Montauk: Alien Connection  4
Morgellon's Disease  498
Morning sickness  264
Mucus  486
Muira puama  337
Mulein oil  311, 462
Multiaxial  135
Multiple sclerosis  60, 266, 486, 487
Muscle  25, 70, 91, 105, 108–110, 112, 113, 136, 147, 148, 150–152, 154, 155, 159, 249, 264, 265, 268, 283, 324, 325, 328, 329, 331–334, 337, 399, 404, 406, 423, 425, 453, 472, 487
Muscle groups  150
Muscular atrophy  265
Muscular dystrophy  60
Muscular system  21, 25, 60, 110, 113, 147
Musculoskeletal system  25
Mycoplasmas  235
Myelin sheath  127, 128, 190, 237, 286, 311, 487, 497
Myelin Sheath Deficiency  196, 266, 292
Myrrh gum  191, 194, 262, 269, 309, 310, 319, 326

# N

NADH  279
Nails  267
Narcolepsy  268, 501
Nasal polyps  488
Nattokinase  190, 276, 313, 326
Near-sightedness  10
Neck  37, 46
Neck pain  268
Neem oil  305
Negative  515
Nerve damage  488
Nerves  9, 26, 75, 120, 126, 127, 237, 269, 277, 298, 307, 311, 328, 453, 471, 478, 497, 498
Nervous system  21, 26, 74, 120, 125, 127, 128, 136, 266, 269, 333, 334, 388, 416, 417, 451, 466, 473, 475, 487, 490, 502, 505
Nettles  239, 491

Neutral  513, 518
New World Order (NWO)  515
New World Religion  515
Niacin  30, 31, 117, 199, 200, 473
Niacin flush  30, 117, 200
Nipples  488
Nose  61, 70, 73, 76, 85, 255, 270, 297, 405, 488, 495
Numb fingers  471
Numb limbs  482
Nutrients  97, 107, 400, 416, 440, 461, 472

# O

Obesity  92, 271
Object observation  441
Objective listening  515
Objective observing  516
Obliques  155
Obsessions  352, 353
Obsessive Compulsive Disorder/OCD  488
Obsessive relationships  381
Ocular range  70
Olio Del Re  260, 262
Olive Gold Dental  179, 286, 287, 297, 309, 326
Olive leaf  211, 219, 234–236, 248, 264, 278, 295, 326
Olive oil  127, 128, 266, 294, 301, 302, 416, 490
Omega-3  127, 128, 190, 237, 266, 276, 277, 286, 290, 293, 301, 302, 311, 326, 416, 442, 450, 451, 469, 470, 479, 485, 487, 497, 499, 500
One Source  10
Opposites  515, 516
Oregano  211, 219, 234, 248, 264, 317, 326
Oregano oil  317, 326
Organ donation  489
Osteoporosis  135, 136, 272, 299
Outpicturing  16, 17, 53, 104, 126, 385, 398, 411, 422, 450, 459, 498
Ovaries  101, 102, 165, 166, 272, 282, 489
Over-Eating  508
Over-hydration  107, 273
Overall Healing Archetype  213, 282, 516
Oversoul  27, 53, 64, 66, 83, 105, 170, 178, 181, 182, 185, 186, 189, 193, 197, 213, 222, 238, 239, 240, 242, 246, 265, 286, 296, 299, 304, 321, 345, 349, 350, 360, 361, 369, 389, 394, 395, 397, 403, 405, 409–411, 417, 419, 442, 445, 448, 450, 452, 454, 459, 503, 504, 516, 517
Ozone treatments  256, 261

## P

Palpitations 471
Pancreas 92, 98, 274, 415, 461
Pancreatic glandulars 98
Panic attacks 445
Paralyzation 275
Parasites 108, 182, 321, 423–425, 428, 454, 478, 495, 498
Parathyroid 76, 82, 275
Paratid gland 489
Parents 516
Parkinson's Disease 60, 276, 490
Parotid 76, 80, 291
Pasteurization 326
Pathogens 86, 295, 297, 323–325
Pau d'Arco 166, 213, 261
Peanut oil 127, 194, 266, 301, 302, 309
Pectorals 151
Pelvic girdle 139
Pelvis 37, 40, 138, 277
Peppermint 98, 186, 223, 274, 326, 329–333, 452, 461, 485
Peptic Ulcer Disease (PUD) 278
Perineum 37, 40
Periodontal disease 468
Peripheral Vascular Disease/PVD 276
Peritoneal Dialysis (PD) 273
Personal affirmations 490
Perspiration Glands 278
Petechia 490
PH 279
Pharyngeal tonsils 85
Physical addictions 354
Physical reality 511
Pica disorder 273
Piercings 74, 75, 498
Pimples 495
Pineal 50, 55, 61–64, 67, 70, 196, 233, 250, 266, 279, 288, 289, 292, 293, 327, 354, 363, 442, 474, 485, 508
Pineal Chakra 53, 55, 61, 62
Pineal gland 62, 180, 190, 196, 225, 238, 266, 292, 299, 516, 518
Pineal Gland Archetype 180, 196, 225, 266, 292
Pineapple 224, 248, 269, 309, 326, 454, 485
Pinoline 61, 62
Pituitary 34, 62, 64, 196, 292, 466
Plantar fascitis 490
Plaque 30, 31, 116, 117, 120, 191, 200, 201, 236, 249, 253, 325, 473
Plastic surgery 280, 490
Pneumonia 10, 260, 280, 281

Poison ivy 280, 491
Polio 281, 491
Polycystic Ovary Syndrome (PCOS) 282
Positive 516
Post nasal drip 11
Power 516
Power Archetype 195, 247, 469
Prader Willi Symdrome 282
Prayer 516
Pregnancy 223, 264, 516
Pregnancy Prevention 516
Premature Ejaculation 283
Premenstrual Syndrome (PMS) 283
Prescriptions 355
Present 512
Proactive learning 516
ProArgi9 191, 230, 245, 249, 313, 319, 327
Probiotics 273, 454
Progeria 284
Progesterone 166, 209, 243, 283, 321, 326, 327, 504
Programming 4, 63, 84, 85, 180, 224, 296, 346, 349, 353, 359, 360, 375–380, 386, 388, 389, 407, 411, 427, 464, 475, 477, 478, 485, 488, 492, 502, 511, 512
Programming matrix 511, 512
Pronation 112
Prostate 104, 162, 166, 167, 210, 284, 285, 327, 337, 491
Protein 107, 491
Protraction 112
Psoas 155
Psoriasis 229, 286, 499
Psychedelic drugs 63
Psychic energy 516
Psychological testing 492
Puberty 492
Pumpkin seeds 210, 285, 491
Pyruvic acid 108

## Q

Quadriceps Femoris 155
Quercetin 186, 327

## R

Radiate 112, 113
Radiation treatments 169
Radionic treatments 167, 256, 260, 261
Rash 287
Reactive learning 516
Reality 4, 516

Recipes  329
Rectus Abdominis  155
Red blood cells  99, 100, 324
Red wine  30, 117, 200, 201, 222, 245, 249, 279, 298, 327
Red yeast rice  30, 117, 201, 245, 249
Regeneration  59, 60, 120, 127, 141, 169, 171, 191, 269, 288, 301, 302, 453, 462, 487
Rejuvenation  288, 517
Relationships  517
Release & Resolve Past Issues  517
Renal Failure  479
Reptilian  511, 517
Reptilian brainstem  180, 286, 289, 388
Reptilian Brainstem Archetype  286, 289
Respiratory system  32
Resveratrol  249, 263, 266, 284, 327
Retraction  112
Rhinophyma  290
Rife treatments  260, 423, 483
Right brain  515
Right side  20, 481
Roman chamomile  332
Root canal  79
Root Chakra  55, 104, 294
Rosacea  290, 499
Rosemary  239, 329, 330, 332, 333
Running  110, 251, 492
Rye grass  87, 193, 327, 448

## S

Sacral  49, 55, 125, 126, 469, 485
Sacral Chakra  54, 55, 101, 103, 219, 250
Sacral ulcer  290
Salivary glands  76, 80
Sandalwood  333
Sarsaparilla  239
Sartorius  155
Sauerkraut juice  264, 327
Saw palmetto  167, 210, 285, 327, 491
Scars  499
Schizophrenia  292
Sciatica  494
Scoliosis  126, 301, 492
Sea salt baths  63, 179–181, 193, 196, 208, 215, 218, 229, 235, 237, 242, 250, 256, 261, 279–281, 295, 312, 446, 461, 465, 478, 482, 493, 497, 498, 500, 509
Seasonal Affective Disorder (SAD)  293
Seizures  293
Selective mutism  502
Selenium  285

Self  4
Self-Integration  517
Self-Punishment  367
Self-Reintegration Archetype  180
Self-Sabotage  368
Senses  62
Serotonin  61
Serratus Anterior  154
Setting the Dial Visualization  199, 201
Sexual behavior  65, 296, 357
Sexual Dysfunction  294
Sexuality  55, 242, 466, 471, 493, 509
Sexually Transmitted Diseases  295, 493
Shankhapushpi powder  188, 221
Shapeshifter  517
Shark cartilage  167, 234, 261
Shaving  469
Shilajit  230
Shingles  297, 500
Shoulders  112, 494
Siberian brown seaweed  288
Siberian ginseng  167, 210, 230, 285, 288, 327, 491
Silence  517
Silica  256, 266, 275, 290, 304, 318, 327
Silver Infinity Archetype  180, 299
Silver Oversoul Archetype  213
Simultaneous Existences  17, 195, 273, 282, 388, 517
Sinuses  10, 71, 72, 91, 218, 297, 324, 495
Skeletal system  21, 23, 120, 121, 129, 298
Skin  22, 50, 90, 105, 116, 169, 179, 210, 211, 229, 276, 286, 290, 299, 305, 320, 323, 326, 328, 417, 457, 476, 480, 495–499, 501
Skull  23, 109, 125, 143, 442
Sleep  300, 356, 501
Sleepwalking  299
Small intestine  97, 103
Smell  62, 73, 360
Smoking  83, 300, 354
Snoring  74, 300
Social anxiety  502
Solar plexus  511
Solar Plexus Chakra  49, 54, 92, 184, 219, 223
Soleus  159
Solomon's seal  179, 211, 215, 241, 254, 263, 265, 286, 290, 319
Sore throat  324, 504
Soul-Personality  59, 66, 86, 170, 171, 296, 517
Sperm and Egg Archetypes  250
Spider veins  506
Spinal column  23, 26, 120, 125, 127, 135, 142, 269, 289, 298

Spine 301, 302, 303
Spiritual & Intuition Connection 517
Spiritual addictions 374
Spiritual Mind 352, 353, 361
Spirituality 517
Spleen 92, 99, 256, 298, 299, 303
Splenium 68
Spontaneous combustion 502
Squamous Cell Carcinoma 203
St. John's Wort 196, 222, 237, 292, 300
Starvation 365, 508
Stem cell therapy 223, 244, 266, 281
Stem cells 284, 299
Stevia 98, 274, 327
Stomach 91–93, 99, 109, 123, 211, 214, 224, 303, 304, 317, 320, 324, 326, 399, 418, 419, 452, 455, 487
Stomach stapling 92
Strep throat 85
Stroke 28, 30, 100, 115, 116, 502
Sub-personality 517
Subconscious mind 517
Subluxations 126, 135
Sudden Infant Death Syndrome (SIDS) 304
Sugar 77, 97, 98, 107, 108, 110, 165, 182, 207, 222, 223, 271, 274, 290, 321–325, 327, 352, 363, 416, 419, 425, 454, 499, 502, 509
Suicide 503
Suma 336
Superconscious mind 517
Supination 112
Supplements 323, 357
Sweat glands 63, 105, 304, 305
Swollen glands 476
Sylvestre Gymnema 327
Sympathetic 21, 161, 173, 388, 475
Synapses 127
Synarthrosis 129
Synthyroid 116
Systemic anatomy 21
Systolic 28, 115

# T

T-Bar 177, 180, 196, 225, 246, 247, 260, 283, 289, 292, 293, 311, 317, 442, 443, 462, 463, 485, 506, 518
T-cells 86
Talking 81, 357, 375
Tamarind 62, 235, 327
T-Bar Archetype 225, 247, 260, 283, 289, 311, 317
Tattoos 500
Taurine 216, 245, 266, 275
Tea tree oil 211, 242, 257, 280, 329, 456, 465, 468, 474, 486, 489, 490, 491, 494, 496
Tear ducts 71
Tears 71, 110, 405, 418, 452
Teary eyes 464
Teeth 76, 79, 80, 120, 143, 144, 173, 213, 257, 305–309, 503, 504
Temporomandibular Joint Dysfunction (TMJ) 11, 310
Tendons 25, 136, 147, 328, 479
Tennis elbow 479
Tensor Fasciae Latae 155
Testicular pain 467
Testosterone 243, 294, 321, 327, 335–338
Thalamus 62, 65–67, 311
Thiamine 16
Thoracic region 49, 125, 126, 169
Thorax 37, 38
Thought 512
Thought-bands 51, 53, 54, 55, 56
Throat 76, 312, 504
Thrombosis 313
Thyme 329, 333
Thymus gland 86, 314
Thyroid 34, 49, 53, 65, 76, 80–82, 102, 116, 120, 169, 184, 239, 246, 247, 282, 314, 504
Thyroid Chakra 49, 53, 76
Thyroid gland 314
Tibialis Anterior 159
Tien Shen tea 248, 278, 327
Tienchi tea 97, 218, 317, 459
Tinnitus 310, 311, 462
Toenails 465
Toes 465
Tongkat ali 337
Tongue 76, 193, 212, 215, 310, 315, 316, 327, 413
Tonsils 76, 85
Topographic Anatomy 37
Tourette's Syndrome 317, 387, 505
Toxins 63, 71, 89, 90, 109, 116, 123, 215, 271, 324, 325, 412, 413, 415, 417, 456, 501
Trapezius 150, 268
Trauma 67, 84, 95, 109, 189, 192, 215, 224, 237, 262, 342, 345, 362, 364, 365, 376, 381, 386, 443, 457, 500, 501, 502
Tribulus 198, 230, 243, 247, 250, 283, 321, 327, 335, 336, 337
Triceps 152
Trigger 518

True Reality  4, 20, 357, 369, 380, 427, 467, 509
True Reality of Sexuality  4
True World History  4
Tumors  161, 167, 213, 259, 424, 498
Turmeric  166, 179, 213, 220, 290, 327

## U

Ulcerative colitis  95, 247, 318
Ulcers  303, 317
Ultimate Protection  518
Under-hydration  107
Uniaxial  135
Universal energy  518
Universal law  518
Upper limbs  37, 44
Urinary system  32
Urinary tract  102
Urogenital systems  32
Urticaria  476
Uterus  101, 102, 104, 250, 284, 318, 323, 456, 505
Uva ursi  197, 252

## V

Valerian root  185, 196, 222, 237, 246, 292, 300, 501
Varicocele  468
Varicose veins  319, 506
Vascular system  21, 28, 245, 294
Vascular walls  31, 117, 200
Veneers  79
Ventricle  28, 88, 115
Vertebrae  125, 127, 129, 135, 470
Vertebral subluxations  126
Vertical experience  518
Vertigo  10, 506
Vetiver  334
Vibration  513, 518
Vibratory imprints  518
Victim mentality  429, 430, 431, 483
Victimization  80, 369, 506
Victimization & the Judicial System  506
Virus  161, 167, 219, 242, 256, 297, 452, 454, 493, 494
Viscera  21, 32, 319
Visceral system  32
Vision therapy  180, 183, 193, 464
Visual recognition  57, 58
Visualization  518
Visualizations  177
Vitamin A  293
Vitamin B-3  30, 117, 200
Vitamin B12  266, 328, 487
Vitamin C  167, 184, 187, 188, 190, 211, 213, 215, 218–221, 250, 256, 261, 263, 281, 288, 290, 320, 328, 463, 494, 496, 499, 500
Vitamin D  30, 62, 63, 82, 117, 127, 136, 141, 173, 192, 199, 200, 214, 234, 236, 249, 253, 257, 275, 277, 282, 293, 301, 302, 309, 310, 328, 446, 468
Vitamin E  217, 240, 249, 293, 328, 473
Vitamin K2  188, 191, 199, 217, 221, 272, 301
Vitamins  107, 328, 357, 487
Vitiligo  320, 501
Voice  83, 84, 378
Vulnerability  105, 369

## W

Walking  10, 110, 237, 331, 405
Warts  465, 486
Water  107, 324, 363, 405, 415, 416, 418, 507
Water intake  65, 264
Watermelon  197, 252, 327
Wealth & Prosperity Archetype  518
Weight  320, 321, 322, 507, 513
Weight loss  418, 421, 507
Weight training  110, 141, 239, 253
White birch bark  327
White blood cells  99
White Owl Legends  4
Wild rice  30, 117, 201
Wild yam root  166, 209, 229, 234, 243, 277, 282, 283, 321, 327, 466, 467, 504
Wintergreen  328, 334
Wisdom  518
Wisdom teeth  504
Wolf Frequency  518
Worry  370
Wounds  508

## Y

Yarrow  239, 334
Yeast  199, 508, 509
Yeast infection  509
Yerba matte  230
Yohimbe  230
You  518

## Z

Zinc  198, 230, 243, 247, 250, 285, 287, 294, 321, 468, 491